Career Options in the Pharmaceutical and Biomedical Industry

Josse R. Thomas • Luciano Saso •
Chris van Schravendijk
Editors

Career Options in the Pharmaceutical and Biomedical Industry

An Insider's Guide

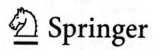 Springer

Editors
Josse R. Thomas
PharmaCS
Merchtem, Belgium

Luciano Saso
Faculty of Pharmacy and Medicine
Sapienza University of Rome
Roma, Italy

Chris van Schravendijk
Faculty of Medicine and Pharmacy
Vrije Universiteit Brussel
Ternat, Belgium

ISBN 978-3-031-14913-9   ISBN 978-3-031-14911-5   (eBook)
https://doi.org/10.1007/978-3-031-14911-5

Cover photo (Under granted copyright of C. van Schravendijk) The cover photo shows a frozen Hogweed flower on an early winter morning. This plant is member of the Apiaceae (or Umbelliferae) family. Many members of this family contain pharmacologically active compounds and hence can be seen as a source of inspiration for pharmacological development. The shape of this flower also symbolizes the many pathways that can be found for a career in the biomedical or pharmaceutical industry.

This Springer imprint is published by the registered company Springer Nature Switzerland AG
The registered company address is: Gewerbestrasse 11, 6330 Cham, Switzerland

Preface

This book is the product of a network of colleagues and scientists active in the pharma/biomed area, network that was initiated about 10 years ago. An important and inspiring framework for collaboration was provided by the much larger UNICA network, which unites the European universities located in the capitals of Europe. The UNICA network made it possible to organize lectures and seminars for students in the life sciences with a focus on medical and pharmaceutical research and development, thereby creating an attractive international environment of speakers and students. With the start of the covid-19 pandemic, organizing academic live meetings was no longer possible and new approaches were needed. In this period of unprecedented hardship especially for students, the UNICA network responded with resilience and creativity by initiating the very successful UNICA webinars. Hundreds of students interested in the pharmaceutical and biotechnological industry took part in these on-line activities, while academic lecture rooms were closed for long periods all over Europe. In the same period, the foundations of this book were laid when the collaborating experts behind the webinars realized that a comprehensive book could also provide strong support to students outside the lecture rooms.

The authors of this book have an extensive inside-experience in their fields of expertise. The editors are very grateful that they took their precious time to write up and contribute their valuable ideas and share their experience for the next generation of workers in the pharmaceutical and biomedical area.

The targeted readership of this book are young university graduates and professionals educated in the life sciences as well as other interested readers. The objective is based on the observation that the employment potential of the pharmaceutical and biomedical industry is largely unknown among young graduates and therefore these readers deserve an insider's view upon the wide variety of job opportunities. The book was written to increase the general understanding of the whole industry by shedding light on the various roles of key-players, our authors, involved in this field. Although a number of skills for job searching, currently taught at the universities, are also described, this book is not written as a comprehensive job seeker's manual that guides each young graduate to his/her job of interest. Rather, to

increase general understanding, the chapters are ordered along the product development life cycle.

Although pharmaceutical and biomedical industry is at the centre stage in this
book, the benefit of the patient is and should be the primary objective of all activities
in the Pharma-Biomed industry. It should thus be understood that this sector is not an
aim in itself, but rather a powerful means to achieve better healthcare. On the other
hand, the fact that the industry is concentrated on developing better medicinal
products makes it necessary that it is primarily product-oriented. This means that
the vast majority of opportunities presented in this book occur along the product life
cycle. Although all the activities from product discovery to marketing are relevant
and necessary, they are finally aimed at the benefit of the patient. The fact that this is
not always obvious and that this requires a healthcare dedication of all actors in the
field is an integral assumption but not a separate chapter in this book. It will become
clear that in the long chain of development of new medicines, rules and regulations
protect the interest and safety of the patient. In the final link between new products
and the patient, such as present in clinical studies or in prescribing and preparing new
treatments, medical doctors and pharmacists must not only have excellent product
knowledge but also be patient-oriented, meaning that they put the interest of the
patient centre stage. This gives these two legally regulated professions special roles
and responsibilities, hence unique job opportunities in the pharmaceutical and
biomedical industry.

The focus of this book is on the pharmaceutical industry. It is composed of five
parts each with several of all together 19 chapters.

In the introductory chapters of part 1 entitled "setting the scene", we first take a
general look at life after academia and what it means to prepare—during your final
university years—for a life in the pharmaceutical industry. To support a better
understanding about what exactly belongs to this industry and what is outside of
it, we will then take a closer look at other fields of the pharmaceutical sector. While
the pharmaceutical industry attracts a broad range of graduates from different
academic disciplines, we will undertake this delineating look from the perspective
of a close academic discipline of the sector, pharmacy education. The pharmaceutical industry will offer a broad range of possibilities, also for graduates in Pharmacy;
depending on which final specializations they choose in their study. This is elaborated in Chap. 2 on competences of pharmacists. Subsequently, we will direct our
focus on the industry, starting in Chap. 3 with a general overview of career
opportunities in the pharmaceutical industry.

Part 2 is organized over seven chapters (Chaps. 4–10) that highlight the various
opportunities in the industry along the drug/product life cycle. Part 3 then continues
with three chapters (Chaps. 11–13) highlighting the various opportunities in supportive functions. Part 4 subsequently presents other opportunities in the pharmaceutical and biomedical sector in three chapters (Chaps. 14–16). The book finalizes
with three chapters that give practical tips, tricks and training opportunities to find
your way towards the pharmaceutical and biomedical industry (Chaps. 17–19). In
the Epilogue, we reflect and give the reader some afterthoughts about this fascinating
field and its career perspectives.

This book is the first edition of a new approach to structurally support graduates in the life sciences in their efforts to find a job in the pharmaceutical and biomedical industry. It would never have been there without the driving force of the authors willing to write about their passion, their life job in terms of a career perspective for the next generation; once again a big thank you for this great generosity! The editors also want to express their gratitude for the editorial assistance provided by prof. Sibel Süzen (U. Ankara—TR) during the busy take-off months of this book.

In this first edition, not all possible topics were covered. Nevertheless, the current set of topics will already significantly support many possible orientations in the pharmaceutical and biomedical industry. We hope and expect that future editions will broaden this rich perspective even further and last but not least, we hope that our readers will find their way through this book, towards their dream job.

Ternat, Belgium   C. van Schravendijk
1 September 2022

Authors' Professional Information

L. Aldrovandi   Senior Project Manager at Science & Technology Park for Medicine, Italy

J. Atkinson   Director at Pharmacolor Consultants Nancy, France

L. M. Azzopardi   Head of Department of Pharmacy at University of Malta, Malta

B. Cahill   Research Scientist at Leibniz Information Centre for Science and Technology, Germany

A. Chalfoun   Senior Director Clinical, Medical & Regulatory Department (CMR) at Novo Nordisk Italy, Italy

A. I. Chiesa   Senior Director Communication & Sustainability at Novo Nordisk Italy, Italy

F. Conicella   Chief Executive Officer at Life Science District, Italy

M. Cornet   European Registered Toxicologist (ERT), Director Nonclinical Safety Evaluation at UCB Biopharma, Belgium

A. Dhoore   Former Human Resources Lead at Amgen Belgium & Luxemburg, and currently Self-employed Mentor and Coach, Belgium

A. Emmerechts   Head of Regulatory Science Benelux and Switzerland/Austria at Bristol Myers Squibb, Belgium

E. Galligan   Former Senior Business Development Manager at Aarhus University Technology Transfer Office, Denmark

A. Gattoni   Human Resources Business Partner at Novo Nordisk Italy, Italy

M. Gons   Associate Director Quality Systems at Merus, The Netherlands

I. Gorter de Vries   Former Director Quality Assurance at SGS-Life
                                Sciences, Belgium
M. Györffi   Senior EU Affairs Analyst at Eötvös Loránd
                                Research Network, Hungary
H. K. Kleinman   Guest Researcher at NIDCR/NIH and Industry
                                Consultant, USA
G. Lastoria   Medical Advisor Diabetes at Novo Nordisk Italy,
                                Italy
R. Manfroni   Medical Science Liaison at GW Pharmaceuticals,
                                Italy
M. Martens   European Registered Toxicologist (ERT), Former
                                Vice-President of Nonclinical Development at
                                Tibotec (J&J) and Consultant in Preclinical
                                Development and Toxicology, Belgium
S. Paeps   Managing Director at HR One Group, Belgium
V. Palatino   Commercial Director Italy ConvaTec, Italy
C. Peters   Founder of HR One Group, Belgium
L. Salvi   Associate Director CMR and Obesity Medical
                                Manager at Novo Nordisk Italy, Italy
S. Sbardelatti   Project Manager at Science & Technology Park for
                                Medicine, Italy
C. van Schravendijk   Former Biomedical Doctoral School Director at
                                Brussels Free University (VUB), Belgium
J. R. Thomas   Former Managing Director at Servier R&D
                                Benelux and currently Independent Senior
                                Pharma Consultant at PharmaCS, Belgium
A. Van den broeck   Former Medical Director at Amgen Belgium &
                                Luxemburg and currently Medical Director at
                                AstraZeneca BeLux, Belgium
V. Van den Nieuwenhuyzen   Marketing Director at Servier Benelux, Belgium
B. Van Nieuwenhove   Managing Director at European Centre for Clinical
                                Research Training, Belgium
D. Vuina   General Manager at Novo Nordisk Italy, Italy

Contents

About the Editors

Josse R. Thomas graduated as a Pharmacist and holds a postgraduate and a PhD degree in Medical Sciences (experimental and clinical pharmacology) from the University of Leuven, Belgium. He is certified as a Clinical Pharmacologist and has more than 30 years of experience in clinical drug development in the pharmaceutical industry. In addition, he held or holds various academic and consulting positions, including former Visiting Professor at KU Leuven (clinical drug development), former member of the Medical Research Ethics Committee of UZ/KU Leuven, member of the Clinical Trials Board of the Belgian Health Care Knowledge Centre (KCE), National Expert participating in the European Commission DG SANTE Union Controls within the framework of the Clinical Trials Regulation (CTR), and Senior Consultant at PharmaCS. He is also co-author of the book 'Global New Drug Development: An Introduction', published by Wiley-Blackwell, and a reference in its field.

Luciano Saso (Faculty of Pharmacy and Medicine, Sapienza University of Rome, Italy) is author of more than 350 scientific articles published in peer-reviewed international journals (H-index Google Scholar 58, Scopus 48). He coordinated several research projects and has been referee for many national and international funding agencies and international scientific journals in the last 30 years. Prof. Saso has extensive experience in international relations and he has been Deputy-Rector at Sapienza University of Rome in the last 7 years. In the last 20 years, he participated in several projects and has been speaker and chair at many international conferences organised by the UNICA network of the universities from the Capitals of Europe (http://www.unica-network.eu/) and other university associations. Prof. Saso is currently President of UNICA (2015-2023) and Member of the Steering Committee of CIVIS (https://civis.eu/en).

Chris van Schravendijk is Emeritus professor at the Faculty of Medicine and Pharmacy of the Vrije Universiteit Brussel, Brussels, Belgium. His research domain is focused on cellular biology, prediction and prevention of type-1 diabetes. As faculty professor he was responsible for the introductory course on Scientific Thought and Evidence-Based Medicine in the first Medical Bachelor year and for the Bachelor course on Formulation and Development of a Scientific Hypothesis in the third Bachelor year of Medicine and Biomedical Sciences. Between 2008 and 2016, he was the Director of the Doctoral School of Life Sciences and Medicine, with more than 200 PhD students. He has a long-standing interest in international benchmarking and harmonization in the area of Higher Education (MEDINE, MEDINE-2, ORPHEUS, UNICA) with focus on the place of the research component in the undergraduate medical curriculum as well as on career perspectives of academic graduates. As emeritus, he is particularly interested in PhD workshops promoting better awareness of research integrity as well as the promotion of job opportunities in the pharma-biomed-medtech sector.

Abbreviations

3D	Three-dimensional
ABPI	Association of the British Pharmaceutical Industry
ABT	American Board of Toxicology
ACCP	American College of Clinical Pharmacy
ACRP	Association of Clinical Research Professionals
ADME	Absorption, Distribution, Metabolism and Excretion
AI	Artificial Intelligence
AIFA	Agenzia Italiana del Farmaco (Italian Medicines Agency)
ANSM	Agence Nationale de Sécurité du Médicament et des produits de santé
API	Active Pharmaceutical Ingredient
ATMP	Advanced Therapy Medicinal Products
ATS	Academy of Toxicological Sciences
BD	Business Development
BI	Business Intelligence
BM	Biometrics or Brand Manager
BMS	Biomedical Sciences
BPS	Bio-Pharmaceutical Sciences
©	Copyright symbol
CA	Competent (regulatory) Authority
CADD	Computer-Aided Drug Design
CAPA	Corrective And Preventive Action
CBPE	Competence-Based Pharmacy Education
CCDS	Company Core Data Sheet
CDMO	Contract Development and Manufacturing Organisation
CEO	Chief Executive Officer
CFO	Chief Financial Officer
ClinOps	Clinical Operations
CLP	Classification, Labelling and Packaging (chemicals)
CMC	Chemistry, Manufacturing and Controls
CME	Continuing (or Continuous) Medical Education

CMO	Chief Marketing Officer
CMO	Contract Manufacturing Organisation
CMR	Clinical, Medical and Regulatory
CO	Clinical Operations
COO	Chief Operations Officer
COVID-19	Coronavirus Disease 2019
CP(T)	Clinical Pharmacology (and Therapeutics)
CPD	Continuing Professional Development
CPU	Clinical Pharmacology Unit
CR	Clinical Research
CRA	Clinical Research Associate
CRF	Case Report Form
CRISPR-Cas9	Clustered Regularly Interspaced Short Palindromic Repeats and CRISPR-associated Protein 9
CRO	Contract Research Organisation
CS	Clinical Services
CSO	Chief Scientific Officer
CTA	Clinical Trial Agreement or Application or Authorisation
CTA	Clinical Trial Assistant
CTD	Common Technical Document
CTO	Chief Technology Officer
CTR	Clinical Trials Regulation
CVD	Core Value Dossier
DABT	Diplomate American Board of Toxicology
DDI	Drug-Drug Interaction
DG SANTE	Directorate-General for Health and Food Safety of the European Commission
DI	Data Integrity
DIA	Drug Information Association
DOI	Digital Object Identifier
DSO	Drug Safety Officer
DSRU	Drug Safety Research Unit
DSUR	Development Safety Update Report
EAFP	European Association of Faculties of Pharmacy
EAHP	European Association of Hospital Pharmacists
EC	European Community or European Commission
ECCRT	European Centre for Clinical Research Training
ECHA	European Chemicals Agency
eCRF	Electronic Case Report Form
EEA	European Economic Area
EFGCP	European Forum for Good Clinical Practice
EFPIA	European Federation of Pharmaceutical Industries and Associations
EFSA	European Food Safety Authority

EIC	European Innovation Council
EIPOD	EMBL Interdisciplinary Postdoctoral programme
EIT	European Institute of Innovation & Technology
EMA	European Medicines Agency
EMBL	European Molecular Biology Laboratory
EMBLEM	EMBL Enterprise Management Technology Transfer GmbH
EMEA	Europe, Middle-East and Africa
EMR	Electronic Medical Record
EOP2	End-Of-Phase 2
EORTC	European Organisation for the Research and Treatment of Cancer
EPCF	European Pharmacy Competence Framework
EPO	European Patent Office
ePRO	Electronic Patient Reported Outcomes
ERC	European Research Council
ERT	European Register of Toxicologists
EU	European Union
Eu2P	European programme in Pharmacovigilance and Pharmacoepidemiology
EUFEMED	European Federation for Exploratory Medicines Development
EUROTOX	Federation of European Toxicologists & European Societies of Toxicology
FATS	Fellow of the Academy of Toxicological Sciences
FDA	Food and Drug Administration (USA)
FIH	First-In-Human
FIP	International Pharmaceutical Federation
FIPCo	Fully Integrated Pharmaceutical Company
FMEA	Failure Mode(s) and Effects Analysis
FWO	Fund for Scientific Research (Belgium)
GCP	Good Clinical Practice
GDP	Good Distribution Practice
GDPR	General Data Protection Regulation
GHTC	Global Health Training Centre
GLP	Good Laboratory Practice
GMP	Good Manufacturing Practice
GVD	Global Value Dossier
GVP	Good Pharmacovigilance Practice
HCP	Health Care Professional
HEOR	Health Economics Outcomes Research
HER2	Human Epidermal growth factor Receptor 2
HIPO	High Potential (employee)
HMA	Heads of Medicines Agencies
HR	Human Resources
HSE	Health, Safety & Environment
HTA	Health Technology Assessment

IARC	International Agency for Research on Cancer
IASP	International Association of Science Parks and Areas of Innovation
IB	Investigator's Brochure
IBM	International Business Machines Corporation
ICH	International Council (formerly Conference) for Harmonisation of Technical Requirements for Pharmaceuticals for Human Use
ICSR	Individual Case Safety Report
IEC	Independent Ethics Committee
IFPMA	International Federation of Pharmaceutical Manufacturers and Associations
IIT	Investigator Initiated Trial
ILAP	Innovative Licensing and Access Pathway
IMI	Innovative Medicines Initiative
IMP	Investigational Medicinal Product
IMPD	Investigational Medicinal Product Dossier
IND	Investigational New Drug
IP	Intellectual Property
IPR	Intellectual Property Rights
iPSC	Induced Pluripotent Stem Cells
IR	Infrared Spectrometer
ISMS	Information Security Management Systems
ISO	International Organization for Standardization
ISoP	International Society of Pharmacovigilance (or alternatively Pharmacometrics)
IST	Investigator Sponsored Trial
IT or ICT	Information (and Communications) Technology
IUCLID	International Uniform ChemicaL Information Database
IUPHAR	International Union of Basic and Clinical Pharmacology
JECFA	Joint FAO/WHO Expert Committee on Food Additives
JMPR	Joint FAO/WHO Meeting on Pesticide Residues
KEE	Key External Expert
KIC	Knowledge and Innovation Community
KOL	Key Opinion Leader
KPI	Key Performance Indicator
KTL	Key Thought Leader
LBS	Learning By Simulation
LPLV	Last Patient Last Visit
M&S	Modelling and Simulation
MA	Marketing Authorisation or Approval
MA	Medical Affairs or Medical Advisor
MAB	Monoclonal Antibody
MAB	Applied Microscopy and Cellular Biology (at TPM)
MAD	Multiple Ascending Dose
MAH	Marketing Authorisation Holder

MBA	Master in Business Administration
MBDD	Model-Based Drug Development
MD	Doctor of Medicine
MDR	Medical Device Regulation
MHRA	Medicines and Healthcare products Regulatory Agency
MIDD	Model-Informed Drug Development
ML	Machine Learning
MOOC	Massive Open Online Course
MPharm	Master of Pharmacy degree (UK)
MR	Medical Review
mRNA	Messenger Ribonucleic Acid
MS2	Materials, Sensors and Systems
MSC	Mesenchymal Stem Cells
MSL	Medical Science Liaison
NBE	New Biological Entity
NCE	New Chemical Entity
NDE	New Drug Entity
NGO	Non-Governmental Organisation
NIH	National Institutes of Health
NVKFB	Nederlandse Vereniging voor Klinische Farmacologie en Biofarmacie (Dutch Society for Clinical Pharmacology & Biopharmacy)
OECD	Organisation of Economic Co-operation and Development
OOS/OOT	Out of Specification or Out of Trend
OTC	Over-The-Counter
PASS	Post-Approval Safety Study
PBPK	Physiologically Based Pharmacokinetic (modelling & simulation)
PBRER	Periodic Benefit-Risk Evaluation Report
PD	Pharmacodynamic
PDCA	Plan-Do-Check-Act
PET	Positron Emission Tomography
PGEU	Pharmaceutical Group of European Union
PharmD	Doctor of Pharmacy
PHARMED	Post-graduate Programme in Pharmaceutical Development Sciences
PhD	Doctor of Philosophy, doctoral degree
PhRMA	Pharmaceutical Research and Manufacturers of America
PI	Principal Investigator
PK	Pharmacokinetic
PK-PD	Pharmacokinetic-Pharmacodynamic
PM	Project or Product Manager
PMDA	Pharmaceutical and Medical Devices Agency (Japan)
PMS	Post-Marketing Surveillance
PMx	Pharmacometrics

POC	Proof-Of-Concept
POM	Proof-Of-Mechanism
PPP	Public-Private Partnership
PQS	Pharmaceutical Quality System
PRG	Pharmacometrics Research Group
PV or PhV	Pharmacovigilance
QA	Quality Assurance
QALY	Quality-Adjusted Life Year
QC	Quality Control
QMR	Quality Management Review
QMS	Quality Management System
QP	Qualified Person (for batch release)
QPPV	Qualified Person responsible for Pharmacovigilance
QR (code)	Quick Response (code)
QS	Quality Systems
QSP	Quantitative Systems Pharmacology
R&D	Research and Development
RA	Regulatory Affairs
RAC	Regulatory Affairs Certification
RAPS	Regulatory Affairs Professionals Society
RCA	Root Cause Analysis
RCT	Randomised Controlled Trial
REACH	Registration, Evaluation, Authorisation and Restriction of Chemicals
REC	Research Ethics Committee
RIP	Responsible for Information and Publicity
RMA	Regional Medical Advisor
RMP	Risk Management Plan
RNA	Ribonucleic Acid
ROI	Return On Investment
RPS	Royal Pharmaceutical Society
RSRN	Regulatory Science Research Needs (EMA)
RWE	Real World Evidence
SA	Scientific Advice
SAD	Single Ascending Dose
SAR	Structure-Activity Relationship
SCM	Supply Chain Manager
SDV	Source Data Verification
SmPC	Summary of Product Characteristics
SOCRA	Society of Clinical Research Associates
SOP	Standard Operating Procedure
SOT	Society of Toxicology
SP	Systems Pharmacology
SPARK	Sharing and Promotion of Awareness and Regional Knowledge

STEM	Science, Technology, Engineering and Mathematics
STP	Science and Technology Park
SWI	Standardised Work Instruction
TAE	Therapy Area Expert
TK	Toxicokinetic
TOP	Toxicology and Proteomics Laboratory (at TPM)
TOPRA	The Organisation for Professionals in Regulatory Affairs
TPM	Technology Park for Medicine "Mario Veronesi"
TPP	Target Product Profile
TRL	Technology Readiness Level
UK	United Kingdom of Great Britain and Northern Ireland
ULLA	European University Consortium for Pharmaceutical Sciences
UNICA	Network of Universities from the Capitals of Europe
URL	Uniform Resource Locator
US	United States (of America)
USA	United States of America
UV-Vis	Ultraviolet/Visible region (in UV spectroscopy)
WHO	World Health Organization

Part I
Setting the Scene

Chapter 1
Life After Academia: Launching Your Pharma/Biotech Career

Chris van Schravendijk

Abstract This chapter will have no references, because it is based on personal experience. After being responsible for a 2-year international Master programme in Medical and Pharmaceutical Research and later Cell and Gene Therapy for 25 years, the author became Director of the Doctoral School of Life Sciences and Medicine of the Vrije Universiteit Brussel (VUB, Belgium) in 2008. In this capacity, he became responsible for support and training of ±200 PhD students per academic year. Most of these students had to leave university after graduation to find a job outside academia. We will take a look at the special contextual setting in Europe for starters of a pharma and biotech career and explain why job seekers benefit more from their specific knowledge and preparation when applying for their dream job, than from their academic talents and mark sheets.

1.1 Introduction

Over the last few decades, our European academic learning places have differentiated towards the American three-cycle system of Bachelor, Master and PhD, in which all serious participants can obtain at least one, but often more than one, academic degree. During the same decades, the enrolment numbers in European universities significantly increased, and it became hard to imagine how to start any career without a university degree. For those who were students in the three cycles, residence in the arms of academia will have extended to a decade. Nevertheless, the prospects of staying inside academia after such a long study period remained rather poor, because academic staff numbers did not increase at the same rate as student intake. As a consequence, less than 5% of PhD holders would have the chance to become full professor. For PhD holders moving out of academia, their specialist knowledge may not always be an asset for fruitful competition with Bachelors or Masters that started their life after academia at lower qualifications, but many years earlier. For those that look back at their university years, life inside academia often

C. van Schravendijk (✉)
Faculty of Medicine and Pharmacy, Brussels Free University (VUB), Brussels, Belgium

© The Author(s), under exclusive license to Springer Nature Switzerland AG 2023
J. R. Thomas et al. (eds.), *Career Options in the Pharmaceutical and Biomedical Industry*, https://doi.org/10.1007/978-3-031-14911-5_1

feels like a safe harbour continuous with the earlier school years. Meanwhile, the world outside the ancient buildings of the beloved university is raging on and presenting ever more specific requirements making a post-academic start of life seem hard. The growing stream of job seekers, each with their own academic degree (s), makes competition more complex. The notion has emerged that academic knowledge from the completed studies is simply no longer sufficient to stand out in competition with the many other candidates.

If knowledge and understanding are not enough to become a successful job seeker, then it is better to directly anticipate and solve this issue inside academia. Today, university is the place where candidates for jobs in society or industry should be prepared on a daily basis. While all students know that their courses and exams are calibrated at the highest possible quality standards, there is no such thing as 'optimal standard knowledge'. Each student will have assimilated his/her own knowledge in a personal way and will have added specific elements according to personal preferences and ideas. Moreover, students gain and develop unique insights and attitudes and become outstanding in more than their own academic discipline, some in sports, some in the arts and others in amateur clubs or youth organisations. This is what head-hunters and human resource specialists actually want to know during a job interview: who are you beyond your academic qualifications and will these additional characteristics contribute to your effectiveness in the vacant role? To what extent are you ready for the unexpected and will you be inspired to solving completely new problems? How interested are you really in this job? It may well be that in the decades to come, some job vacancies will just remain open, not because there are no candidates, but because the postulating candidates do not meet the requirements. How can you become that one person that really fits in the vacancy? Reflecting on questions like these is the topic of this chapter.

1.2 Timing, Skills and Strategy

Preparation for life after academia should typically start before the second cycle, become more intense during the second and continue during the third cycle. There are (or should be) university courses enhancing general competencies that are applicable in a wide range of jobs. Relevant topics are communication skills, presentation skills, creating slide shows, writing impactful short texts, running a brainstorm session with several participants, language capabilities, etc.

There are also more targeted courses to prepare for your life after academia in the second cycle. Weekly seminars with invited speakers from various areas in medical or pharmaceutical research, healthcare, biotechnology or drug development are a good example. It is no problem that such activities are organised for both Master and PhD students together. To broaden the job perspective, universities should preferably organise these learning activities in English; invited speakers and guest lecturers will also have an international profile. Students can train their language skills by asking a question to the speaker after the presentation. All this is consistent with the important fact that your dream job will not necessarily be located in the street where you live. If you are motivated to leave your hometown for that job, then this is a valuable addition to your profile. Speaking at least one additional European language is a major asset as a job seeker.

The impact of language skills is hard to overestimate for the effective job seeker in the area of healthcare, pharmaceutical activities and biotechnology. Increased language abilities can become a real advantage when you are fluent in three or more European languages. A non-European language can give a unique advantage; some job seekers, for example, can not only speak German but also Japanese, or Korean, and should mention such ability in bold in their printed and online curriculum vitae. They will of course pay extra attention to job vacancies in companies that are collaborating with, or have affiliations in, for example, Japan, Germany or Korea. Some universities organise language courses for students willing to seek a job abroad. Students who are not fluent in a second language should consider taking such courses, depending on their long-term strategy for job seeking; is there a country with a high frequency of dream jobs for you in Europe or elsewhere? Successful job seekers are often crossing borders.

Students can—and should—be trained in writing job applications and curriculum vitae and in oral interview techniques. Often, these activities require a combination of generic and specific competencies. Training activities of this kind should be part of the yearly regular curriculum of the second and third cycles in each faculty. If faculties have no staff to organise these activities, they can be contracted out to consultants or external companies. Doing a successful job application, job interview or elevator pitch is a real skill that each student can and should learn. Ignoring this simple reality can lead to very demotivating experiences that no student deserves. Nevertheless, at university there are only a few time windows during which you can actually follow such a course, and it may be too late when you realise you should have done that. Thus, a good planning is vital for taking the available opportunities for training. Many faculties have study advisors, if you are not sure about what to choose and when.

The importance of computer (IT) skills can only be underestimated, and this is also true for the job seeker leaving university. Many students have fairly good computer skills; in most cases, these were developed by activities in the social media. The increased physical isolation due to the Covid-19 crises may have amplified your skills; the experience of following university courses and webinars via Zoom or similar technology may also be helpful in future job interviews.

There are many presentations available on YouTube that can be helpful in increasing the skills needed in job seeking. LinkedIn supports professional networking and may also be instrumental in finding future peers and knowing how they look at certain positions and vacancies. Communicating with persons who have similar challenges or made similar choices, as you want to make, can be helpful. However, networking is necessary, but not enough.

The rapid expansion of the Internet has not only increased the possibilities for students to prepare for job interviews by gathering relevant information or contacting helpful people. It also increased the expectations that companies or institutions have of the specific knowledge of the candidates. However, finding key information about a company is difficult and time-consuming because it may not be easily traceable in the public domain. Reading papers and communicating with experienced people can provide crucial support. We know from experience that when during a job interview it becomes clear you are knowledgeable about, for example, the company's development strategy or a certain drug trial, this will significantly add to your authenticity and success as a job seeker.

In addition to the previously discussed approach, job seekers will benefit from having a special knowledge or skill, something standing out of the ordinary. Patent law might be such an extra, or data analysis or biostatistics. People with an appetite for more complex techniques and skills have an advantage. Collecting knowledge in your particular area of interest requires perseverance and a strategy. The knowledge can be collected within academia during the final years, but the student then has to apply what was learned to his/her situation in order to understand how it will contribute to the effective filling of the position.

What can you do in terms of your academic knowledge when preparing for a specific job interview? Everyone knows PubMed/Medline (which is still free of charge, thanks to Nobel Peace Prize 2007 winner Al Gore, when he was vice-president in 1997). Suppose you apply for a job in a drug company that is particularly famous for its antihypertensive drugs. It would then be smart to use PubMed to find a recent review on that topic. You read the paper and see if there is an opportunity for you to use this knowledge during the interview.

Media such as YouTube provide excellent preparative short courses with free access, such as those given by the late MIT professor Patrick Winston (1943–2019). This famous formula of his hand is directly applicable to this chapter as presented so far:

$$Q = f\,(K, P, t)$$

where Q is the quality (of, e.g. your job interview), which is the function (f) of three elements, namely, knowledge (K), preparation (P) and talent (t). The relative importance of these factors are $K > P \gg t$. Surprisingly, talent (not in capital T) can hardly help you during a job interview, and counting on it (or on your academic mark sheets) is a mistake. In the long run, your talents will of course contribute to your job success.

In the previous paragraphs, we have underlined the importance of specific knowledge, just because your extra knowledge relevant for this position is what makes you the outstanding candidate for that job. Sometimes your valuable extra knowledge even locates outside the area of the job description sensu stricto, making K even larger. Preparation (P) is what gives you extra knowledge over your competitors, but P could also stand for passion. If the job is in, for example, optical isomers and that part of chemistry happens to be your passion, you should prepare a way to briefly illustrate your passion. Another point that all applicants should realise in advance is that job interviews normally do not take very long (although you may have to wait a bit before it all really starts). It may be good to keep in mind that you should be able to express in 5 min why this job is so interesting for you. Also this has to be prepared (*P* not *p*) in advance, because if you do not succeed, your chances are over. So, knowledge and preparation are most important for a job interview. More about the special capabilities for job seeking and interviews is presented elsewhere in this book (see Part 5: Practical tips and tricks).

1.3 Contextual Issues and Job Offers in the Pharmaceutical Sector

There are some important contextual issues that need to be addressed briefly because they can directly affect your start of life after academia:

- Different academic profiles can prepare for jobs in the pharmaceutical sector.
- Specific pharma- or biotech-related activities are often geographically clustered.
- Work styles and cultures vary between companies, sectors and countries.
- Rules and legislation/regulation are a sector for jobs.
- Pharmaceutical sector has a developing role in global healthcare.
- How the most attractive vacancies are (never) advertised.

1.3.1 Academic Diversity in the Pharma and Biotech Sector

There is an enormous array of academic disciplines that can actually lead to a job in pharma/biotech. Pharmaceutical sciences, medicine, biology, biomedical sciences, biochemistry and veterinary sciences belong to the core set of disciplines. Engineering, mathematics, law, economy and finance and even communication sciences and languages can provide key competences for some vacancies. There is always a balance in each company between the research and development (R&D) segment of that company and the financial and marketing segment. In companies with a large R&D segment, the above-mentioned core set of academic disciplines will have more open positions than in companies that focus on marketing and generic drugs. As already mentioned, knowledge of different disciplines, even if only via a few well-chosen courses, can give applicants a significant advantage. A whole year of extra study is even better (although not always necessary). For example, the first year after your graduation as a pharmacist might be an ideal opportunity to add another competency to your portfolio, for example, data analysis or biostatistics or a 1-year Master in Business Administration (MBA) or international patent law. Best do this abroad, not in your alma mater (own university). In this way, you internationalise you educational portfolio and CV. How you do it and what you do is up to you: it all depends on your personal preferences.

1.3.2   Science Parks and Hubs

Regions and clusters of companies will compete for intake of new generations of employees and developing specialists. Companies are often represented in umbrella organisations with other similar companies, and they are also represented in organisations promoting hub regions for a particular type of biotech of pharma innovation. So clustering can be both conceptual and geographical. In this way, they are better able to reach out to future employees and there can be several positions to choose from. If this is the case, you should follow the activities of these organisations and see what is going on. The author of this chapter lives in Belgium, where we have FlandersBio as umbrella organisation, which represents ±350 pharma and biotech organisations, often located in science parks located close to our main university cities. In terms of job vacancies, such environments create a multiplication effect for opportunities.

Thus, in Belgium, the UK, Germany, France, Italy, etc., you have these hubs, but they are different in each location and science park. You should investigate if there are interesting things for you in these hubs, first geographically nearby, if not, then further away. Science parks abroad will offer you several possible positions: it is necessary to make up your mind in advance to avoid doing many applications for very different positions where each time your preparation will have to be quite different. If you make several applications for jobs that are rather similar, you will start growing in your role of applicant for that type of job. In any case, your willingness to move for a job is already a reliable indication that you are a serious applicant. More about job and training opportunities in science parks is presented in Chaps. 14 and 19.

1.3.3   Work Styles and Cultures

Work styles and cultures may differ dramatically between people, between countries but also between companies. Some companies will inactivate their mail servers during weekends, to avoid that staff is constantly checking mails and working on during the off-days, as these are behaviours now generally recognised as promoting burnout. Knowing in advance what is expected from you in a certain type of job will give you a major advantage over those completely ignorant about such issues. The quality of a job is also in the remuneration, the opportunities for training and conferences, the policy for promotions, the (low) amount of job-hopping (i.e. colleagues applying for internal or external vacancies) and so on. During an interview for a job, it is not advisable to start discussing these issues in the first interview of your application, where job content and your extra competencies should come first. Knowing people in a company may be an advantage, but they don't have to be your best friends; they could be a LinkedIn contact. Looking at how a company presents itself to the outside world can help you understand if you really want to join them. If that company has policies and staff to manage work-life balance, gender issues, etc., this is a reliable indicator of that company's attitude towards these topics. Female applicants, for example, should be certain that their career is not ruined by taking maternity leave, even if this topic was not brought up during their job interview. Companies with the best work styles and cultures certainly deserve the best employees: competent employees means better growth potential.

1.3.4 Rules and Regulations

Especially in the European culture, consumers are protected against bad and falsified products by a strong legal framework, and this is certainly true for the pharmaceutical and biotechnological sector. Even medicines (partly) produced outside Europe will have to be investigated and approved before they are allowed to access the European market (Falsified Medicines Directive of the European Commission, activated on 2 January 2013). Activities around, for example, regulatory issues and quality assurance in companies, are presented in depth in Chaps. 11 and 12. The only remark that has to be made here is that this area of quality, rules and regulations for pharmacology and biotechnology development implies that there is a whole job market with various specialist fields and different types of academic preparation, where legal, linguistic and administrative knowledge becomes more important. For example, the European Medicines Agency (EMA) recently moved from London to Amsterdam (2019); it has ± 900 employees and a 358 million euros budget (2020).

1.3.5 Pharmaceutical Sector and Global Healthcare: New Perspectives

The Covid-19 pandemic and the unseen success of rapid vaccine development and its deployment by the pharmaceutical sector in 2021 and 2022 have been an impressive demonstration of the enormous importance of this sector for global healthcare. Nevertheless, the worldwide roll-out of RNA vaccines is now hindered by the classical financial structure behind inventions with a ± 10-year on-market protection period by patent law. This creates a healthcare paradox: while the existing financial structure of the sector was at the basis of its recent successes, protecting new inventions could become an obstacle for the worldwide implementation of vaccines in less developed regions of the world. Evidently, European prices are too high for these regions and local production could be the solution if patent law would not stand in the way. WHO projects in South Africa now try to reinvent the Covid-19 RNA vaccine. This is done by 'reverse engineering', which is reconstructing the vaccine by analysing the active product to reveal its original (and patented) formulation. This might offer a solution, but is time-consuming and risky. There are no simple solutions for this problem, and the world might be better off with a new breed of experts for responsible price setting of 'global medicines'. Such experts need to combine their pharma knowledge with financial and economic expertise and with negotiation skills to develop responsible solutions for all stakeholders. About 70 years ago, the Constitution of the World Health Organization stated that health is a fundamental human right. Today, new generations of graduates will understand that pharmaceutical and biotechnological development means not only the discovery of new molecules and formulations but also the development of a global roll-out strategy for new medicines, to improve global access to healthcare for all.

1.3.6   Visibility of the Best Vacancies

There is an old wisdom in real estate that says that the best houses are never advertised on the market. This is also true for the best jobs, be it your dream job, or not. Some jobs are so difficult and challenging that finding the right person to do them becomes a challenge in itself. Expensive head-hunters try to find the right candidate and advertisements appear month after month for that job. This is even truer for jobs higher in the hierarchy within an organisation, because there is much at stake in such a leading position that also creates opportunities for many others. Even if you hold a PhD, this may not be the best type of position you should apply for. Such positions often require a lot of sectorial experience and networking. An alternative approach is to start at a lower level in an organisation and work your way up through training and experience. Companies often provide in-house training programmes that help you grow while already being an employee and on the payroll. Some of these programmes are even open for external job seekers, but it takes an active interest in that company to find such opportunities.

1.4   Closing Remarks

When leaving academia for the pharmaceutical sector, one could wonder whether it is better to be a specialist or a universalist. By doing a Master or even a PhD research project in your final year(s), you inevitably became some kind of specialist. However, very often, it is not possible to continue your line of academic research specialisation in industry. People who could do so are more the exception than the rule. Although you may have loved your academic topic very much, switching is not a problem at all for your post-academic chances, especially if you keep an open mind for the sector as a whole. It is thus advisable to keep your professional interests rather broad and open, for example, keep reading outside your field of specialisation. In doing so, ideally, you become *both a specialist and a universalist*. Keeping an open mind is, in the first place, a matter of attitude. Sincere interest in the field in which you will seek a job is certainly appreciated and quickly recognised, but general awareness of what happens in pharma/biotech is also very much appreciated. If over the past few Covid-19 years your family and friends were already picking your brains about vaccine development, expectations for vaccinations and what other Covid medicines are in the pipeline, then this is an indication that you are already doing the right thing, being both a specialist and a universalist. If you are seriously interested in your field in the pharmaceutical sector and you discover how attractive this type of work can be, there is the perspective of a lifelong job satisfaction and a dynamic career in the service of healthcare.

Chapter 2
Competences for Pharmacists

Jeffrey Atkinson and Chris van Schravendijk

Abstract This chapter examines first of all the development of competences for traditional pharmacy practice throughout the ages to those of the present day. It reviews the changes in pharmacy practice notably in industrial pharmacy with an evolution from chemistry-based therapy to therapy based on biotechnology, and the changes involved in the switch from medicine-based to patient-based care, in community and hospital pharmacy. These transitions are occurring very rapidly and necessitate education and training that can adapt rapidly and incorporate the changes in the competences needed for evolving practice. We present the Delphi-based method used in the European Union "Pharmacy education in Europe" project for the definition of competences required. Finally, factors that may influence the evolution in the future competences are reviewed with the reports on the evidence of the beneficial effects of such changes that will also affect the job perspectives for future generations of pharmacists.

We will first of all look at traditional pharmacy competences. We will then present the European Union "Pharmacy education in Europe" project for the definition of competences (Atkinson et al. 2013, 2014). Finally, we will examine factors that may influence future changes in the competences.

2.1 The Traditional Competences of Pharmacists

Preventive and curative healthcare practice can be divided into two phases:

J. Atkinson (✉)
Pharmacolor Consultants Nancy, Villers, France

C. van Schravendijk
Faculty of Medicine and Pharmacy, Brussels Free University (VUB), Brussels, Belgium

© The Author(s), under exclusive license to Springer Nature Switzerland AG 2023
J. R. Thomas et al. (eds.), *Career Options in the Pharmaceutical and Biomedical Industry*, https://doi.org/10.1007/978-3-031-14911-5_2

1. Decisional

    (a) Risk assessment
    (b) Clinical and clinical biology examination
    (c) Monitoring

2. Therapeutic

    (a) Chemical substances (medicines)
    (b) Physical interventions (surgery, etc.)
    (c) Socio-psychological acts

Healthcare practice has developed over the ages. The advances in the science of healthcare occurred essentially within academia, as witness the studies of Pedanius Dioscorides, Aelius Galenus, Ibn Sina and Claude Bernard, to quote but a few; the evolution of the practice of healthcare took place within the world at large. Within this context, the pharmacist developed specific competences essentially related to chemical substances or medicines.

After centuries of shamanism and other primitive forms of "therapy" (Stone 1932), which were based on a mixture of potions of more or less unknown composition (with plants such as figs and castor oil, minerals such as copper and magnesium salts), and of pseudo-medical and socio-psychological rituals, remedies based on identified chemical substances (or "medicines") emerged as essential to therapy.

Medicines became the trade of grocers, herbalists, apothecaries, local chemists and human and veterinary doctors—and, subsequently, the licensed domain of pharmacists (Zebroski 2016). For instance, in the years immediately following the French Revolution, the law of 21 Germinal year XI (revolutionary calendar, corresponding to 11 April 1803) regulated the dispensation of medicines in France. It was valid for more than a century, until 1941 (Faure 2014). The monopoly of the sale of medicines was restricted to pharmacists. Everything was done to ensure that pharmacists were to be few in number. The law provided for six higher schools of pharmacy but only three were established in Paris, Montpellier and Strasbourg. Moreover, the studies were long and expensive. In the United Kingdom, the Apothecaries Act of 1815 delimited the pharmacists' profession, and the creation of a specific guild separating them from grocers and the like.

Today, the Merriam-Webster American English dictionary defines the pharmacist as "a health-care professional licensed to engage in pharmacy with duties including dispensing prescription medicines, monitoring medicine interactions, administering vaccines, and counselling patients regarding the effects and proper usage of medicines and dietary supplements" (Merriam Webster Dictionary 2022).

Pharmacists have competences—to be defined as capabilities associated with legal responsibilities – in the following domains:

1. Patient-oriented competences:

    (a) Dispensation of medicines
    (b) Diagnostic procedures and clinical biology guiding the use of medicines
    (c) Patient counselling on medicines

2. Medicine-oriented competences:

   (a) Research and development of active medicines and studies on dose and formulation

   (b) Evaluation of fitness for purpose (efficacy, safety) of medicines in preclinical and clinical evaluation

   (c) Post-administration monitoring of medicinal actions and interactions

   (d) Production and distribution of medicines (storage and logistics)

   (e) Marketing of medicines

   (f) Economics and policy of the use of medicines

The above roles are undergoing constant evolution.

We will now describe a tool to determine the competences for pharmacists, competences to be delivered in education and training, and then transcribed into outcomes for present and future practice.

2.2 The EU "Pharmacy Education in Europe" Project for the Definition of Competences

2.2.1 Introduction

Competences required of pharmacists are changing rapidly. To illustrate the urgency of this, we take an example from industrial pharmacy. Over the last decades, millions of patients in Europe have benefited from medicines, manufactured by the biotechnological and pharmaceutical industries for the treatment of a broad range of diseases ranging from diabetes and stroke to cystic fibrosis, cancer and various infectious diseases. The driving force behind this enormous success in healthcare has been the increase in our understanding of human pathophysiology, genetics and pharmacology.

This has coincided with the growth of the pharmaceutical/biotechnological industry in which new drugs were developed, produced and followed-up after approval, by integrated teams of experts with various academic backgrounds. Along with this development, it became clear that the discovery, development and marketing of completely new drugs will become an even greater key element for improving the health status of an ageing population in Europe, both in terms of treatment and prevention, diagnosis, individualisation and follow-up.

However, the increasing speed at which new insights in human biology are translated into treatments with newly discovered drugs poses a major challenge in the transfer of knowledge from discovery to application and practice. More than ever, there appears to be a knowledge transfer time gap between industry, the performance of which depends on new staff for innovation and implementation, and academia responsible for education and training that are behind the timely delivery of new competent staff.

The timescales in which universities can adjust their educational content and training procedures to the latest developments are too long. The university system of educational boards and external evaluation produces updates every 3–5 years, whilst the pharmaceutical/biotechnological world evolves on a yearly basis—or even faster. That this speed of pharmaceutical/biotechnological development is a major advantage has become even clearer during the Covid-19 pandemic with vaccines and medication developed faster than ever before. However due to the time gap with education, there is a risk that industrial vacancies remain open—simply because the required expertise is not yet available amongst the candidates postulating—and research and development are hindered.

To overcome this time gap, the two sides at each end of this dilemma have to adopt a common vocabulary to articulate the requirements of the innovation and production and to make these understood by the higher education institutes responsible for training and education. This vocabulary consists of a specific set of competences that newly graduated individuals in the fields of pharmaceutical/biotechnological education will need to have.

Similar arguments to those developed in the above example from industrial pharmacy can be drawn from community and hospital pharmacy where switch to patient care and competence-based education are occurring. In a review of the literature between 2000 and 2013, Nash and co-workers (Nash et al. 2015) noted a steep rise in the number of publications per year for competence-based assessment in pharmacy education from 2004 onwards. Interest has not waned since.

The major requirement is that both ends of the gap (educators and innovators) mutually understand and agree upon the competences required to form the competence framework. The development and formulation of competences frameworks for pharmacy practice in industry, community and hospital settings involve the relevant stakeholders, working together towards a consensus in an iterative process. This overview will describe the methodology behind this process. We will define a competence as the ability to fulfil a certain task.

2.3 Methods

One important tool for the development of a competence framework is the Delphi method, elaborated in the 1950s by the RAND Corporation for the American air force (Dalkey 1967). It uses quantitative statistical methods to reach consensus amongst predefined groups of experts, independently answering questionnaires on the competences required. In a stepwise manner, competences are ranked according to their perceived importance for outcomes. Consensus is typically reached after two or three rounds.

In our study, six groups of experts were selected: those involved in education (one group of university staff and one group of students), those involved in practice (three groups: community, hospital and industrial pharmacist), and one group of organisations that represented practitioners (societies, orders, chambers and associations).

The choice of the groups influences the ranking of the outcomes thus possibly inducing bias in a study. One group of experts may select competences related to practice of that specific group. Were different groups to rank means or medians differently, this would lead to a distortion of variance and an increase in group variances. This was not the case: we showed that the distributions of the ranking data were not statistically significantly different across all groups (Mircioiu and Atkinson 2017). Furthermore, the Leik ordinal consensus values were similar in all groups showing that the degree to which individuals of a group agreed upon a certain ranking was not significantly different from one group to another (Atkinson et al. 2016a, b, c, d).

In our study, we restricted ranking to predefined competences. Some useful competences may have been ignored. However, in the study, practitioners and all other groups had the opportunity to comment on any insufficiencies in the list of competences. Their comments did not reveal any new competences that may have been missed (Atkinson et al. 2016a, b, c, d).

Comments mainly centred on the apparently recondite nature of the questions. This is understandable given that the English version of the survey was sent out to all EU member states, and thus (probably) to many whose first language was not English. Other comments concerned organisational aspects of the educational process behind the acquirement of the competences such as whether a given competence should be taught at an early or advanced stage of formation.

It can also be questioned whether the inclusion of administrative, governmental bodies in the ranking would have increased the value of our study. Such institutions are concerned with the regulation of the outcomes of competences, viz. safe and effective therapy, and this within a given social, economic and political context, rather than with the evaluation of the competences themselves.

This is important in international organisations such as the EU. The governing bodies of the EU are charged with assuring an identical level of safety and efficacy of medicines and therapy, within the context of the free movement of healthcare professionals from one member state to another. This is of prime importance when healthcare professionals move from one member state in which they received their education and training to another member state within which they are to practice. In order to ensure the equality of care within the context of interstate free movement of healthcare professionals, it is necessary that all member states accept a common, fundamental competence level in education and training of such professionals. Education and training constitute the first step in the triad: education → competences → outcomes (practice).

The directives of the EU prompt the different member states to implement such competence requirements for the sectoral profession of pharmacy (EU directive 2013). EU directives guide the education and training of pharmacists in the different member states. The fact that the different EU member states were all represented, and in statistically significant numbers, in each of the three expert groups emphasises the pan-European nature of the competence framework produced.

It is interesting to note the similarities amongst our EU framework and the Australian, Canadian, UK and US pharmacy learning outcome frameworks suggesting that this work could have a more global impact (Nash et al. 2015; Stupans et al. 2016) and that competence frameworks represent an essential element in the equation between pharmacy education and training and pharmacy practice.

2.4   Results and Discussion

In Fig. 2.1 is shown a radar plot of competences proposed in our study.

For definition of 50 competences, see appendix (Atkinson et al. 2016a, b, c, d; Volmer et al. 2017).

Overall our study showed that pharmacists, regardless of their career path, rank competences in a similar fashion. They thus have a great deal in common; all are seeking improvements in their services to patients.

The different perspectives in various areas represent a solid starting point for steering the necessary changes in the profession. An initial fundamental curriculum can be based on the clusters of competences with the highest ranking scores like "need for drug treatment", "drug interactions" and "provision of information and service".

Further specialisation in an advanced curriculum (master, residency, second degree in biomedical sciences or whatever) can occur in three areas, where only the first two will lead to the degree of licensed pharmacist:

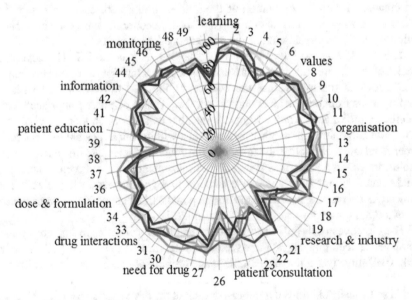

Fig. 2.1 The European Pharmacy Competence Framework (EPCF). Scores for the 50 competences of the six expert groups (vertical scale, score; circumference, competence number; and cluster, 1. academics, yellow; 2. students, blue; 3. community pharmacists, green; 4. hospital pharmacists, orange; 5. industrial pharmacists, red; 6. pharmacists in other professions, purple

- Community pharmacy with emphasis on competences like "ability to identify and prioritise drug-drug interactions and advise appropriate changes to medication" and "ability to identify and prioritise drug-disease interactions (e.g. non-steroidal anti-inflammatory drugs in heart failure) and advise on appropriate changes to medication".
- Hospital pharmacy with emphasis on competences such as "ability to recommend interchangeability of drugs based on in-depth understanding and knowledge of bioequivalence, bio-similarity and therapeutic equivalence of drugs" and "ability to contribute to the cost effectiveness of treatment by collection and analysis of data on medicines' use".
- Industrial pharmacy with emphasis on competences like "knowledge of good manufacturing practice and of good laboratory practice" and "knowledge of drug registration, licensing and marketing". There are currently no EU standards for training in industrial pharmacy. Some pharmacy students follow industrial specialisation courses and will be well prepared for work in the pharmaceutical industry, but they will have no immediate access to the sectorial profession and legal framework of the community/hospital pharmacist.

This list of specialisation areas in pharmacy is not exhaustive and can be completed with specialisation in clinical biology, national and governmental institutions (armed forces, police forces, etc.), education of health sciences, etc.

Our study showed that the perception that pharmacists have of specialisation is double. Whilst they recognise the importance of the biotechnological revolution in medicines and of the advances in hospital pharmacy, they are perplexed as to the everyday applications of this in the community pharmacy. For instance, we found that although the rankings of industrial pharmacists for competences in the areas of "research and industry" and "dose and formulation" were high, the rankings of the other five groups were much lower (Atkinson et al. 2016a, b, c, d).

The evolution of outcomes for pharmacy practice depends on a balance between socio-economic, political and market factors (e.g. the economics of transition from small molecule, chemical medicines to biotechnological medicines). Such factors operate within the framework of the legal requirements for the exercise of the sectoral profession of community pharmacy. Pharmacy education and training can be divided into two domains. Fundamental education and training is primarily centred on preparing for community pharmacy practice. More specialised studies focus on advanced community and hospital pharmacy practice; industrial pharmaceutical research; development, production and regulation of medicines; and research into health sciences. It can be expected that changes will occur in both domains. This could provoke some organisational difficulties.

Many universities have a state-imposed numerus clausus admissions system wherein the number of students accepted is determined by the number of community pharmacists that the healthcare system requires. Even if a numerus clausus is not applied, the number of pharmacy graduates is limited by the number of student practice and residency placements available, i.e. the number of work experience assignments where students can improve their competences within the established legal framework.

As pharmaceutical sciences develop, more graduates above and beyond those for community pharmacy practice may be needed. These could be found by opening up pharmacy studies to studies in industrial pharmacy and hospital pharmacy, for example. Such a move would require a substantial revision of the legislative status of the sectoral profession of a pharmacist. The pharmacist is legally responsible for his/her acts. The license to practice issued by a supervisory, governmental body is based on an appropriate pharmacy degree and, in some cases, a preregistration training period. Licensing bodies oversee the competence requirements for practice.

In Europe such supervision occurs within the context of the EU commission directives. It is unlikely that within the foreseeable future a student who had followed a long, predominately "industrial" pharmacy course, for instance, could obtain registration and a licence to practice as a community pharmacy practitioner.

This could imply that pharmacy (and medical?) faculties develop parallel courses in pharmaceutical specialisation to produce pharmaceutical specialists that do not qualify to be licensed sectoral healthcare professionals. Another alternative is that basic and applied science faculties "pharmaceuticalise" or "medicinalise" their degree courses with courses in physiology, pathology and pharmacology as well as molecular biology, molecular genetics, immunology, biotechnology, etc.

Pharmacology faculties, for instance, should be able to easily modernise their degree courses in this direction. The paradigms involved in the research and development of biotechnological drugs are not basically different from those involved in the research and development of small molecule drugs, viz. receptor theory, screening, preclinical expertise and so on. The main difference is in the tools used (Ritter et al. 2019).

One final comment on industrial pharmacy specialisation: licenced pharmacists are preferentially employed in certain areas of drug development and production, for instance, as "qualified persons" responsible for assuring the quality of medicines.

The EU directive (EU/EC directive 2001) stipulates that the holder of an authorisation to manufacture medicines has at his/her disposal the services of at least one qualified person. It goes on to state that a "qualified person shall be in possession of a diploma, certificate or other evidence of formal qualifications awarded on completion of a university course of study. . . extending over a period of at least four years of theoretical and practical study in one of the following scientific disciplines: pharmacy. . ." In some EU member states, e.g. Germany, only those with a pharmacy degree can meet the requirements set down in the directive on qualified persons (Atkinson et al. 2016a, b, c, d).

2.5 How to Use the Competence-Based Pharmacy Education (CBPE) Framework

We will now look at how competences can be used as educational tools. CBPE can be used for analysis, development and structuring of a curriculum (Nash et al. 2015).

The implementation of CBPE has been described by Koster and his group (Koster et al. 2017). Implementation follows a stepwise process starting with the choice of whether or not to adopt CBPE. CBPE is often adopted as an alternative and improvement on discipline-based teaching (based on subject matters like medicinal chemistry, pharmaco-therapeutics, etc.). It accompanies simultaneously the switch from product-based to patient-based pharmacy. This step also includes a decision as to which CBPE to adopt as several possibilities are available with CBPE becoming more and more dominant throughout the world (Nash et al. 2015). All implementation steps benefit from a collaborative effort involving academia, students, practitioners, societies, chambers and others working to produce consensual decisions. It is important that such a consensual approach is adopted from the very start. The second step involves the definition of the intended learning outcomes; at this stage, representatives of the pertinent government agencies should be recruited into the process given that the main drive is to prepare pharmacists for their specific role in the promotion and improvement of healthcare. The next steps embrace the trajectory of development and the appropriate assessment methods. The final steps focus on the design of the teaching/learning environment, and evaluation followed by adjustment of individual courses and the curriculum as a whole.

The European Pharmacy Competence Framework (EPCF) has been used in Finland (Katajavuori et al. 2017) and Estonia (Volmer et al. 2017), to evaluate existing curricula and to construct new ones.

In Estonia, it was revealed that the traditional discipline-based way of teaching suffered from the lack of involvement of pharmacy practitioners and the lack of collaboration within the pharmacy sector (academia, industry, community and hospital pharmacy). It failed to reply to questions on person-centred health especially regarding chronic conditions and polypharmacy in ageing populations. These require self-care consultation and counselling as well as medicine management services. The Tartu group considered that a competence-based approach to teaching could improve critical thinking, information analysis and communication in these and other matters. CBPE can stimulate the ability to think on a higher, wider level and assess connections in different situations.

CBPE was introduced in 2019 in Estonia and a survey in 2020 showed that in most aspects students were satisfied with the change; for (almost) all evaluation criteria, a Likert score > 3 out of 4 was obtained. Students also considered that yet further progress could be made in transferable and digital skills (Volmer et al. 2021).

The CBPE was also used in Helsinki (Katajavuori et al. 2017). In reports on their experience, the Helsinki group emphasises the need to include all relevant stakeholders from the early stages onwards and to take sufficient time to define the intended learning outcomes before starting on the consideration of the competences required, and the teaching process by which they can be acquired. This emphasises the need for the constructive alignment of learning outcomes and the competences required with real-life teaching practice throughout the curriculum.

The above are interesting experiments in pharmacy education and training. It will be fascinating to follow these substantive changes in teaching and other new developments in this area. In the EU, these changes appear for the moment to be pioneered by relative small EU member states. In the future, when larger states such as France and Germany are more involved, certainly new opportunities and new challenges will arise.

We will now examine several ways in which the pharmacy profession may evolve in the EU and elsewhere in the world.

2.6   Career Options Following the Evolution in Medicines

The issue concerning the evolution in medicines is complex. Since the 1940s, prescription drugs have been primarily small molecules such as aspirin and paracetamol, researched, developed and produced mainly by pharmacological and chemical methods. In the future, large biomolecules may replace (most or some of?) these medicines. These are peptides and nucleic acids, researched, developed and produced mainly by pharmacological, biomolecular, immunological sciences, genetic engineering, biotechnological and other methods.

As the pharmaceutical and biotechnological companies producing these new medicines operate within a free market economy, this evolution will be to some extent economically driven. Already today, the most profitable (expensive) drugs on the market are all of biomolecular/biotechnological origin (Chen et al. 2021). They are all peptides; the top three therapeutic classes are anti-rheumatics, anticoagulants and anticancer drugs (LEEM 2021a).

However, in the immediate future, the vast majority of prescription drugs dispensed by community (and hospital) pharmacists will be (relatively) cheap, small, chemical molecules. In 2006–2009, British academics and National Health Service specialists developed a core list of the 100 most commonly prescribed medicines. This was revised in 2018. The list was relatively stable over the decade concerned. The top three drug classes were small molecular weight oestrogens and progestogens, phosphodiesterase inhibitors and serotonin receptor agonists (Audi et al. 2018).

2.7 Career Options Following the Evolution in Responsibilities and Interaction with Others

Whilst pharmacists are licensed with a responsibility in their fundamental domain (medicines), this responsibility is shared in several specialised domains with others from areas such as chemical and biotechnological engineering, basic biological sciences, etc. This is the case for qualified persons as seen before. This underlines the fact that one essential competence of the pharmacist is the ability to work with others.

Pharmacists interact with other healthcare professionals, such as doctors, nurses and others, in the prescription and dispensation of medicines. Several changes are underway as regards the prescription of dispensed medicines. Already today in some cases, pharmacists can provide patients with drugs without a doctor's prescription. One example is the dispensation of naloxone, an opioid antagonist that rapidly reverses opioid overdose (Puzantian and Gasper 2018; California State Board of Pharmacy 2022).

Pharmacists also interact with doctors in the usual prescription and follow-up process. One example of this is the modification by pharmacists of prescription errors (Buurma et al. 2004). In this Dutch study, 0.49% of prescriptions contained errors that were picked up by pharmacists, 72% of these were unclear prescriptions (illegible or with omissions) and 22% contained errors such as wrong dose, wrong medicine or contraindication. The authors concluded that the pharmacists' interventions led to a modification of the prescription, solved a whole array of drug-related problems in prescriptions and contributed positively to the quality of the pharmacotherapy.

Another example comes from hospital pharmacy in Australia where it is estimated that one of the most frequent clinical incidents in hospitals is medication-related error (Beks et al. 2021). These errors often occur during admission and discharge of patients, so questioning the interaction of the hospital pharmacist with other hospital staff, and the interaction between the hospital pharmacist and the patient's community pharmacist. The study showed that pharmacists with a special training in medication charting and interaction with other healthcare professionals can play a major role in improving this situation.

Finally, it should be noted that although in most cases the dispensation of prescription medications is the prerogative of community (and hospital) pharmacists, this is not always so as human and (even more so) veterinary doctors may play a more or less important role.

Competences for pharmacy practice will develop in the future within this context of an interactive, global healthcare complex of responsibilities. One aspect of this is the creation of healthcare centres grouping the activities of pharmacists and other professionals (doctors, nurses, etc.) (LEEM 2021b). This could allow a more in-depth examination and management of therapy of the patient with a reduction in the multiplication of visits to different healthcare specialists.

Whether the integration of pharmacists into primary care general practice clinics can improve treatment has been studied in a meta-analysis of 38 studies (Tan et al. 2014). Most (29/38) studies recruited patients with specific medical conditions (15 on cardiovascular disease and 9 on diabetes). Pharmacist interventions usually involved medication review delivered collaboratively with the general practitioner. These interventions were favourable in 19 studies with, for instance, significant improvements in blood pressure, glycosylated haemoglobin and cholesterol.

2.8 Career Perspectives Following Evolution in Diagnosis

Pharmacists are becoming more and more involved in clinical biology (blood sugar analysis, etc.) and other procedures (blood pressure measurement, etc.) for diagnosis and monitoring of treatment. This increasing involvement poses the question of whether clinical biology measurements performed by pharmacists are reliable enough in the detection of disease and the monitoring of treatment.

This question was studied by a Canadian group in respect to blood pressure measurement where the measurement error is frequently greater than the size of the effect of therapy or of modification of lifestyle (Chambers et al. 2013). In this trial on 275 adults (mean age 76 years), there were no differences in systolic and diastolic blood pressures measured by pharmacists compared to those measured by physicians. They concluded that automated measurement of blood pressure by pharmacists provides accurate and valid information that can be used in the diagnosis and management of hypertension. With the development of more automation in this area, the role of the pharmacist will take on greater importance.

Pharmacists are also involved in other areas such as the handling of radio-chemicals in imaging procedures performed by medical practitioners. It is accepted that the nuclear medicine team includes doctors, radiographers, technologists, physicists, nurses, administrators and pharmacists (EANM 2006). The radio-pharmacist, in this case, essentially fulfils the role of the qualified person.

2.9 Evolution in Physical Interventions: The Example of Vaccination

Although physical interventions are still largely recognised as the domain of medical doctors, in recent years, pharmacists are more and more involved in physical procedures such as injection of vaccines (Kirkdale et al. 2017; Paudyal et al. 2021).

There are various reasons why the implication of pharmacists is beneficial: pharmacies are open for longer periods and often situated in more deprived areas and especially in medically deprived areas. They see patients with comorbidity that are likely to be on poly-medication thus accessing their pharmacists on a regular basis and hence providing multiple opportunities for acts such as vaccination. Furthermore, access to pharmaceutical services is relatively unhindered (lack of need to have an appointment). This is backed up by a recent American study (Berenbrok et al. 2020) on the access to community pharmacists. The study showed that the ratio of pharmacist to primary physician encounters was 13:8 in metropolitan areas and even higher at 14:5 in rural areas.

Pharmacist-led influenza vaccination campaigns have become a commonly utilised tool to reach vaccination targets. This alternative option for delivery helps to increase the vaccination coverage rate. In 2012–2013, attempts to reach the EU target for influenza vaccination of 75% stood at only 53% for over 65 s and 39% for those with comorbidity (Mereckiene et al. 2014). In areas where community pharmacists are commissioned to vaccinate, rates in over 65 s were much higher (Howard 2015).

Another example of the importance of pharmacists in vaccination programmes has been seen in the rapid response measures needed all over the world to mitigate the spread and impact of Covid-19 (Paudyal et al. 2021). The Paudyal et al. study in 13 European countries showed that the pharmacists' involvement in vaccination involves logistics, reconstitution of vaccine preparations, patient education and vaccination. Pharmacists are on the front line of the aim to hit vaccination targets, not only in community pharmacies but also alongside general medical practitioners, and in hospitals and vaccination centres.

2.10   Evolutions in Patient/Pharmaceutical Care

In recent years, the psychological element, whilst remaining a prerogative of medical doctors, has developed a pharmacist facet with the creation of the discipline of pharmaceutical care. This is within a context of the evolution of the roles of community pharmacists from product-oriented services (dispensation of prescribed medicines and sale of over-the-counter preparations) to patient-centred services (management of medication therapy).

Their new roles include preventive services such as administration of vaccines and identifying patients at high risk for disease. They also include management—in the form of patient consultations and education—of chronic diseases such as diabetes, arterial hypertension, HIV/AIDS, hyperlipidaemia, asthma and depression. All this is occurring in parallel with changes in pharmacy education and trading from a chemical/medicine orientation to a treatment/medical orientation.

One example of the effectiveness of pharmacists in the above changes is seen in a recent meta-analysis of reviews published from 2007 to 2017 on the impact of community pharmacist-led interventions in chronic disease management (Newman et al. 2020). This showed that pharmacist interventions produced significant reductions in haemoglobin A1c, total cholesterol and low-density lipoproteins, blood pressure, etc. They also improved adherence to medication, for example, in

HIV/AIDS, reduced admission rates for heart failure and improved lung function in patients with respiratory conditions.

2.11 Evolution in Public/Private Financing, National/International Healthcare Policy and Economics

Given the in-depth knowledge of pharmacists coming from their 5–6-year degree course, governments are looking more and more into the possibilities for economically driven repartition of outcomes (and therefore competences). This is occurring in a context of exploding healthcare budgets. One future aspect of this could be the increased role that pharmacists play in screening for certain diseases (LEEM 2021a).

The role of pharmacists in other governmental policies is also changing with greater involvement in surveys of general health of the population and in health improvement campaigns against smoking, excessive alcohol consumption, obesity and high blood pressure. A future development in this area may be the heightened involvement of pharmacists in telemedicine (LEEM 2021b).

Finally, it should be noted that the economic status of pharmacies and pharmacists is changing in some countries with the private sector becoming more and more involved. This is seen in changes in the national law regarding the ownership of a pharmacy. Ownership is often no longer uniquely and wholly the domain of the pharmacist. Another recent example of such changes is seen in changes in national laws brought on by the Covid-19 situation with the possibility for supermarkets and other outlets, which do not always have a registered pharmacist on their premises, to sell products such as face masks.

2.12 Career Options in Response to Global Change in the Environment, Climate and Illness

Urbanisation, climate change, increased mobility, etc. induce population movements with ensuing changes in disease profiles and the appearance of previously unknown zoonoses. This raises the subject of specialisation in veterinary pharmacy. Such practitioners already have a critical role to play treating the ever increasing numbers of domestic pets in urban practice. Pharmacists are the only healthcare professionals legally allowed to provide care for both human and non-human patients. Zoonotic pandemics caused by viruses such as HIV/AIDS, severe acute respiratory syndrome and influenza originate in animals displaced by ecological, behavioural and/or socio-economic changes (Morse 2012).

So far no pandemic has ever been predicted before infection of human beings sets in. The challenges in the future are to predict epidemics, target surveillance and identify prevention strategies. Veterinary pharmacists have a unique knowledge of human and non-human physiology, pharmacology and other subjects. They would be ideal partners for teams involved in prediction, preventive and therapeutics of zoonoses.

Another important aspect of global change is the ageing of populations with the increasing complexity of multiple comorbidities and subsequent poly-medication. All this leads to decreased compliance to therapy, loss of contact with the healthcare system, etc. (LEEM 2021b). The increase in life expectancy, with growing numbers of people 100 or more years old, together with ever-increasing number of tools emerging from the IT and biology revolutions (such as the application of genomics to diagnosis and subsequent choice of therapy), will lead to a new form of "5P" care: predictive, preventive, personalised, participative and proven. The ways in which such care is delivered will also evolve with a change towards home support and telemedicine. Pharmacists will have an important role to play in such progress.

2.13 Conclusion

This chapter describes the historical development of the practice of product-/medicine-based pharmacy and the traditional competences and legal responsibilities of the pharmacist practising this profession. It then turns to the future and the substantial changes occurring in all areas of pharmacy practice such as the biotechnological revolution in the research, development and production of medicines and the switch to a more patient-based community and hospital pharmacy practice.

It presents an iterative Delphi-based methodology capable of allowing universities to rapidly respond to these changes and to produce teaching programmes capable of providing the framework of competences required. It presents examples of how this European Pharmacy Competence Framework (EPCF) is practically applied in curricula. Competence-based education can provide a response to the new and stimulating avenues for future practice and the new competences for pharmacy practice they require. Its ongoing implementation in academia will support further growth of the career options for all graduates in pharmacy in the EU.

Appendix

The European Pharmacy Competence Framework (EPCF)

	Personal competences: learning and knowledge
1	Ability to identify learning needs and to learn independently (including continuous professional development (CPD)
2	Ability to apply logic to problem solving

(continued)

3	Ability to critically appraise relevant knowledge and to summarise the key points
4	Ability to evaluate scientific data in line with current scientific and technological knowledge
5	Ability to apply preclinical and clinical evidence-based medical science to pharmaceutical practice
6	Ability to apply current knowledge of relevant legislation and codes of pharmacy practice

Personal competences: values

7	A professional approach to tasks and human relations
8	Ability to maintain confidentiality
9	Ability to take full responsibility for patient care
10	Ability to inspire the confidence of others in one's actions and advice
11	Knowledge of appropriate legislation and of ethics

Personal competences: communication and organisational skills

12	Ability to communicate effectively, both oral and written, in the locally relevant language
13	Ability to effectively use information technology
14	Ability to work effectively as part of a team
15	Ability to implement general legal requirements that impact upon the practice of pharmacy (e.g. health and safety legislation, employment law)
16	Ability to contribute to the training of staff
17	Ability to manage risk and quality of service issues
18	Ability to identify the need for new services
19	Ability to understand a business environment and develop entrepreneurship

Personal competences: research and industrial pharmacy

20	Knowledge of design, synthesis, isolation, characterisation and biological evaluation of active substances
21	Knowledge of good manufacturing practice and of good laboratory practice
22	Knowledge of European directives on qualified persons
23	Knowledge of drug registration, licensing and marketing
24	Knowledge of the importance of research in pharmaceutical development and practice

Patient care competences: patient consultation and assessment

25	Ability to interpret basic medical laboratory tests
26	Ability to perform appropriate diagnostic tests, e.g. measurement of blood pressure or blood sugar
27	Ability to recognise when referral to another member of the healthcare team is needed

Patient care competences: need for drug treatment

28	Ability to retrieve and interpret information on the patient's clinical background
29	Ability to compile and interpret a comprehensive drug history for an individual patient
30	Ability to identify non-adherence to medicine therapy and make an appropriate intervention
31	Ability to advise to physicians on the appropriateness of prescribed medicines and, in some cases, to prescribe medication

Patient care competences: drug interactions

32	Ability to identify and prioritise drug-drug interactions and advise appropriate changes to medication
33	Ability to identify and prioritise drug-patient interactions, including those that prevent or require the use of a specific drug, based on pharmacogenetics, and advise on appropriate changes to medication

(continued)

34	Ability to identify and prioritise drug-disease interactions (e.g. NSAIDs in heart failure) and advise on appropriate changes to medication

Patient care competences: drug dose and formulation

35	Knowledge of the biopharmaceutical, pharmacodynamic and pharmacokinetic activity of a substance in the body
36	Ability to recommend interchangeability of drugs based on in-depth understanding and knowledge of bioequivalence, bio-similarity and therapeutic equivalence of drugs
37	Ability to undertake a critical evaluation of a prescription ensuring that it is clinically appropriate and legally valid
38	Knowledge of the supply chain of medicines thus ensuring timely flow of quality drug products to the patient
39	Ability to manufacture medicinal products that are not commercially available

Patient care competences: patient education

40	Ability to promote public health in collaboration with other professionals within the healthcare system
41	Ability to provide appropriate lifestyle advice to improve patient outcomes (e.g. advice on smoking, obesity, etc.)
42	Ability to use pharmaceutical knowledge and provide evidence-based advice on public health issues involving medicines

Patient care competences: provision of information and service

43	Ability to use effective consultations to identify the patient's need for information
44	Ability to provide accurate and appropriate information on prescription medicines
45	Ability to provide evidence-based support for patients in selection and use of non-prescription medicines

Patient care competences: monitoring of drug therapy

46	Ability to identify and prioritise problems in the management of medicines in a timely and effective manner and so ensure patient safety
47	Ability to monitor and report adverse drug events and adverse drug reactions (ADEs and ADRs) to all concerned, in a timely manner, and in accordance with current regulatory guidelines on good pharmacovigilance practices (GVPs)
48	Ability to undertake a critical evaluation of prescribed medicines to confirm that current clinical guidelines are appropriately applied
49	Ability to monitor patient care outcomes to optimise treatment in collaboration with the prescriber
50	Ability to contribute to the cost-effectiveness of treatment by collection and analysis of data on medicines' use

References

Atkinson J, Rombaut B, Sánchez Pozo A, Rekkas D, Veski P, Hirvonen J, Bozic N, Skowron A, Mircioiu C (2013) A description of the European pharmacy education and training quality assurance project. Pharmacy 1:3–7. https://doi.org/10.3390/pharmacy1010003

Atkinson J, Rombaut B, Sánchez Pozo A, Rekkas D, Veski P, Hirvonen J, Bozic N, Skowron A, Mircioiu C, Marcincal A, Wilson K (2014) The production of a framework of competences for pharmacy practice in the European Union. Pharmacy 2:161–174. https://doi.org/10.3390/pharmacy2020161

Atkinson J, de Paepe K, Sánchez Pozo A, Rekkas D, Volmer D, Hirvonen J, Bozic B, Skowron A, Mircioiu C, Marcincal A, Koster K, Wilson K, van Schravendijk C, Wilkinson J (2016a) What is a pharmacist: opinions of pharmacy department academics and community pharmacists on competences required for pharmacy practice. Pharmacy (Basel) 4:12–20. https://doi.org/10.3390/pharmacy4010012

Atkinson J, de Paepe K, Sánchez Pozo A, Rekkas D, Volmer D, Hirvonen J, Bozic B, Skowron A, Mircioiu C, Marcincal A, Koster K, Wilson K, van Schravendijk C (2016b) A study on how industrial pharmacists rank competences for pharmacy practice: a case for industrial pharmacy specialization. Pharmacy (Basel) 4:1–15. https://doi.org/10.3390/pharmacy4010013

Atkinson J, Sánchez Pozo A, Rekkas D, Volmer D, Hirvonen J, Bozic B, Skowron A, Mircioiu C, Sandulovici R, Marcincal A, Koster A, Wilson KA, van Schravendijk C, Frontini R, Price R, Bates I, De Paepe K (2016c) Hospital and community pharmacists' perceptions of which competences are important for their practice. Pharmacy 4:1–21. https://doi.org/10.3390/pharmacy4020021

Atkinson J, De Paepe K, Sánchez Pozo A, Rekkas D, Volmer D, Hirvonen J, Bozic B, Skowron A, Mircioiu C, Marcincal A, Koster A, Wilson K, van Schravendijk C (2016d) The second round of the PHAR-QA survey of competences for pharmacy practice. Pharmacy (Basel) 4:1–7. https://doi.org/10.3390/pharmacy4030027

Audi S, Burrage DR, Lonsdale DO, Pontefract S, Coleman JJ, Hitchings AW, Baker EH (2018) The 'top 100' drugs and classes in England: an updated 'starter formulary' for trainee prescribers. Br J Clin Pharmacol 84:2562–2571. https://doi.org/10.1111/bcp.13709

Beks H, McNamara K, Manias E, Dalton A, Tong E, Dooley M (2021) Hospital pharmacists' experiences of participating in a partnered pharmacist medication charting credentialing program: a qualitative study. BMC Health Services Res 21:251–255. https://doi.org/10.1186/s12913-021-06267-w

Berenbrok LA, Gabriel N, Coley KC, Hernandez I (2020) Evaluation of frequency of encounters with primary care physicians vs visits to community pharmacies among Medicare beneficiaries. JAMA Netw Open 3:e209132. https://doi.org/10.1001/jamanetworkopen.2020.9132

Buurma H, De Smet PAGM, Leufkens HGM, Egberts ACG (2004) Evaluation of the clinical value of pharmacists' modifications of prescription errors. Br J Clin Pharmacol 58:503–511. https://doi.org/10.1111/j.1365-2125.2004.02181.x

California State Board of Pharmacy. Cal. Code Regs. Tit. 16, § 1746.3 - Protocol for pharmacists furnishing naloxone hydrochloride (2022). https://www.pharmacy.ca.gov/licensees/naloxone_info.shtml. Accessed 26 Jan 2022

Chambers LW, Kaczorowski J, O'Rielly S, Ignagni S, Hearps SJC (2013) Comparison of blood pressure measurements using an automated blood pressure device in community pharmacies and family physicians' offices: a randomized controlled trial. CMAJ Open 1:E37–E42. https://doi.org/10.9778/cmajo.20130005

Chen Y, Monnard A, Santos da Silva J (2021) An inflection point for biosimilars. Mackinsey Life Sciences, New York. https://www.mckinsey.com/industries/life-sciences/our-insights/an-inflection-point-for-biosimilars. Accessed 26 Jan 2022

Dalkey NC (1967) The Delphi method an experimental study of group opinion. Rand Corporation, Santa Monica. https://www.rand.org/pubs/research_memoranda/RM5888.html. Accessed 26 Jan 2022

EANM. European Association of Nuclear Medicine. Best practice in nuclear medicine (2006). https://www.eanm.org/publications/technologists-guide/best-practice-nuclear-medicine-part-1/. Accessed 26 Jan 2022

EU/EC. Directive. Directive 2001/83/EC of the European parliament and of the council of 6 November 2001 on the Community code relating to medicinal products for human use https://eur-lex.europa.eu/legal-content/en/TXT/?uri=CELEX%3A32001L0083. Accessed 26 Jan 2022

EU. Directive. Directive 2013/55/EU of the European parliament and of the council of 20 November 2013 amending Directive 2005/36/EC on the recognition of professional qualifications and Regulation (EU) No 1024/2012 on administrative cooperation through the Internal Market Information System ('the IMI Regulation'). https://eur-lex.europa.eu/legal-content/EN/ALL/?uri=celex%3A32013L0055. Accessed 26 Jan 2022

Faure E (2014) Le médicament en France au XIXe siècle. Un triomphe inattendu 21:119–130. https://doi.org/10.3917/bhesv.212.0119

Howard P (2015) Antimicrobial stewardship in community pharmacy – what do commissioners need to know? https://www.google.com/url?sa=t&rct=j&q=&esrc=s&source=web&cd=&ved=2ahUKEwiGs9jB1c_1AhUF5OAKHTiMDTAQFnoECAcQAQ&url=https%3A%2F%2Fwww.england.nhs.uk%2Fwp-content%2Fuploads%2F2015%2F04%2F10-amr-brim-antimicrobial-stewardship-com-pharm.pdf&usg=AOvVaw2hpSQ07F2PaDqk2Pd48p1q. Accessed 26 Jan 2022

Katajavuori N, Salminen O, Vuorensola K, Huhtala H, Vuorela P, Hirvonen J (2017) Competence-Based Pharmacy Education in the University of Helsinki. Pharmacy (Basel) 5:29–37. http://www.mdpi.com/2226-4787/5/2/29

Kirkdale CL, Nebout G, Megerlinc F, Thornley T (2017) Benefits of pharmacist-led flu vaccination services in community pharmacy. Ann Pharm Fr 75:3–8. https://doi.org/10.1016/j.pharma.2016.08.005

Koster A, Schalekamp T, Meijerman I (2017) Implementation of competency-based pharmacy education (CBPE). Pharmacy (Basel) 5:10–16. https://doi.org/10.3390/pharmacy5010010

LEEM: les entreprises du médicament. Bilan économique (2021a). https://www.leem.org/publication/bilan-economique-2020-des-entreprises-du-medicament-edition-2021. Accessed 26 Jan 2022

LEEM: les entreprises du médicament. Santé 2030, une analyse prospective de l'innovation en santé (2021b). https://www.leem.org/publication/sante-2030-une-analyse-prospective-de-linnovation-en-sante. Accessed 26 Jan 2022

Mereckiene J, Cotter S, Nicoll A, Lopalco P, Noori T, Weber JT, D'Ancona F, Lévy-Bruhl D, Dematte L, Giambi C, Valentiner-Branth P, Stankiewicz I, Appelgren E, O'Flanagan D, the VENICE project gatekeepers group. Seasonal influenza immunisation in Europe (2014) Overview of recommendations and vaccination coverage for three seasons: pre-pandemic (2008/09), pandemic (2009/10) and post-pandemic (2010/11). Euro Surveill 19:16–50. https://doi.org/10.2807/1560-7917.es2014.19.16.20780

Merriam Webster Dictionary. Merriam Webster Company, Springfield. https://www.merriam-webster.com/dictionary/pharmacist. Accessed 26 Jan 2022

Mircioiu C, Atkinson J (2017) A comparison of parametric and non-parametric methods applied to a likert scale. Pharmacy (Basel) 5:26–36. https://doi.org/10.3390/pharmacy5020026

Morse SS (2012) Prediction and prevention of the next pandemic zoonosis. Lancet 380:1956–1965. https://doi.org/10.1016/S0140-6736(12)61684-5

Nash RE, Chalmers J, Brown N, Jackson S, Peterson G (2015) An international review of the use of competency standards in undergraduate pharmacy education. Pharmacy Educ 15: 131–141. https://pharmacyeducation.fip.org/pharmacyeducation/article/view/324/295. Accessed 26 Jan 2022

Newman TV, San-Juan-Rodriguez A, Parekh N, Swart ECS, Klein-Fedyshin M, Shrank WH, Hernandez I (2020) Impact of community pharmacist-led interventions in chronic disease management on clinical utilization and economic outcomes. Res Social Adm Pharm 16:1155–1165. https://doi.org/10.1016/j.sapharm.2019.12.016

Paudyal V, Fialová D, Henman MC, Hazen A, Okuyan B, Lutters M, Cadogan C, Alves da Costa F, Galfrascoli E, Pudritz YM, Rydant S, Acosta-Gómez J (2021) Pharmacists' involvement in COVID-19 vaccination across Europe: a situational analysis of current practice and policy. Int J Clin Pharm 43:1139–1148. https://doi.org/10.1007/s11096-021-01301-7

Puzantian T, Gasper JJ (2018) Provision of naloxone without a prescription by California pharmacists 2 years after legislation implementation. JAMA 320:1933–1934. https://doi.org/10.1001/jama.2018.12291

Ritter J, Flower R, Henderson G, Loke YK, MacEwan D, Rang H (2019) Rang & Dale's pharmacology, 9th edn. Elsevier, London. https://www.elsevier.com/books/rang-and-dales-pharmacology/ritter/978-0-7020-7448-6. Accessed 26 Jan 2022

Stone E (1932) Medicine among the American Indians. Clio Medica, Hoeber, P.B., New York. https://sfu-primo.hosted.exlibrisgroup.com/primo-explore/search?query=lsr31,exact,Clio%20medica%20%20a%20series%20of%20primers%20on%20the%20history%20of%20medicine, AND&query=any,contains,indians,AND&tab=default_tab&search_scope=default_scope&vid=SFUL&mode=advanced&offset=0. Accessed 26 Jan 2022

Stupans I, Atkinson J, Meštrovi'c E, Nash R, Rouse MJ (2016) A shared focus: comparing the Australian, Canadian, United Kingdom and United States pharmacy learning outcome frameworks and the global competency framework. Pharmacy (Basel) 4:26–36. https://doi.org/10.3390/pharmacy4030026

Tan ECK, Stewart K, Elliott RA, George J (2014) Pharmacist services provided in general practice clinics: a systematic review and meta-analysis. Res Social Adm Pharm 10:608–622. https://doi.org/10.1016/j.sapharm.2013.08.006

Volmer D, Sepp K, Veski P, Raal A (2017) The implementation of pharmacy competence teaching in Estonia. Pharmacy 5:18–30. https://doi.org/10.3390/pharmacy5020018

Volmer D, Sepp K, Raal A (2021) Students' feedback on the development of a competency-based pharmacy education (CBPE) at the university of Tartu. Estonia 9:45–55. https://doi.org/10.3390/pharmacy9010045

Zebroski B (2016) A brief history of pharmacy. Routledge, New York. https://www.routledge.com/A-Brief-History-of-Pharmacy-Humanitys-Search-for-Wellness/Zebroski/p/book/9780415537841. Accessed 26 Jan 2022

Chapter 3
Job and Career Opportunities in the Pharmaceutical Industry: An Overview

Josse R. Thomas

Abstract The pharmaceutical industry offers a wealth of job and career opportunities for talented graduates and (young) professionals in the life sciences, i.e. Bachelors, Masters, PhDers and Post-docs in pharmaceutical sciences, medicine, biomedical sciences, biotechnology, bioengineering, bioinformatics, data science, biostatistics, veterinary medicine and many more. This chapter gives an overview of the many possibilities, often poorly known to young graduates.

The core of the chapter is structured in three parts.

The introductory part explains what is understood by the pharmaceutical industry and its place within the broader life sciences sector, with key data on its employment potential; and describes the essential phases of the drug life cycle, i.e. discovery research, development (pharmaceutical, non-clinical and clinical), and commercialisation.

The main part overviews the different job opportunities throughout the drug life cycle, possibilities in overarching supportive functions (e.g. regulatory affairs, quality management, pharmacovigilance, medical/scientific writing, project planning) as well as in more general business management roles (e.g. business intelligence, portfolio management, business development and even human resources, information technology, finance and legal affairs).

The final part focuses on career perspectives in the pharmaceutical industry and beyond: first describing what is needed for a successful start, then following with a few thoughts about career development, and finalising with some information on the wide range of potential career paths within this fascinating sector.

For more detailed information, the reader is often referred to the other chapters of the book or the list of references.

J. R. Thomas (✉)
PharmaCS, Merchtem, Belgium

3.1 Introduction

A lot of undergraduate students and young graduates or researchers in the life sciences do not have a sufficiently precise idea of the employment potential of the pharmaceutical industry, to seriously consider such a start or move for their professional career. This chapter is written to give them an initial overview of the myriad of job and career opportunities in this attractive sector.

3.2 The Pharmaceutical Industry

3.2.1 What Is Meant by the Pharmaceutical Industry?

As a general term, the pharmaceutical industry is defined as the industrial sector oriented to the research, development, production and commercialisation of medicinal products (medicines, drugs, pharmaceuticals) to treat, prevent or diagnose diseases in humans or animals. The current definition of medicines (EUR-Lex 2001) is not limited to the classic world of small molecules, but also includes the more recently widely introduced biologicals or biopharmaceuticals (produced by living organisms), vaccines, in vivo diagnostics, radiopharmaceuticals and advanced therapy medicinal products (ATMPs) such as gene, cell and tissue therapies. Therefore, the term pharmaceutical industry is currently often replaced by biopharmaceutical industry.

Drug research, development, production and commercialisation are highly regulated. The pharmaceutical industry has to comply with a vast array of legislation, issued by government bodies worldwide, and various sets of (inter)national guidelines and standards. Guidelines, guidance or recommendations are mostly related to scientific and technical topics and can be issued by regulatory authorities, such as by the European Medicines Agency (EMA) or the Food and Drug Administration (FDA in the USA), or the International Council for Harmonisation of Technical Requirements for Pharmaceuticals for Human Use (ICH). ICH issues guidelines on scientific and technical aspects of drug registration, by consensus between experts of regulatory authorities and the pharmaceutical industry from various world regions. International standards are agreed by the International Organization for Standardization (ISO) and 'describe the best way of doing something, e.g. making a product, managing a process, delivering a solution, or supplying materials'. Some (sets of) standards are highly relevant for the pharmaceutical industry, such as ISO 9000 intended to embed a quality management system (QMS) in an organisation, and ISO 27000 related to information security management systems (ISMS). Overall, a lot of regulations to comply with.

The pharmaceutical industry spans a wide range of companies, either involved in innovative original brand medicines, or generics (copies of small molecules), or biosimilars (versions of biologicals), or either active in several of these branches.

Most companies are into human medicines, but some are specialised in veterinary medicines. Some are big companies operating worldwide (big pharma), and others are smaller and more focused on discovery research and early clinical development (often biotech companies), either licensing their products out to big pharma or finally being acquired by them. In addition, the pharma companies who finally sell medicines often appeal to different types of pharmaceutical service providers and outsourcing companies all along the drug life cycle, from contract research organisations (CROs) to contract manufacturing organisations (CMOs), creating a whole world of extra employment possibilities.

3.2.2 Employment Potential

According to EFPIA (European Federation of Pharmaceutical Industries and Associations), the research-based pharmaceutical industry in Europe directly employed about 830,000 individuals in 2020, and a number that is still growing (EFPIA 2021). The International Federation of Pharmaceutical Manufacturers and Associations (IFPMA) estimates that the biopharmaceutical industry employs approximately 5.5 million people worldwide, including the manufacturing of generics (IFPMA 2021).

Of course, not all of these positions are occupied by graduates in life sciences, but the vast majority of employees in pharmaceutical research and development (125,000 in Europe in 2020) probably are, thus indicating that number-wise it constitutes a particularly attractive occupational sector.

The public at large perceives the reputation of the pharmaceutical industry as poor, largely because of its 'unethical practice of making large profits on the back of the misery of patients'. Nevertheless, its reputation within healthcare professionals (HCPs) is a lot better and is even improving since the COVID-19 pandemic (ABPI-IPSOS 2021).

According to BioSpace (Zahid 2021), there are six good reasons why a career in the pharmaceutical industry can be very rewarding: (1) the salary range, i.e. it pays well; (2) learning opportunities, i.e. you constantly learn, gain knowledge and discover new things; (3) job and career satisfaction, i.e. you help to save lives; (4) scope for flexibility, i.e. although the pharma industry has to deal with some regulatory rigidity, innovation stimulates thinking outside the box; (5) diversity, i.e. in the sense of operating worldwide, but also in being able to work in a multidisciplinary environment; and (6) access to latest technology, i.e. allowing you to stay up-to-date with the newest innovative technologies.

And finally, there is certainly also room to start one's own company. Entrepreneurship merits more attention in the curricula of life scientists at the university, and especially during their doctoral training. To close this gap, several initiatives have recently been taken to launch life sciences entrepreneurship programmes. Moreover, outside academia there seem to be adequate ways to find help for start-ups and scale-ups. More detailed information on these matters can be found in Chap. 15.

3.2.3   Place Within the Life Sciences Sector

The pharmaceutical industry is part of the broader life sciences sector, wherein you can further find similar job and career opportunities.

The life sciences sector comprises mainly the following sub-sectors:

1. The life sciences industries, incl. the (bio)pharmaceutical industry (human and veterinary), but also related industries operating in, e.g. biotechnology or biotech (medical/red, industrial/white, environmental/green, marine/blue), medical technology or medtech (medical devices, in vitro diagnostics, digital health and care), e-health data management, healthy food and food supplements (nutraceuticals) or personal care (cosmeceuticals).

   A lot of the job and career opportunities that are described in this book for the pharmaceutical industry have similar options in these related industries and widen further the wealth of possibilities. On top of that, all these industries have national or international member associations or federations, with interesting positions to further your career.

2. The vast array of stakeholder organisations within the sector, such as the following:

   • Regulatory authorities, e.g. the European Commission/DG SANTE, national and regional medicines agencies (EU member state agencies, EMA, FDA, etc.), notified bodies and patent offices. They also need talented professionals in the life sciences, e.g. to set up and guide the regulatory framework; to give scientific advice to the industrial partners; to evaluate the drug/product clinical trial applications, the marketing authorisation applications and the pharmaco- or other vigilance dossiers; and to perform inspections related to regulatory compliance.

   • Health technology assessment (HTA) bodies, especially looking for clinicians and pharmacists who are experts in rational (pharmaco)therapy, as well as health and pharmaco-economists.

   • Research ethics committees (RECs), having amongst their members various types of clinicians, hospital pharmacists, clinical pharmacologists, clinical research methodologists, biostatisticians, ethicists, legal advisors and patient representatives.

   • Academic research institutions, active within the wide range of life sciences mentioned earlier. As an alternative to a full academic career as researcher, a move from academia to industry, with then a switch to a regulatory body, and ending back in academia, can be evenly attractive.

   • Other types of stakeholders, such as clinical investigation sites (phase 1 units, hospitals, private practices), non-profit organisations (e.g. the European Organisation for the Research and Treatment of Cancer, EORTC), science parks, tech transfer offices, incubators and accelerators, consulting companies, venture capitalist and investment management companies as well as (bio)defence and bioterrorism research organisations, are all also keen to find motivated professionals in the various life sciences.

Most of these institutions, bodies or organisations cited above are looking for similar profiles as the pharmaceutical industry and also offer a wide variety of interesting job positions. More detailed information on the possibilities in science and technology parks can be found in Chap. 14 .

3. Within the pharmaceutical and medical sub-sectors, the primary and hospital healthcare settings both offer rewarding job and career opportunities closer to patients. Here, various healthcare professionals (HCPs), such as general practitioners and medical specialists, community and hospital pharmacists, nurses, physio- or psychotherapists, lab technicians, etc., may all find their way. More detailed information on the competences of pharmacists can be found in Chap. 2, and on how to become a successful community or hospital pharmacist in Chap. 16.

And finally, let's not forget the central role of patients, patient organisations and patient advocacy groups in this sector. As the search for new medicines becomes more patient-centric, these organisations will be more solicited, and they'll need to organise themselves better. Therefore, in their quest for independence from industrial sponsors, they too are looking for motivated and enthusiastic people with expertise in their domain.

3.3 The Drug Life Cycle

In healthcare interventions, the life cycle of a drug (or medicinal product, or medicine, or biopharmaceutical) or a product (e.g. a medical device or an in vitro diagnostic) is commonly divided in three phases: discovery research, development and commercialisation. They run roughly consecutively, but for a substantial time also in parallel. Along the timeline of the drug/product life cycle, there are a number of important milestones, i.e. securing a patent, the start of the first-in-human (FIH) study, obtaining the first marketing authorisation, the end of the patent protection and finally, market withdrawal, which signals the end of the life cycle. Figure 3.1 shows a schematic representation of the drug life cycle.

The development phase is usually subdivided in three sub-streams: chemical/ pharmaceutical development (or technical development for a medtech product or solution), non-clinical development, and clinical development.

The duration of the different phases can be highly variable, but usually ranges between 3 and 5 years for research (R), and between 5 and 8 years for development (D), easily adding up to about a decade of R & D to bring a new drug to the market. The mean cost of R & D investment, based on publicly available data, has recently been estimated at 1.3 billion US dollars (Wouters et al. 2020). In order to recoup

The Drug Life Cycle

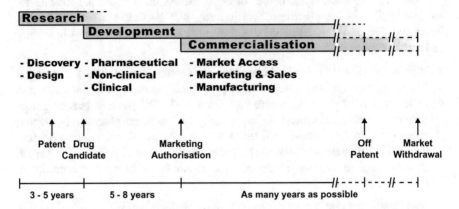

Fig. 3.1 Schematic representation of the drug life cycle.
© 2016 Josse R. Thomas et al. Adapted from *Job and Career Opportunities in the Pharmaceutical Sector*; originally published under CC BY 3.0 licence. Available from: DOI 10.5772/66422

these upfront costs and get a fair return on investment (ROI), the commercialisation of a new drug is intended to last as long as possible.

In this section, the different phases of the drug life cycle will be briefly summarised. More detailed information can be found in 'Global New Drug Development: An Introduction' by Rosier et al. (2014). This typical life cycle and its different phases and sub-streams are similar for medtech or related healthcare products.

3.3.1 Drug Discovery Research

Although the search for medicines has been going on since many centuries, the medical need for new drugs in some disease areas is still very high today.

For many years, drugs were mainly *discovered* by serendipity, thus finding (parts of) organisms or products to be pharmacologically active in nature (e.g. the discovery of poppies and later morphine as potent pain killers) or in large sample collections of existing or newly synthesised chemical substances. Discovering new drugs by synthesis of a series of new chemical compounds is still very popular today, using automated combinatorial chemistry and high-throughput screening as modern tools.

Since a number of decades, the rational *design* of medicines has come to the forefront as a more powerful and more successful method for drug discovery. This is mainly due to a better understanding of the biology, biochemical molecular structures, mechanisms and defects that underlie the causes and pathophysiology of diseases. This then led to the identification of 'drug targets', i.e. macromolecules such as proteins (e.g. ion channels, enzymes) or nucleosides (nuclear receptors, mRNA) that can interact with the drug to sort a desired pharmacological activity, but also unwanted toxicological side effects. Modern techniques, such as detailed 3D structure-activity relationship (SAR) analysis, computer-aided drug design (CADD, either structure- or ligand-based), modelling and simulation (M & S) and bioinformatics, all play a crucial role in this rapidly evolving field of drug research.

More recently, drug research has been revolutionised by developments in the biotechnology field. In the past, drugs were mostly *small molecules* (usually less than 1 kilodaltons in molecular weight), interacting with a docking site or a pocket in the larger biological target molecules. Since the advent of genetic engineering techniques, such as recombinant DNA technology and CRISPR-Cas9 gene editing, more complex and larger *biologicals*, *biopharmaceuticals* or *ATMPs* can now be produced by living organisms (bacteria, yeasts or mammalian cells or tissues) and used as therapeutics (e.g. human insulin, humanised monoclonal antibodies or MABs, nucleosides), vaccines (e.g. COVID-19 mRNA vaccines) or diagnostic agents (e.g. recombinant antigens). In 2020, already half of the ten top-selling medicines worldwide were biopharmaceuticals, and this trend is still increasing (Fierce Pharma 2021).

Finally, a few words about the drug discovery process itself.

The target-based approach is commonly divided into the following steps: (1) identification and validation of the target, and whether the target is 'druggable'; (2) bioassay development for screening of interesting compounds; (3) high-throughput screening to identify 'hits' (first proof of interaction with the target); (4) hit-to-lead phase, wherein medicinal chemists iteratively synthesise new molecules to improve their in vitro pharmacologic activity, with acceptable basic in vitro pharmacokinetic properties and toxicological effects, in order to identify a limited number of 'lead compounds' (e.g. 10); and (5) lead optimisation, with an early phase, wherein in vivo animal models are used to narrow down the leads to a few best proposals to proceed to late lead optimisation, wherein more extensive results are produced on pharmacologic activity, kinetics and toxicity, to finally deliver one or two candidate drugs found suitable for further development.

3.3.2 Drug Development

The initial objective of drug development is to gather sufficient sound evidence of the quality, the efficacy and the safety of a new drug to allow authorities to grant it a marketing authorisation. Once on the market though, its development continues to prove its clinical effectiveness in real-world conditions; to study new indications, formulations and combinations; and to continue gathering information on its safety profile.

As the development process is complex and long-lasting, it is useful to describe it here in a bit more detail.

3.3.2.1 Functional Drug Development Disciplines

Successful drug development is the result of the interplay between three essential groups of disciplines, each responsible for generating their specific part of the evidence needed, i.e. chemical/pharmaceutical development, non-clinical development and clinical development.

Chemical/Pharmaceutical Development
The chemical (or biotechnological) development focuses on the production of the active pharmaceutical ingredient(s) (API), whereas the pharmaceutical development is concentrated on the production of the end product or pharmaceutical formulation (e.g. a tablet or a solution for injection or inhalation). These activities are also referred to as chemistry, manufacturing and controls (*CMC*, more in the USA) or *chem-pharm*. Both should guarantee that throughout the drug life cycle, sufficient *quantities* of the active ingredient and the end product are available for development and commercialisation (supply chain management), all with the appropriate *quality specifications* according to regulatory standards, e.g. the International Council for Harmonisation quality guidelines (ICH Qx), and good manufacturing practice (GMP). The chemical/pharmaceutical development also relies heavily on the (bio)-analytical chemistry discipline, responsible for developing the assay methods to test the identity, quality and stability of all the products involved in manufacturing a medicinal product (e.g. starting material, API, excipients, intermediates, degradation products, end product).

Non-clinical Development
Non-clinical development studies the efficacy, safety and kinetics of the candidate drug in a laboratory setting, e.g. in animals and in animal and human bodily material, and by computer modelling and simulation. The scientific disciplines specifically involved are pharmacology, toxicology, pharmacokinetics and (bio)analytical chemistry.

The specific *pharmacology* part generates evidence related to the intended on-target effects, i.e. 'what the drug is doing with the body', known as its pharmacodynamic activity and efficacy.

Thorough off-target safety is studied in short- and long-term general *toxicology*, genotoxicology, reproductive toxicology, carcinogenicity and more specific regulatory toxicology studies. The *safety pharmacology* completes the evidence by studying more general safety effects on the cardiovascular, neurobehavioral, respiratory and gastrointestinal systems.

Pharmacokinetics investigates the kinetic behaviour of the parent drug and its metabolites, i.e. 'what the body does with the drug', but also drug-food and drug-drug interactions (DDI), and pharmacokinetic-pharmacodynamic (PK-PD) relationships. Today, these disciplines rely heavily on modelling and simulation (M & S).

Final note: Non-clinical development is often referred to as *preclinical development*. This is only partly correct. Some of its activities are indeed preclinical in nature, i.e. their results are a prerequisite before clinical development (in humans for human medicines, or targeted animals for veterinary medicines) can even start or progress. But some of it continues when the clinical development is already ongoing. That is why, since the introduction of ICH guidelines, the term non-clinical development is preferred and is becoming more widely used.

Clinical Development

For human medicines, their clinical development encompasses all experiments involving human subjects, be it healthy volunteers or patients, human bodily material or human data.

For veterinary medicines, it involves clinical studies in animals for which the drug is targeted.

It is the most complex part of the drug life cycle, absorbing considerable financial and human resources.

The core activity in humans is conducting clinical trials to assess the kinetics, efficacy and safety of the drug. Clinical drug development is usually divided in several phases that will be discussed in somewhat more detail below.

3.3.2.2 Drug Development Phases

Drug development is classically divided into an early and a late phase. Early drug development is essentially exploratory, whereas late drug development is confirmatory. The clinical part is traditionally split up in four phases: phase 1, 2, 3 and 4. The definition and the relationship between the two categorisations are briefly described below.

Drug development is ideally presented as a simple successive linear process, but that is seldom the case. It is rather characterised by continuous feedback loops and repetitive reiterations.

Early Drug Development

Early drug development can be subdivided into a preclinical and a clinical phase.

During the *preclinical phase*, still two or three candidate drugs can be in the running for further development. The final choice to decide which one will progress to full clinical development is then usually based on the results of so-called phase 0 studies in humans, small exploratory or microdose studies that prerequire less extensive datasets from the chempharm and non-clinical teams. Their main objective is to explore, at very low subtherapeutic doses, the initial pharmacokinetic characteristics of a few candidate drugs (e.g. are they at all bioavailable in humans) and their pharmacodynamic potential (e.g. how do they engage with the intended receptor, which can be explored by modern medical imaging techniques, in so-called early 'proof-of-mechanism' or POM studies).

The candidate with the best potential will then be taken forward to the *clinical phase* of early drug development, where it is typically first administered as single ascending doses (SAD) to human healthy volunteers (*phase 1a*), and then in repeated or multiple ascending doses (MAD, *phase 1b*), followed by a proof-of-concept

(POC) study or an exploratory dose-response trial in a selected patient population (*phase 2a*). These different clinical trials can only be started when sufficient prerequisite data are available from the chempharm and non-clinical streams.

Late Drug Development

Late drug development is usually subdivided into a pre-approval and a post-approval phase, separated by the milestone of obtaining the first marketing authorisation or approval (MA) for the drug, also known as its registration by the competent authorities (e.g. the EMA or FDA).

The *pre-approval phase* is further subdivided into *phase 2b*, i.e. medium-sized trials in patients with the target indication, to confirm the optimal dose regimen to be used on a larger scale, and *phase 3*, i.e. large-scale pivotal therapeutic benefit trials to provide the necessary evidence to support the drug's marketing authorisation. This pre-approval phase is considered to be the most complex and most expensive of all drug life cycle phases, especially when you want the drug to become available worldwide, and the company has to consider the diversity in medical practice, regulatory requirements and the potential pharmaceutical market in different world regions.

The *post-approval phase* of late drug development is typically an open-end phase that runs in parallel with drug commercialisation and can last for many years.

One of the main objectives is to gather real-world evidence of the drug's true place in the therapeutic arsenal for a given disease. Pre-approval clinical trials, with their limited numbers of highly selected patient populations (with strict inclusion and exclusion criteria, limited to a few thousand patients), can only demonstrate with some confidence the *efficacy* of a drug, often against placebo, and give only a rough idea about its safety profile. Therefore, large pragmatic post-approval studies in real-world patients, with concomitant diseases and concomitant therapies, are needed to demonstrate the comparative (cost-)*effectiveness* of the new drug versus existing (standard) therapies. Likewise, large post-approval safety studies (PASS) are conducted, and both general and specific pharmacovigilance activities are set up to get a better idea of the drug's real safety profile in day-to-day clinical practice.

A second important goal of the post-approval development is to further explore new potential indications for the drug, innovative new formulations and new combinations, in order to expand its market potential or to defend its market share once competition becomes fierce.

Also during the whole late development phase, the interdisciplinary interaction between the three development streams (chempharm, non-clinical and clinical) remains of utmost importance.

3.3.3 Marketing Authorisation

Obtaining a first marketing authorisation (MA) is the principal milestone in the drug life cycle. It is an absolute prerequisite for pharmaceutical companies to be allowed to market and sell the new drug. Once the new drug is on the market, additional MAs can be applied for new indications, new formulations or new drug combinations.

Drug marketing authorisations are granted by regulatory medicines agencies for a certain territory, either regional (e.g. the European Economic Area or EEA, by the European Medicines Agency or EMA) or national (e.g. the United States of America or USA, by the Food and Drug Administration or FDA, or any other national agency).

The MA procedures (from application to approval) vary widely and will not be discussed here. For more details, the reader is referred to the textbook already cited above (Rosier et al. 2014). Suffice to state here that the standard procedures can take up to 1 year or longer, whereas some of the accelerated procedures (more recently installed to speed up market access to patients in real need of innovative disease-modifying drugs) can be much faster.

A MA is granted on the basis of three criteria: impeccable quality, adequate efficacy and sufficient safety. Evidence that the new drug demonstrates appropriate quality, and that the benefit-risk ratio is positive, is provided by the applicant in the MA file or registration dossier, according to an internationally standardised document: the ICH Common Technical Document or CTD.

3.3.4 Drug Commercialisation

This is the final phase of the drug life cycle, the time to generate return of investment (ROI).

This section briefly describes some important aspects of drug commercialisation: e.g. market access, marketing, sales, and manufacturing.

3.3.4.1 Market Access

Obtaining a marketing authorisation in different parts of the world for a new drug is a regulatory prerequisite, but only the first step for successful drug commercialisation. Getting real worldwide market access also needs a correct price setting and fair reimbursement by the social security systems, often very different from region to region or country to country.

Real market access is conditional to an extra criterion for success, i.e. value, *the fourth hurdle*. The (high) price setting of innovative drugs and its impact on total healthcare costs for the society are currently hot debate topics. Pharmaceutical companies are responsible for their drug pricing, but national health technology assessment (HTA) bodies have to accept it, together with reasonable reimbursement conditions. To gain real market access, the health economic evaluation of the cost-effectiveness of the new drug is crucial. Therefore, during the late development phase, pharmaco-economic data are collected to calculate the total cost of the drug per quality-adjusted life year (QALY), and its impact on the social security budget, with the final objective that both should remain fair and feasible.

3.3.4.2 Marketing

Pharmaceutical marketing can be described as the process of promoting the sales of medicines. As it is the case for all marketed products, its strategy and tactics should be adapted to the different phases of the commercial life cycle of a product: the prelaunch period, the market launch period, the ascending phase, the mature phase and finally the end-stage phase. One of the specificities of pharmaceutical marketing is that sales promotion of prescription drugs is legally not at all (or only very restrictively) allowed to address itself to the end consumer, i.e. the patient. Therefore, for prescription drugs, pharmaceutical marketing focuses on prescribing physicians and their influencers or key opinion leaders (KOLs), whereas over-the-counter drugs can be promoted directly to patients.

The toolbox of the drug marketer mainly includes detail aids to sales representatives, advertisements in medical journals, sponsoring continuous medical education (CME), provision of drug samples and more recently, the use of digital media and e-marketing tools.

3.3.4.3 Sales

The sales department of a pharma company is responsible for concluding the ultimate goal of having drugs on the market, i.e. selling the drugs to generate income that can be reinvested in research and development of new drugs. As most currently developed innovative drugs are available by prescription only, their sales can only be boosted by targeting intermediate healthcare professionals, such as the prescribing physicians and the dispensing community or hospital pharmacists.

3.3.4.4 Manufacturing

Although pharmaceutical manufacturing is important throughout the entire drug life cycle, it merits special attention during the commercialisation phase. During drug R & D, manufacturing is a relatively small-scale activity. But once the new drug is on the market, both the continuous production of the API and the end product are running at full industrial scale, implying huge investment in the creation of production plants all over the world. Some drug formulations are high-tech products and require sterile, dust-free or cold-chain production and distribution environments, which poses extra burden and costs to companies.

3.3.5   The End of the Drug Life Cycle

Even when a drug has been successful on the market, its sales usually start to decline sharply when it goes off-patent, the 'patent cliff'. When the patent protection and market exclusivity period expires, generic or biosimilar competitors are allowed to enter the market, cutting sales of the originator branded medicine by two thirds or more in only 3 months. For blockbuster drugs, i.e. with a sales revenue exceeding 1 billion US dollars annually, this can be quite dramatic, although it can generally be well anticipated. Some drugs are less successful, in that they have to be withdrawn from the market early because of (relatively) rare but life-threatening side effects that surface only once the drug is used in a large number of patients. Others come to be obsolete when a more efficient novel drug or intervention becomes available and replaces the old ones as the new standard of therapy.

3.4   Operational Jobs Along the Drug Life Cycle

In this section of the chapter, the focus is on job opportunities for life sciences graduates in the biopharmaceutical industry, all along the different phases of the drug life cycle. In addition, similar positions are also available in the medtech and related industries.

These jobs are also more specifically known as 'operational' positions (the daily core business operations), in contrast to the more general 'supportive' positions (helping the operations running smoothly) that will be presented in Sect. 3.5.

As an introduction, two organisational aspects will be discussed, i.e. the role and composition of the drug project team, as well as the variety of positions and job titles mainly used. In the core part, the various possibilities will be briefly presented with a focus on the major life sciences disciplines involved; the qualifications, skills and experience needed to be successful; and a brief description of the usual workplace. More general aspects of the wanted qualifications and key employment assets will be further discussed in Sect. 3.7.

More detailed information on job options in specific subsegments of the drug life cycle can be found in Chaps. 4–10.

3.4.1   The Drug Project Team

In most pharmaceutical companies, the activities along the drug life cycle are coordinated by and fall under the responsibility of *a globally operating project team*, led by a project team leader, pilot, manager or director. The team is generally composed of several scientific experts in a particular drug life cycle segment, complemented by representatives of the supporting functions such as regulatory

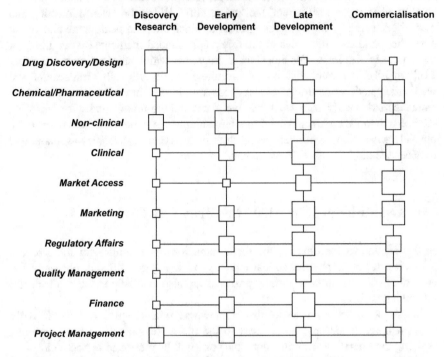

Fig. 3.2 Functional input in the drug project team along the drug life cycle.
The dimension of the squares indicates the relative importance of the major implicated function groups in the drug project team in each major phase of the drug life cycle (vertical lines), as well as the evolution of their contribution all along the drug life cycle (horizontal lines). Chemical/pharmaceutical also includes manufacturing, and project management also includes project planning. Early development is exploratory; late development is confirmatory and continues partly during commercialisation (see Fig. 3.1). Adapted from *Global New Drug Development: An Introduction*, by Jan A. Rosier, Mark A. Martens, Josse R. Thomas, 2014, Wiley-Blackwell. © 2014 by John Wiley & Sons Ltd. Adapted with permission

affairs, quality management, finance and marketing, often supported also by an expert in project planning and management. The composition of the team changes as the drug progresses along its life cycle, which is illustrated in Fig. 3.2.

The drug project team leader, an experienced manager reporting to higher management, may switch from an experimental pharmacologist or a medicinal chemist during drug discovery and design to a toxicologist, pharmacokineticist or clinical pharmacologist during early development, then to a medical specialist during late development, and finally to a marketer in the commercialisation phase.

3.4.2 Variety of Positions and Job Titles

Biopharmaceutical companies use a wide variety of function names and job or position titles to describe what their employees are responsible for. Their exact tasks are more precisely detailed in a job description. Although names and titles for similar jobs can vary substantially, and finding its way in this employment jungle can be tricky, some general trends can be summarised as follows:

- At entry, most young graduates start in a position as Junior, Assistant or Associate. With experience, that prefix is dropped and can later progress to Senior.
- Most job titles also reflect what the person does on the job, e.g. research scientist, lab technician, non-clinical safety lead, clinical project manager, regulatory specialist, drug safety officer, product manager, medical science liaison, sales representative, production technician or operator, etc.
- When some form of coordination, supervision or leadership of several staff members or a team is required, then a qualification such as Lead(er), Supervisor, Pilot, Manager, Director or Chief is added. A team can be composed of members with the same expertise, which is often the case in supportive functions, but in operational functions, the teams are highly multidisciplinary, which is also strongly the case in the overall drug project team.
- Sometimes, the title can also reflect the geographic coverage of the function, with specifications such as Country Manager, General Manager Benelux, Sales Manager EMEA (Europe, the Middle East and Africa), Global Medical Affairs Manager or International Clinical Project Manager (both operating worldwide).
- Corporate organisational units, sites and departments are led by top managers, such as General Managers, Chief Officers or (Senior) Vice Presidents (e.g. Chief Operations Officer, Chief Scientific Officer, Senior Vice-President R & D, Chief Marketing Officer), with on top of the company the Corporate Executive Director or Chief Executive Officer (CEO).

3.4.3 Jobs in Drug Discovery and Design

3.4.3.1 Disciplines Involved

In the biopharmaceutical industry, the decision to start searching for a new drug is usually based on careful consideration of mainly three sets of criteria: strategic criteria (should it be done?), scientific and technical criteria (can it be done?) and operational criteria (can we do it?) (Hill and Rang 2013; Rosier et al. 2014). All these criteria are carefully studied and analysed by a team of top executives in pipeline or portfolio management (see Sect. 3.6), possibly with the help of expert external consultants.

Once this decision is taken, the primary objective of the drug research team is to understand what is going wrong in the targeted disease. Therefore, its pathophysiology and (molecular) biology should be studied in order to identify and validate molecular targets which are druggable. This is an area of expertise of various basic biomedical scientists such as (patho)physiologists, (molecular, cellular or systems) biologists and (bio)chemists; but also of people specialised in various disease areas or mechanisms, such as epidemiologists, medical specialists, immunologists, microbiologists as well as bioinformaticians, geneticists, specialists in genomics, transcriptomics, proteomics and metabolomics; and experts in precision medicine, rare diseases, disease modelling, etc. A large amount of this 'preparatory' disease research is done in academia, but the pharmaceutical industry is also an important player in this biomedical research area.

When an interesting target has been picked out, and its molecular structure identified, medicinal chemists start synthesising new compounds that could potentially interact with the chosen target. They are supported by subspecialists in, e.g. heterocyclic, combinatorial, biopharmaceutical, protein, nucleotide, nanocatalytic, catalytic, green and analytical chemistry.

The development and validation of the different in vitro, in vivo and in silico biological assay methods and animal models to screen all these compounds for pharmacological activity is primarily done by biologists and experimental pharmacologists. As this screening is highly automated and becoming high-tech (with organoid models, and organs- or body-on-a-chip), other professionals such as (bio-)engineers, data analysts and experts in information technology (IT), artificial intelligence (AI) and machine learning (ML) are also very wanted.

During the final process of lead identification and optimisation, experimental pharmacokineticists, experts in drug absorption or drug metabolism and toxicologists also play an important role.

Although drug discovery research is in nature exploratory and characterised by a high degree of freedom, most experiments are conducted according to international good laboratory practice (GLP) guidelines. Therefore, a research quality management team guarantees compliance with these rules (for additional information, see Sect. 3.5.2).

And finally, as the ultimate goal of drug research is to deliver a patented drug for further development, the biopharma industry also employs intellectual property (IP) specialists and patent lawyers.

3.4.3.2 Required Qualifications and Skills

For lab technicians, a bachelor degree in life sciences can be sufficient, but for most positions, a master degree is required. On top of that, a specialisation or a PhD or a postdoc experience in a relevant discipline mentioned above is certainly an asset, and sometimes a must. For jobs in pharmaceutical IP protection, a double diploma, e.g. in life sciences and law, is definitely an advantage.

Most of these jobs require a strong team spirit in a highly multidisciplinary environment. Although being a team player has become today a prerequisite in many jobs, this is certainly the case in the pharma industry. More specifically, successful drug discovery research requires passion to explore the unknown, out-of-the-box thinking, intense intellectual creativity and resilience to failures.

3.4.3.3 Workplace Setting

Most of the positions described above are performed in laboratories, either at the bench (e.g. hands-on lab work) or in an office (e.g. computer-aided drug design, managerial positions).

In big research-based pharma companies, the workplace is in (one of) their research centre(s), organised in different departments according to specific criteria, e.g. disease, therapeutic area, class of drugs, phases in the discovery or design process or contributing disciplines.

Some smaller (biotech) companies develop specialised (high-tech) drug discovery platforms, e.g. for humanised nanobody engineering and for gene and (stem) cell therapy products, using organoids-on-a-chip, etc. Once they have thus found an interesting drug candidate, they licence it out to a bigger biopharma company for further development while getting upfront and milestone payments, plus royalties once the drug is on the market. These smaller companies have similar interesting positions, often requiring experts in more advanced biotech and high-tech disciplines.

3.4.4 Jobs in Chemical/Pharmaceutical Development

3.4.4.1 Disciplines Involved

The key professions to develop the production of pure active pharmaceutical ingredient(s) are synthetic and analytical chemists, while process (development) chemists are important in scaling up the production (from kilolab to pilot plant, and full-scale factory). The development of the manufacturing of biopharmaceuticals or biologicals is mostly in the hands of biotechnologists or bioengineers, while that of radiopharmaceuticals (like PET tracers) is handled by radiochemists and radiopharmacists.

The development of a suitable pharmaceutical formulation, e.g. an oral tablet, a solution for injection, a dermal patch or an inhaler, is generally assigned to formulation scientists, drug delivery specialists and pharmaceutical technologists. The quality and stability of the end product is guaranteed by analytical and physical chemists, and stability analysts. The scaling up of the manufacturing of the end product is more a task for industrial pharmacists and process (development) (bio)engineers.

As the production of (bio)pharmaceuticals has to comply with international good manufacturing practice (GMP) guidelines, every production site has an appropriate quality management system in place with the necessary staff (see Sect. 3.5.2). Each manufacturing authorisation holder is also legally required to have a qualified person (QP) or responsible pharmacist, usually an industrial pharmacist, who certifies the release of each finished product batch before it is used in a clinical trial or made available on the market.

3.4.4.2 Required Qualifications and Skills

Pharmaceutical production technicians can usually do with a bachelor degree in either chemistry, pharmaceutical sciences, biotechnology or (bio)engineering. Higher positions will require a master degree in those life sciences, sometimes supplemented with a specialisation, e.g. in industrial or radiopharmacy. Here too, a PhD (with postdoc experience) is certainly an asset in the competition for talented people, as well as for further career development.

3.4.4.3 Workplace Setting

During early drug development, these jobs are performed in laboratories and small-scale plants of pharmaceutical and biotech companies, while during late development and commercialisation, they are transferred to full-scale production facilities.

Chem/pharm development and full-scale pharmaceutical production is currently often also outsourced to service providers specialised in the development of innovative formulations, and to contract development and manufacturing organisations (CDMOs).

3.4.5   Jobs in Non-clinical Development

3.4.5.1   Disciplines Involved

The *pharmacology* part of non-clinical development, essentially dealing with the drug candidate's desired pharmacodynamic effects (efficacy) in biological assay systems and animal models, is the workspace of experimental pharmacologists.

The non-clinical *safety pharmacology* team investigates the drug's undesirable pharmacodynamic effects on physiological functions of the cardiovascular, the gastrointestinal, the pulmonary and the central nervous system. In these activities, pharmacologists as well as toxicologists are involved.

Non-clinical *pharmacokinetics* studies the absorption, distribution, metabolism and excretion (ADME) of the drug in different in vitro animal and human models, and in different in vivo animal species. This is the playing field of pharmacokineticists, specialists in drug metabolism, and more recently of experts in quantitative biology and pharmacology, such as systems biology and pharmacometrics, where computer modelling and simulation (M & S) plays an important role in what is now called model-informed drug development (MIDD). All with the ultimate objective to better predict the pharmacokinetics of the drug in human subjects or target animals.

Non-clinical *toxicology* is a vast domain, with different types of studies along the drug life cycle, all performed according to internationally agreed test guidelines and GLP. They are categorised in acute and repeated-dose general toxicity studies, and several targeted toxicity studies, such as genotoxicity; local tolerance; reproductive, immuno-, neuro- and mechanistic toxicity; carcinogenicity; and juvenile toxicity studies. They are roughly performed in that order, some in vitro, others in vivo in several species of laboratory animals, mostly rat and dog, but for some drugs (e.g. biologicals) also in non-human primates. For this battery of tests you need a solid team of toxicologists, supplemented with bioassay and animal model developers from various life science disciplines.

The pharmacokinetic and toxicokinetic development cannot be successful without the help of *bioanalytical chemistry* experts. They are responsible for the separation, detection, identification and quantification of the parent drug and its metabolites in biological samples of animal or human origin, such as whole blood, plasma or serum, urine, saliva, cerebrospinal fluid, sputum, bile, semen, various cells and tissues, tumours, etc.

Non-clinical drug development is par excellence a *multidisciplinary* activity. In the study of the drug's pharmacokinetic-pharmacodynamic (PK-PD) relationship, or its exposure- or dose-response relationship, pharmacokineticists, pharmacometricians and pharmacologists work together. In the toxicokinetic studies, where the drug's systemic exposure is assessed in relationship with its toxicological effects, pharmacokineticists collaborate with toxicologists. In the safety pharmacology studies, pharmacologists team up with toxicologists. To reach the final goal, i.e. propose one candidate drug to be further developed in man (or target animals), they all work together as one team.

In addition, as non-clinical drug development is also highly regulated, e.g. by GLP guidelines and a number of international guidelines on preclinical prerequisites to start or continue the clinical development in humans or target animals, a sound quality management system, properly staffed, should be in place in order to comply with all these regulations (see Sect. 3.5.2).

3.4.5.2 Required Qualifications and Skills

Lab technicians in the different disciplines involved, as well as laboratory animal facility technicians, require at least a bachelor degree or a professional master in the appropriate life sciences segment. For other entry positions, an academic master degree or a specialty post-master degree may be sufficient, but it may take time to progress in your career. In order to start in a position with some responsibility, and to be able to progress more quickly, a doctoral degree (PhD) is a must, and some postdoc experience in a relevant discipline will be highly appreciated.

In non-clinical drug development, there is room for many diverse life science professionals, i.e. the usual suspects such as biologists, pharmacists, biochemists, biomedical scientists, biotechnologists, pharmacologists, toxicologists and bioanalytical chemists. But in addition, there is also room for veterinarians (vets), pathologists, immunologists, mathematicians, data analysts and biostatisticians.

Some attitudes and skills that are particularly valued include ambition, team spirit, a problem-solving mindset, good interactive and communication skills and willingness to learn continuously from others. PK-PD modellers should have a knack for maths and get along well with the relevant software platforms.

3.4.5.3 Workplace Setting

Again, most of these jobs are performed in a laboratory environment, either at the bench or in an office. Some will work in a laboratory animal research facility or animalarium that requires proper staffing assuring animal welfare and biosafety.

Most pharma and biotech companies have their own non-clinical research centres, with sometimes separate but closely interacting departments of pharmacology, toxicology, pharmacokinetics and bioanalytical chemistry. But a lot of the work is also subcontracted to service providers or contract research organisations (CROs) specialised in some specific part of non-clinical drug development. In particular, there is a growing field of job opportunities in smaller companies focusing on modelling and simulation as a service to other companies. This is also an area where independent or freelance consultants can easily find their way.

More detailed information on job and career opportunities in toxicology can be found in Chap. 4.

3.4.6 Jobs in Clinical Development

3.4.6.1 Disciplines Involved

Clinical drug development is the most complex and most expensive part of the drug life cycle. As mentioned before, the process can be split into two main phases, i.e. the pre-approval and the post-approval phase, with the drug's marketing authorisation as a milestone between these two phases.

The success rate of the pre-approval phase of clinical drug development is still very low. From the drug candidates that entered into a first-in-human study during 2011–2020, only 7.9% made it to a marketing authorisation (BIO 2021). Currently, a number of initiatives have been taken to make the process more efficient, thus hoping to improve this disappointing statistic.

In most pharma companies, clinical drug development is jointly run by several teams of separate operational functions or departments that highly interact with one another: clinical research (CR, also called clinical science or therapeutic research), clinical operations (CO or Clin Ops), (clinical) biometrics (BM), medical review (MR), pharmacovigilance (PV or PhV) and clinical services (CS). At the corporate level, these departments are responsible for the whole drug pipeline or portfolio. They are usually organised in different units, either:

- Specialised in a specific disease or therapeutic area (as in CR, BM, MR and PV), e.g. oncology, infectious diseases, neurodegenerative disorders or immunotherapy. Within these units, several drugs can be developed simultaneously, each one assigned to a separate team.
- Responsible for a specific geographic area (as in clinical operations), e.g. a country or a region (e.g. Scandinavian countries), or operating worldwide.
- Focusing on a particular service (as in clinical services), e.g. clinical supplies, central lab support and study material logistics.

Clinical Research is responsible for the overall clinical development strategy, as well as for the planning, the design and the oversight of all clinical trials with the drug. These teams also pilot the entire clinical development of the drug, with the help of members from the other departments.

During early clinical development, the team is usually led by a clinician, mostly a medical specialist with experience in the therapeutic area under study, supported by experts in human or clinical pharmacology, clinical pharmacokinetics or pharmacometrics as well as other physicians, pharmacists or biomedical scientists. During late clinical development, the team is more specifically composed of clinicians, pharmaceutical physicians, (clinical or hospital) pharmacists, population pharmacokineticists and pharmaco-epidemiologists. In addition, these teams can get extra support from experts in clinical trial methodology, biostatistics, disease modelling and simulation and medical writing.

As most of these functions have an international character, and are limited to a specific disease area, the title of the positions is often preceded by the prefix International and a suffix indicating the disease domain concerned, e.g. International Clinical Project Leader/Manager/Director Oncology.

Clinical Operations is responsible for coordinating the practical implementation, smooth running and monitoring of clinical trials. Common Clin Ops activities cover a wide range of work, and include:

- Evaluation, selection and management of clinical investigation centres or sites, i.e. either a single phase 1 unit (monocentric study), or more often, tens or hundreds of clinical investigators in hospitals, or medical specialists in private practice, or general practitioners, in several countries (national or multinational multicentre trials).
- Evaluation, selection and management of contract research organisations (CROs) or vendors to whom a lot of its own activities can be outsourced.

- Monitoring the overall quality of the trials, by checking its compliance with (inter)national regulations and good clinical practice (GCP) guidance, and by performing the quality control (QC) of the collected patient data. Some of this work is done during on-site visits, e.g. verification of the data collected in the electronic study case report forms (eCRFs, with all the data needed from one study participant) versus the original source data in the patients' (electronic or paper) medical files. This is currently more and more done off-site or remote, either by the study monitor working at his office or at home, and having access to both the eCRFs and the electronic medical records (EMR), or either by data managers having access to the central study database, by running proper algorithms to search for possible inconsistencies that can then be verified by the study monitor on-site if needed. This is known as the risk-based or risk-adapted approach to study monitoring, instead of wanting to do 100% source data verification (SDV) on-site, which is much more resource intensive.
- Management of the study timeline and deadlines, e.g. study and site start-up, recruitment progress of study participants (healthy volunteers or patients), last patient last visit (LPLV) and site closures.
- Control over the site budgets, the CRO budgets and the overall trial budget.
- As well as, various study site staff training on topics such as the study protocol, CRF completion, GCP rules, pharmacovigilance obligations, etc.

The bulk of this work is done by many study monitors or clinical research associates (CRAs), while the managerial positions are occupied by clinical trial managers, clinical operations managers and a clinical operations director.

Clinical Biometrics is responsible for clinical data management (e.g. CRF design, set-up and maintenance of the database, data quality control, database lock), clinical trial methodology (e.g. trial design, blinding, treatment allocation, endpoint selection) and biostatistics (e.g. writing the statistical analysis plan, performing the pre-specified and additional statistical analyses, interpretation of the results together with the CR team and the investigators).

This is the world of (big) data analysts, data scientists, clinical data managers, information technology (IT) and artificial intelligence (AI) experts, clinical trial methodologists and (bio)statisticians.

Medical Review is responsible for periodic critical review of the medical data collected in the study eCRFs and database, focusing on the participants' medical history, demographics (respect of the in- and exclusion criteria), concomitant medications, clinical endpoints and lab results, in view of detecting inconsistencies or protocol deviations, which are then fed back to the study CRA or the clinical trial manager, and finally to the investigator for verification and correction if appropriate.

This QC activity is mostly performed by physicians (or pharmacists) with clinical practice experience, i.e. medical specialists, general practitioners or clinical pharmacists.

Pharmacovigilance is responsible for the management of drug safety issues during clinical trials. In many companies, this team is embedded in the operational team of the Pharmacovigilance Department. Its roles will be discussed in Sect. 3.5.3.1.

Clinical Services is responsible for the management of:

- Clinical supplies, i.e. the drugs studied in clinical trials, including the drugs in development, the corresponding placebos or comparator drugs.
- Other study materials, e.g. from lab kits for biospecimen collection (such as the different types of blood tubes), handheld tablets for study participants to record electronic patient reported outcomes (ePROs) or an e-diary, home blood pressure monitoring devices and wearable activity trackers, to standardised software to be used in medical imaging equipment at the participating sites.
- Central laboratory or clinical assessment services, e.g. central clinical biology labs, central reading facilities for medical images and central clinical endpoint adjudication committees.

Managing these services means to evaluate the internal or external service providers, decide which one to choose for a particular trial, see to it that all user manuals are ready and organise the shipments to the investigator sites worldwide (with respect of the cold chain if needed), as well as the return shipments of leftovers, and their disposal as toxic, radioactive or simple waste. All this requires a good knowledge of the import and export rules and customs formalities of these different materials for various countries.

Jobs in clinical services are very diverse, including supply chain, distribution or logistics managers, lab technicians, clinical biology/pathology/imaging experts, software engineers, clinical evaluators, etc.

3.4.6.2 Required Qualifications and Skills

As the job opportunities are manifold and varied, most life scientists with a bachelor or master degree might find a suitable job in this sector. A PhD is not a must here, but can be an asset for later career development. For some jobs, clinical practice experience is mandatory, thus creating openings for physicians and clinical pharmacists. Some other postgraduate specialisation may be helpful, e.g. industrial pharmacists in supply chain management, medical specialists in clinical research and pharmaceutical physicians in clinical research or clinical operations.

As a lot of these professionals are operating on a regional or worldwide level, willingness to travel and to stay abroad, as well as a good command of English, is certainly a plus.

3.4.6.3 Workplace Setting

Most of the available positions in clinical drug development are typically office jobs, either at the headquarters of a pharma company or a CRO or in their national or regional subsidiaries. Today, some of these jobs can also be (partly) performed at home (e.g. clinical project managers, CRAs or medical reviewers), while others will work in a lab environment, a production site or a warehouse (e.g. positions in clinical supplies).

Especially professionals in clinical operations, but also those working in clinical research, will have to travel a lot to visit investigator or service provider sites and might thus spend several hours or even days in foreign locations.

More detailed information on jobs and careers in clinical development can be found in Chap. 5 (Job Possibilities in Clinical Research), Chap. 8 (Working in Medical Affairs and Clinical Operations) and Chap. 10 (Career Development for Physicians in the Biopharmaceutical Industry).

3.4.7 Jobs in Market Access

3.4.7.1 Disciplines Involved

Obtaining a marketing authorisation (MA) is a prerequisite but not enough to put a new drug on the market and make it a success story. Real market access is conditioned by getting a correct price, and by obtaining a fair reimbursement status.

Even when a MA can be secured on a regional level, e.g. at the European Medicines Agency (EMA), price setting and reimbursement have to be negotiated at country level. These processes can be painstakingly complex and slow, involving reiterative interactions with multiple price setting and health technology assessment (HTA) bodies, operating within national Ministries of Economics, Health or Social Security under various political influences.

Biopharmaceutical companies conduct these negotiations based on the global or core value dossier (GVD or CVD), containing comprehensive information on the value drivers of the new drug, e.g. the societal impact of the targeted disease, the therapeutic benefits of the drug, its cost-effectiveness and its budget impact on the social security system.

This document is prepared and defended by the market access team, mainly composed or making use of market access analysts/managers or advisors/consultants, epidemiologists and pharmaco-epidemiologists, economists and health or pharmaco-economists, HTA or reimbursement experts, clinicians, health economics outcomes research (HEOR) managers, marketers, public policy experts and lobbyists.

3.4.7.2 Required Qualifications and Skills

Market access jobs are mostly occupied by professionals with a life sciences degree with high-level understanding of the business. Relevant industry experience is important and can also be acquired after some internship period. Otherwise, a master in business administration (MBA) is certainly a plus. If your background is outside life sciences, e.g. economics, then you might need a postgraduate specialisation or a PhD in health or pharmaco-economics in order to be able to make substantial career progress in this field.

Otherwise, a broad skill set is needed, but the importance of excellent communication and negotiation skills across many different cultures and politics cannot be underestimated.

3.4.7.3 Workplace Setting

The market access teams in biopharmaceutical companies tend to be rather small and rely heavily on external advisors or consultants. Therefore, there are probably more job opportunities with market access service providers or as independent freelance consultants.

More detailed information on market access jobs and careers in the medical devices industry can be found in Chap. 6.

3.4.8 Jobs in Medical Affairs

3.4.8.1 Disciplines Involved

The primary role of the medical affairs department is to bridge the gap between drug R & D and the commercial activities of marketing and sales. It is responsible for the credible communication of the scientific and medical evidence gathered on the drug to key opinion or thought leaders (KOLs or KTLs) and various healthcare professionals (HCPs).

Other activities include the following: organise continuous or continuing medical education (CME) for HCPs, set up and follow up post-approval clinical studies in day-to-day clinical practice, support marketing to formulate convincing but credible marketing messages and take part in the training of marketing and sales staff members.

One of the cornerstone positions in medical affairs is medical science liaisons (MSLs), often with a territory or a therapeutic area added to their title. They mainly interact with influential KOLs, academics and other HCPs. Other positions in the team include medical information managers, project leader CME or CME manager and medical director or director of medical affairs. An additional task is to participate in the training of marketing and sales staff, providing them with up-to-date scientific and medical information about the drugs they will have to work with.

3.4.8.2　Required Qualifications and Skills

Medical affairs departments in the pharma industry are primarily populated by physicians, either with a master degree in medicine, a medical specialist degree or a PhD in a relevant discipline, or an extra diploma in pharmaceutical medicine. As they have to communicate deeply with high-level experts, pharma companies want them to have advanced degrees, and preferably some experience in clinical research or marketing. However, as the number of available positions has been booming since a number of years, other profiles are also getting a chance, such as pharmacists and biomedical scientists with or without a PhD.

Skills-wise you need to combine the skills of a clinical development expert with the mindset of a commercial champion and act as an all-rounder.

3.4.8.3　Workplace Setting

In the pharma industry, medical affairs professionals operate mainly from their office, and spend a lot of time interacting with KOLs and other HCPs, either in their professional habitat, at CME events and at medical congresses or satellite symposia. These contacts suppose some travel, but with the pleasure of working in a true international environment.

Some medical affairs professionals prefer to work as a service provider, i.e. as freelance medical advisor.

More detailed information can be found in Chap. 8 (Working in Medical Affairs and Clinical Operations), Chap. 9 (The Role of Medical Science Liaison) and Chap. 10 (Career Development for Physicians in the Biopharmaceutical Industry).

3.4.9　Jobs in Marketing

3.4.9.1　Disciplines Involved

In pharmaceutical marketing, there is a central role for product or brand managers (PMs or BMs). They are responsible for the promotional strategy and tactics to convince prescribers (for prescription medicines) or consumers (for over-the-counter or OTC products) to prescribe or use their drug (instead of a competitor drug).

They do market research and market analysis to identify the audience they want to target with promotional material for their drug, and they develop and oversee marketing campaigns to boost its sales. At company headquarters, marketers develop a global marketing strategy for each drug, while at regional or country level, this global strategy is translated into local tactics adapted to local market specificities.

Other common marketing positions are marketing research assistant, market development manager, digital marketing manager, sales support specialist and (key) account manager. Group product managers supervise a number of product managers and other staff members, usually within a therapeutic area or business unit.

3.4.9.2 Required Qualifications and Skills

In fact, all types of graduates in life sciences can become successful in a pharmaceutical marketing job, but a degree in marketing or an (additional) MBA is also a much appreciated qualification.

What you need in the first place is a passion for commercial awareness, and a good understanding of the pharmaceutical business. Other skills, like strategic thinking, creativity, a sound research and analytical mindset and above all excellent communication skills, are of paramount importance to be successful in this field.

3.4.9.3 Workplace Setting

In pharma companies, these jobs are performed either at corporate headquarters or in local subsidiaries. They are mostly office jobs, but frequent outside contacts with key opinion leaders (KOL), who might act as expert advisors and influencers of other prescribers, are also part of the job.

More detailed information on job opportunities in pharmaceutical marketing can be found in Chap. 7.

3.4.10 Jobs in Sales

3.4.10.1 Disciplines Involved

The operational drug sales activities are performed by sales representatives ('sales reps' or the sales force). According to the type of drug to sell, they may target primarily prescribers, i.e. general practitioners (medical reps) or medical specialists (hospital reps or specialty reps), but also community (pharmacy reps) and hospital pharmacists (hospital pharmacy reps). Many pharmaceutical companies still prefer face-to-face meetings, but digital and virtual interaction is gaining momentum.

Key account managers, mostly operating from corporate headquarters, target the most important customers. Territory managers (area, regional and national sales managers) manage the activities of a group of sales reps, setting individual and group sales objectives, and motivating the teams to reach or surpass them.

3.4.10.2   Required Qualifications and Skills

Pharmaceutical sales positions are usually occupied by people with a very diverse background. A bachelor or master degree in life sciences is certainly appreciated, but not a must. All newcomers, regardless of their background, receive an intensive initial training, then gain experience by accompanying senior sales colleagues, and continue to receive regular sales training each time a new promotional campaign is launched.

Important skills are a flair for sales, a detailed knowledge of your product(s), great persuasiveness and influencing skills and a knack for time management and self-discipline.

3.4.10.3   Workplace Setting

The field sales force works in various healthcare facilities, e.g. private practices, hospitals or pharmacies. Sales management positions are primarily office jobs, although managers might sometimes accompany the sales reps on the road in order to coach them or do a part of their performance assessment.

3.4.11   Jobs in Manufacturing

3.4.11.1   Disciplines Involved

The major activities involved in pharmaceutical manufacturing can be categorised in:

- Chemical, biotechnological and pharmaceutical development of new drugs.
- Small-, mid- and large-scale production of the API and finished product, used in clinical trials and once on the market.
- Operational quality control of starting materials, production processes and production equipment.
- Supply chain management (SCM) and distribution logistics.

These activities are guided by specific legislation and good manufacturing or good distribution practices (GMP and GDP).

A wide variety of jobs are available, such as chemistry, manufacturing and controls (CMC) scientist or manager; pharmaceutical technology project leader, engineer or manager; production operator, supervisor or manager; and operational quality specialist or production process quality controller.

In the EU, each MAH should legally have at least one qualified person (QP) designated responsible for the certification and release of each batch of its drugs manufactured for use in clinical practice or in clinical trials. The QP is responsible for compliance of the production with all relevant legislation and regulations, including good manufacturing practice (GMP).

Of note is the fact that a lot of the pharmaceutical manufacturing of small molecule drugs and biologicals is outsourced to specialised service providers, i.e. contract (development and) manufacturing organisations (CMOs or CDMOs), some being big global players with many job opportunities worldwide. This was recently particularly the case with the expedited mass production of COVID-19 vaccines. Equally important are manufacturers of generics and biosimilars, both currently being booming businesses.

3.4.11.2 Required Qualifications and Skills

Pharmaceutical manufacturing offers a lot of job opportunities for professional bachelors, especially as production technicians, technologists or operators. Graduates with a master degree in life sciences such as pharmacy, biotechnology or (bio)engineering easily find their way as production supervisor or manager, as quality controller or operational quality specialist or as project engineer. For more developmental jobs and senior management positions, an advanced master degree in industrial pharmacy or a PhD in pharmaceutical technology is preferred.

In the EU, the qualified person (QP) for batch release is preferentially someone with a master degree in pharmacy, plus adequate experience in a number of topics. However, other holders of a life sciences master degree (e.g. medicine, veterinary medicine, chemistry or biology) can also be certified provided that they take some extra courses and gain adequate experience.

In a pharmaceutical production environment, candidates for a job should be team players, possess trouble-shooting skills and be flexible as some jobs require working in shifts, during nights and weekends.

3.4.11.3 Workplace Setting

Small-scale production of APIs (small molecules or biologicals), or pharmaceutical technology development and manufacturing, can take place in a laboratory; but mid- and large-scale manufacturing of medicines for clinical trials and the market is done in factories present in several countries worldwide. Therefore, a majority of the jobs available in manufacturing are performed on the work floor, and only a minor fraction in an office.

As already mentioned before, a lot of these activities can be outsourced to service providers.

3.5   Jobs in Overarching Supportive Functions

This section will give an overview of the most representative overarching supportive functions to operations, important throughout the entire drug life cycle. More detailed information can be found in Chaps. 11–13.

The functions described here are available in pharmaceutical companies as well as in CROs or specialised service providers, and some can be performed as independent freelance advisors. They are essentially office jobs.

3.5.1   Jobs in Regulatory Affairs/Science(s)

3.5.1.1   Essential Functions

Preamble: In the pharmaceutical industry, the term regulatory affairs is more common and stands more for the practical implementation of the pharmaceutical legislation and regulations. The term regulatory science(s) is in principle more reserved for the study of the scientific and technical foundations of legislation and regulations, as it is applied in academia and regulatory agencies. Legislation is defined as laws enacted by legislative bodies (that must be complied with), while regulations stand for the implementation of legislation, with rules and guidelines or guidance to clarify matters.

Regulatory affairs professionals have several important tasks:

- They define the regulatory strategy within a company, e.g. should scientific advice (SA) be asked to a medicines agency, and if yes, which one(s); which marketing authorisation (MA) procedure will best be used for a particular drug; etc.
- They manage regulatory procedures ('core operations'), e.g. prepare the necessary documents for clinical trial applications (CTAs), or for SA or MA applications.
- They interact with competent regulatory authorities, e.g. national medicines agencies (such as the FDA or others), or regional medicines agencies (such as the EMA), or the European Patent Office (EPO).
- They keep other departments up-to-date about (changes in) legislation and regulations in their area of interest, e.g. the recently introduced EU Clinical Trials Regulation (CTR) or the UK Innovative Licensing and Access Pathway (ILAP), the various good practice guidelines (GxPs) or the rules for communication of medical and scientific information by medical affairs and marketing.

Their perimeter of responsibility can be defined by geographic extent (national, regional or global), by type of operations (e.g. clinical trials or marketing authorisations, or both), by therapeutic area (e.g. oncology, cardiovascular), by location (in a subsidiary or in headquarters) or simply covering it all as vice-president regulatory affairs.

Much used titles are regulatory affairs specialist, manager or director, plus the specification of the perimeter of activity.

3.5.1.2 Preferred Qualifications and Skills

At least a bachelor degree in any of the life sciences is needed, but preferably a master degree. Having had some (extra) courses on regulatory affairs is a plus. A doctoral degree is not a must, but can help in career progression. Work experience can be gained on the job, possibly during an internship.

A sound knowledge of the pharmaceutical legislation and regulations is of paramount importance. Otherwise, good communication skills and a good command of English are valuable assets.

More detailed information can be found in Chap. 11.

3.5.2 Jobs in Quality Management

3.5.2.1 Essential Functions

Preamble: Total quality management (TQM) of a drug, product or process supposes four essential elements that constitute the pillars of any quality management system (QMS) (Rose 2005):

- Quality planning: building quality into the drug or the process, i.e. quality by design (QbD), and preparing and training the operational teams to execute their work up to the required quality standards ('do it right the first time').
- Quality control (QC): in-process efforts to improve the process output, e.g. by self-inspections and quality monitoring, performed by the operational units and staff members themselves ('quality is everyone's responsibility').
- Quality assurance (QA): by providing confidence that the drug or process complies (or will comply) with requirements. This is essentially done by performing audits of the QMS at relevant points in time by QA professionals (auditors) who are strictly independent from the operational teams. Therefore, audits are performed by either independent internal QA professionals or external auditors from QA service providers. Inspections (or Union Controls by the European Commission in the European Union) have a similar objective as audits, but are performed by regulatory authorities.
- Quality improvement: based on root cause analysis (RCA), learning from identified errors with application of corrective and preventive actions (CAPAs) and by implementing continuously and iteratively the classic 'plan-do-check-act' (PDCA) quality cycles.

In the pharmaceutical industry, the required quality standards are dictated by pharmaceutical legislation and regulations. In this context, the various good practice guidelines (GxPs) are key reference documents.

As every organisation in the pharmaceutical industry (be it a company, a CRO or any other service provider) needs to have a QMS in place, quality management professionals are active in these four domains.

Quality planning tasks, often integrated in the QA department, include writing quality documents such as standard operating procedures (SOPs) and more detailed standardised work instructions (SWIs), training operational staff in the relevant regulatory requirements and advising operational departments in implementing QbD (already well developed in manufacturing, but also making its way in clinical drug research).

Quality control professionals are embedded in the operational teams to continuously monitor their day-to-day activities for quality aspects. In the drug life cycle, this is particularly prominently present in:

– Clinical development, i.e. the essential role of clinical research associates (CRAs) or (clinical trial) monitors, and clinical data managers (more details in Sect. 3.4.6.1).
– Manufacturing, i.e. the essential role of process controllers and 'self-inspections'.

Quality assurance professionals are predominantly auditors, but in some organisations, they also do (some of the) quality planning activities. Auditors check the compliance of a specific part of the operations with the corresponding regulatory rules and the goals of the QMS, according to a predefined auditing programme or 'for cause' (because a potential deviation has been signalled by the QC team). Audits give a snapshot of the situation at a certain point in time and give rise to findings and suggestions for CAPAs in order to improve the quality of the operations or system. Audits can be internal (on operations within the QA unit's own company) or external, performed either by an external QA service provider or, alternatively, by the own QA unit on operations outsourced, for example, to a CRO or a CMO, or at a certain software vendor before deciding whether to use his technology in, for instance, a clinical trial.

Quality improvement processes like CAPA management and change management are owned by the QA department, although all departments with regulated activities will use such systems to correct and improve their processes and drive the level of compliance.

3.5.2.2 Preferred Qualifications and Skills

As the spectrum of quality management functions is very diverse, and spread across the entire drug life cycle, the required qualifications can vary widely. For most of the functions described above, a master degree in one of the life sciences will do. However, in specific areas such as manufacturing, a degree in (bio)engineering or an advanced degree in industrial pharmacy may be preferred, while auditing the currently widely used digital technologies in the pharma industry would rather require a degree in computer sciences or information technology (systems).

A couple of years of experience in drug life cycle operations is certainly an interesting asset.

Some skills may be particularly appreciated, such as an excellent knowledge of the required quality standards, attention to details and good communication skills (oral as well as written). Auditors may especially benefit from some diplomatic skills and emotional intelligence, as their interventions are sometimes perceived as policing or patronising.

As a side note, it is also worth mentioning that audits may last for several days on external sites and abroad, such as in a clinical investigation centre, in a manufacturing site or in the facilities of a service provider or (digital) technology vendor. Some people might find this an attractive prospect, while others might perceive it as burdensome.

More detailed information can be found in Chap. 12 (Job Opportunities in Clinical Research Quality Assurance) and Chap. 13 (Job Opportunities in Quality Assurance Related to Manufacturing of Medicinal Products).

.

3.5.3 Jobs in Pharmacovigilance

3.5.3.1 Essential Functions

Pharmacovigilance (PV or PhV), also known as drug safety, is legally defined as the science and activities relating to the detection, assessment, understanding and prevention of adverse drug effects. Drug safety focuses in fact more on the product safety, while pharmacovigilance focuses more on patient safety.

Across the drug life cycle, pharmacovigilance is particularly important during drug development and once the drug is on the market (post-marketing surveillance or PMS).

Its activities include:

– An operational part, i.e. collection of the individual case safety reports (ICSRs) from investigators, healthcare professionals (i.e. prescribing physicians or dentists, pharmacists and nurses), as well as from patients, evaluation of their seriousness, their possible causal relationship with drug exposure (causality assessment) and—whenever required—their expedited reporting to the concerned competent (regulatory) authorities (CAs) and research ethics committees (RECs).
– A surveillance part, including proactive risk management (e.g. drafting and updating the drug's risk management plan or RMP); the mining, detection and assessment of new safety signals in a drug safety database that is continuously increasing in size as the drug is successfully marketed; and the drafting of

periodic aggregate reports, such as the development safety update reports (DSURs) for drugs in development, as well as the periodic benefit-risk evaluation reports (PBRERs) for drugs on the market, that are also to be sent to the concerned CAs and RECs.

Common titles in these functions are drug safety or PV analyst, officer, scientist, specialist, or consultant, PV (project) manager or director, with responsibilities at country, regional or global level, or in operations, surveillance or systems.

In the European Union (EU), every marketing authorisation holder (MAH) is legally required to have a single qualified person responsible for pharmacovigilance (QPPV) at corporate level. This is usually a high-level senior PV manager with extensive prior PV experience who will represent the company in interactions with the competent authorities. The QPPV is also responsible for the creation and maintenance of a well-performing PV system compliant with relevant international legislations and good pharmacovigilance practice (GVP). National or regional drug safety officers (DSOs) report to this central person.

3.5.3.2 Preferred Qualifications and Skills

Pharmacovigilance positions requiring clinical experience are preferably held by physicians (general practitioners or medical specialists) or clinical pharmacists. Physicians may benefit from an extra diploma in pharmaceutical medicine.

The administrative tasks, such as adverse event coding and the expedited or periodic safety reporting, can be delegated to a wider range of masters in life sciences, including pharmacists and biomedical scientists.

For clinical work, good analytical and problem-solving skills, critical thinking and sound clinical judgement are assets. For the more administrative jobs, attention to details, as well as good writing and reporting skills, is appreciated.

Pharmacovigilance managers will also need excellent negotiating and crisis management skills, as they will have to interact regularly with the competent authorities on drug safety issues, sometimes in complex and difficult circumstances.

3.5.4 Jobs in Medical/Scientific Writing

3.5.4.1 Essential Functions

In the pharmaceutical industry, the medical and/or scientific writing function is responsible for creating or reviewing various:

– Scientific/clinical study documents, such as study protocols and study reports, lay summaries as well as articles with the study results for publication in scientific or medical journals.

- Regulatory documents, such as the IMP dossier or investigator brochure (IB) for clinical trial applications, all overview and (overall) summary documents needed for the marketing authorisation application file and the DSURs or PBRERs for pharmacovigilance reporting.
- Educational documents, covering the medico-scientific communication needs mainly used by medical affairs, marketing and sales.

The most used job title is medical or scientific writer, possibly with a prefix as junior or senior, and with the addition of his field of responsibility, such as a part of the drug life cycle, a therapeutic area or specifically supported functions, e.g. regulatory affairs, quality management and pharmacovigilance.

Medical and scientific writing is often performed in collaboration with specialised service providers, such as CROs or individual freelancers, which creates alternative job opportunities.

3.5.4.2 Preferred Qualifications and Skills

Basically, all graduates with a life sciences degree qualify, but masters in communication or (scientific) journalism are also good candidates. Prior experience in the field concerned can be an asset.

Some important skills are: analytical capacity, excellent written communication skills for different audiences (for some documents strictly factual, for others somewhat more engaging or promotional), an excellent command of English, getting along with literature search and publishing software, ability to interact with different disciplines, and resilience to the stress of tight deadlines.

3.5.5 Jobs in Project Planning

3.5.5.1 Essential Functions

Defined in general, project planning is a part of project management. It defines how to prepare, execute and complete a project within a certain timeframe. It is a function in support of project managers, department heads, pipeline or portfolio managers as well as corporate strategy executives.

The deliverable is a project plan with details on the scope of the project, the different stages to go through, the resources needed (manpower, materials, equipment, facilities), the timeline and the financial budget to be respected. In the project plan, a number of potential scenarios are presented, such as the best-case and the worst-case scenario, with a couple of scenarios in-between.

In the context of drug life cycle management, it concerns either a specific operational part of the process (e.g. planning a single research study or a clinical trial, or the whole non-clinical drug development), or a specific support function (e.g. preparing an audit programme plan), or either the entire drug life cycle.

Project planners create these project plans by using specific planning software, which will also deliver a visually attractive overview of the project activities displayed against time, e.g. the widely used Gantt charts.

Common job titles are either very specific (e.g. lab planner, production planner or scheduler) or more general, such as (drug) project planner followed by the specification of the scope.

3.5.5.2 Preferred Qualifications and Skills

Again, essentially all graduates with a life sciences degree will qualify for these jobs, but (supply-chain) engineers and IT specialists will also find their way as project planners. In fact, a good knowledge of the field of interest is more important. Therefore, some years of experience in the operations concerned are usually an asset, or even a prerequisite.

Essential skills are able to collaborate cross-functionally and connect people, having an analytical and solution-oriented mindset and good mastery of specific project planning software.

3.6 Jobs in Other Essential Business Roles

Up to now, this overview focused on job opportunities in operational and supportive functions all along or spanning the entire drug life cycle.

As in any other business, pharmaceutical companies have several general business departments. Because of the specific nature of the biopharmaceutical industry, some of these functions and positions can be of particular interest to life sciences graduates.

For the sake of completeness, they will be briefly presented here.

3.6.1 Business Intelligence

The corporate business intelligence (BI) department collects and analyses key business data and information from the company as well as competitors (competitive intelligence, CI), compares them and makes recommendations to the executive committee, in order to facilitate informed corporate strategic planning and operational decision-making. The ultimate goal is to improve corporate business performance and the competitive positioning of the company, as well as to anticipate future market developments that may affect these.

As the amount of information to be treated is enormous, BI uses different IT and management tools to make the information more digestible and meaningful, such as big data analytics, artificial intelligence (AI)-powered market intelligence platforms, key performance indicators (KPIs) and data dashboards (the visual representation of KPIs).

BI professionals need an excellent understanding of the business. Therefore, several years of experience in an operational job and at a mid-managerial level, even with different companies, are definitely much appreciated assets.

3.6.2 Portfolio Management

Portfolio management in a biopharmaceutical company is about selecting which projects in the drug pipeline should be started or proceeded, which ones should be adapted and which ones should be abandoned or killed.

Because of the huge financial risks and high failure rates typical for the pharmaceutical business, it seeks to reduce these risks by diversification of the portfolio (e.g. in different therapeutic areas with diverse risk scores) and risk minimisation (e.g. by having various drug projects neatly distributed along the different phases of the drug life cycle) or risk sharing (e.g. by creating partnerships and alliances). All this should be done in line with the near-, mid- and long-term corporate strategic objectives.

Candidates for a job in this function will preferentially have some years of experience in one or more operational positions before being eligible to move into portfolio management.

3.6.3 Business Development

Business development (BD) includes various activities making a business grow in the long run. Growth can mean increase in market share, revenue or profit, but can also be obtained by business expansion or partnerships.

It impacts every organisational department in a company, from research to sales, human resources, finance and service provider management. Within the biopharmaceutical industry, it is focused on strategic issues such as in- and out-licensing of products, choice of service provider partnerships (either outsourcing activities to a CRO or temporarily insourcing external staff), mergers and acquisitions.

Again, in order to be successful in this function, candidates should have spent some years in the pharmaceutical industry, or benefit from a similar experience in another business.

3.6.4 Human Resources

The human resources (HR) function of a company is responsible for recruitment, retention and dismissal of staff, their training and development, their remuneration and benefits package and stimulating a pleasant working environment or company culture.

As the competition for talented people is high ('the war on talent'), pharmaceutical companies invest a lot in recruiting and retaining high-potential employees ('HIPOs'), who are keen to pursue leadership opportunities.

The educational background of HR professionals varies widely. Although it is primarily (and also in the pharma industry) the domain of graduates in HR or industrial-organisational psychology, life sciences graduates with experience in people management acquired as team manager in an operational function can also progress to an interesting HR position.

Smaller company units, such as a research centre, a production plant or a subsidiary, as well as corporate headquarters, have openings for HR professionals.

3.6.5 Training and Development

Both educational activities are designed to improve the performance and productivity of company employees. Training is meant to enhance the job-specific knowledge and skills of individuals or teams in their present job, while development refers to preparing individuals for future higher-level positions.

Most pharmaceutical companies have their own in-house training (or learning) and development department or academy, but there are also numerous service providers active in this field. They operate in close collaboration with human resources.

Most newcomers receive induction training, focused on general information on the business, the company's mission and organisation as well as more specific training on the job's operational aspects. According to the job, this can take a few days to several weeks. Later on, these individuals or teams can be offered additional continuous training.

Job titles in this function can be very general, e.g. trainer or training manager, or very specific, e.g. training and development specialist—quality assurance. Trainers have widely different backgrounds, but some experience in the field of interest is of course mandatory. Above all, they should have excellent communication and teaching skills.

3.6.6 Information Technology

Information (and communications) technology (IT or ICT) is all about digital hardware, software and data management (and transmission) systems. The importance of ICT in this business cannot be underestimated. Indeed, the biopharmaceutical industry generates enormous amounts of data that need to be analysed to create information, knowledge and value; it needs to plan and monitor complex processes; it interacts with many external partners and stakeholders; and it operates worldwide.

With the advent and further evolutions in digital technologies, automation and robotisation of processes, social media, artificial and virtual intelligence, the Internet of things, the iCloud and the metaverse, the strategic importance of this department will certainly keep on growing in the future.

3.6.7 Finance and Accounting

Finance and accounting is responsible for the management of the incoming and outgoing flow of money in the company. In the biopharmaceutical industry, the financial focus is mainly on the high R & D costs and the price setting of new medicines. As innovative drug prices are currently considered by many as too high, finance managers at country, regional or headquarter level should have tough negotiating skills.

Finance and accounting jobs are typically for masters in accounting, finance or economics. Possible exceptions in pharma are life sciences graduates with an additional master in business administration (MBA) degree.

3.6.8 Legal Affairs

Legal affairs professionals advice the company on legal issues related to business operations. Apart from the usual responsibilities such as drafting and negotiating all types of contracts and agreements (e.g. clinical trial or licensing agreements), in the pharmaceutical industry, their focus is mainly on compliance with patent and intellectual property legislation, data privacy law (such as the General Data Protection Regulation or GDPR in the European Union) and general information security regulation (such as ISO 27000). They also provide litigation support in lawsuits related to severe drug side effects (e.g. class actions) or competition violations.

Legal affair jobs require a law degree, but candidates with a double diploma (life sciences and law) or a specialisation in, for instance, patent or corporate law are one step ahead.

3.7   How to Kick-Start Your Career in This Sector?

Young graduates, be it in the life sciences or other disciplines, often struggle to find their way to start a professional career in the healthcare industry. This is mainly due to a lack of sufficient knowledge about the wealth of possibilities that are out there. The previous sections of this chapter tried to narrow this knowledge gap. The present section offers general information on what is required to start in (one of) these jobs, focusing on wanted qualifications, key employability assets and some practical advice.

3.7.1   Wanted Qualifications

3.7.1.1   Graduates in Life Sciences

Because of its nature, the (bio)pharmaceutical industry, and by extension the related industries as well as the entire biomedical or healthcare sector, has a special interest to employ talented graduates in the life sciences.

The term life sciences refers to the study of living organisms and comprises many disciplines such as the basic 'robust' sciences (e.g. biology, chemistry, physics and their myriad of subdisciplines), human sciences (e.g. psychology, social sciences), applied sciences (e.g. engineering, biotechnology) as well as specialists in disease research or management (e.g. pharmaceutical sciences, biomedical sciences, medicine, veterinary medicine).

3.7.1.2   Other Sought Disciplines

Of course, the employability of the sector is not limited to graduates in life sciences. Other disciplines are also highly wanted, such as graduates in (health or pharmaco-) economics, business administration, (big) data analysis, mathematics and statistics, information technology, finance and accounting, human resources, training and development, (health or patent) law, etc.

3.7.1.3   All Levels of Higher Education Have a Chance

The wide diversity in available positions also guarantees that every level of higher education can find its way.

Professional or academic *bachelors* can find a job in the frontline day-to-day operations, as analyst, scientist, (lab) technician, sales representative, operator in manufacturing, administrative assistant, etc.

A *master degree* is also suited or sometimes required to start in some of the functions cited above, but is definitely a must to qualify for positions at higher-level day-to-day operations or low-level management, e.g. as researcher, data manager, project or product manager, supervisor, team leader, group product manager, etc. At entry, these graduates usually get a job title with a prefix such as Assistant or Junior, which will be dropped after a couple of years, and later eventually replaced by Principal or Senior.

Since a number of years, some universities pioneered with more specific master degree programmes better targeted to the pharmaceutical industry, such as the master in drug development (at KU Leuven, Belgium), the biopharmaceutical sciences master's programme (at Leiden University, the Netherlands), the master's in drug innovation programme (at Utrecht University, the Netherlands) and certainly other initiatives.

A third cycle or postgraduate *research doctorate, such as Doctor of Philosophy (PhD)* in any of the above-cited disciplines, is undoubtedly a must in discovery research and for many positions in drug development (perhaps more so in chempharm and non-clinical development than in clinical development where specialisation may be more wanted).

Other postgraduate or advanced higher education paths are also appreciated, such as:

– Further *specialisation*: either by obtaining a formal advanced master degree (e.g. industrial or hospital or clinical pharmacy, specialist medicine or pharmaceutical medicine), or either by taking extra specialised courses, diplomas or certifications in order to extend your competences in one of the disciplines that are highly wanted in the pharma industry (e.g. clinical pharmacology, pharmacometrics, quality management, regulatory affairs, manufacturing, etc.).
– A *second diploma* in a completely different discipline: e.g. a master in business administration (MBA), a master degree in (patent) law, a master in (health or pharmaco-)economics or a master in engineering.

In general, when postgraduates are in competition with graduates for a job where a graduate degree is sufficient, then the extra educational degree may not be an advantage, except when it might be considered by the employer as an extra asset for future career development.

More detailed information on education and training opportunities for a career in the pharmaceutical and biomedical industry can be found in Chap. 19.

3.7.2 Key Employability Assets

3.7.2.1 Know What You Want

The best road to professional success is to know what you want to do, and where you want to end up in 10 years or more. Some people rather leave it to chance or coincidence, but they are then left at the mercy of the circumstances, instead of having their future in their own hands. But still, keep an open mind to be able to take advantage of interesting unexpected opportunities.

In order to know best where you would fit in or want to land, a good understanding of the pharmaceutical business is of paramount importance. This book helps you to gain knowledge about the processes involved to get a drug/product from bench to patient (the drug life cycle), and all the different disciplines and players involved to make it happen. Only when you have this holistic view will you be able to decide for yourself where you would best fit in to start with, and where you would like to go next in the near future.

3.7.2.2 Soft Skills

In the competition for position openings, your educational qualifications will be a basic requirement. On top of that, employers will be more interested in your personal and interpersonal skills, to find out where you stand out from the crowd. In the war for talent, your soft skills profile can make a decisive difference to finally get the job you want so badly.

A lot of lists of soft skills to be successful in any profession are in circulation. Here, I present my personal set of soft skills that I think are important to be successful in the pharmaceutical industry. They are not necessarily presented in the order of importance, and some are more needed in some particular positions, while others are more suited for other positions.

Personal skills

– First and foremost: passion, drive, enthusiasm and motivation; for the sector you appreciate, the company you admire and the job you long for.
– A creative and problem-solving mindset, as the business is essentially based on innovation. In discovery research and exploratory development, you'll be allowed and even stimulated to think out of the box. And although the rest of the business is highly regulated, innovation means exploring how far you can colour outside the lines.
– Willingness to learn lifelong.
– Professionalism, integrity and strong work ethic.
– Commercial awareness. Even researchers and developers should be constantly aware that their ultimate goal is to get new drugs/products on the market, so that they can benefit patients, but also generate return on investment.
– Management skills. In particular, project, product or strategic management (the core of the business), risk management (it is a particularly high-risk business) and self-management (including time and stress management).
– Flexibility and adaptiveness, as the failure rate of drug R & D is high, and the forced market withdrawal of a successful drug can have very painful consequences.

- For some jobs, willingness to travel, stay a few days abroad or relocate to another country.

Interpersonal skills

- First and foremost, excellent communication skills, both oral and written.
- Being a team player. Because of the complexity of this business, teamwork is important, either in teams of the same discipline, but more so in interdisciplinary teams. In this context, you will need active listening capacities and empathy for others.
- Networking skills, in order to build relationships, both within and outside the company you're working for. Of particular importance when you'll need help from others, or for future career development.
- Leadership, to be inspirational to team or staff members and to motivate them to surpass themselves. The top executive (CEO) should be visionary ('I have a dream'), while lower-level managers should be more down to earth ('Yes we can').
- And last but not least, a good command of English, and openness to other languages and cultures, especially when you want to pursue an international career.

This long list of appreciated soft skills should not discourage you, as you will not need them all for a hundred percent to be successful in your job and career. Some functions require for example more in-depth numeracy, while others require more empathy and communication skills.

3.7.2.3   What About Professional Experience?

The importance of professional experience as an employability criterion in the pharma industry can vary widely.

For some jobs, mostly very specific or higher-level ones, having a specific professional experience in the field of interest may be a prerequisite. For example:

- Even for an entry job as pharmacometrician in a pharmacokinetics department in industry, a couple of years as postdoc in a similar academic environment can be required.
- For the position of a senior regulatory affairs manager, a principal medical writer or a senior pharmaceutical process engineer, several years of relevant (operational) experience may be needed.

For many of the available positions, some professional experience is considered an additional asset, on top of your educational background, your technical competences (e.g. digital literacy or specific software capabilities) and your soft skills profile.

Recent graduates may feel limited by a lack of professional experience. However, this can be compensated for by alternative work experience or other (previous) initiatives that may impress recruiters, such as:

- A curricular internship during your graduate or postgraduate education.
- Part-time or flex job experience as a student.
- Volunteer engagement in community service or charities.
- Involvement or leadership in social activities or hobby clubs, e.g. experience in running meetings, or in organising (big) events, or as leader of a scouts group.

You may also apply for an unpaid 6-month or 1-year internship offered to starters by many pharmaceutical companies, or accept a lower-paid entry job for a couple of years in order to gain work experience before taking your career to the next level.

3.7.3   Some Practical Advice

Mentioned below are a few general tips and tricks that can help you to find and land your (first) job in the pharma industry successfully.

- Start working on it during your studies.
- Do your homework, and prepare yourself.
   Know your own strengths and weaknesses. Learn about the sector, the pharmaceutical industry, the companies that are active in it and the job(s) you are keen on. Attend job search events or career fairs organised by universities, recruiters and employers.
- Build a network of people who can help you.
   Look out for and talk to people who already work in the pharmaceutical industry and the desired job. They will give you valuable information and advice.
   Reach out to your professors who know the industry well. They are acquainted with your competencies and capabilities and might support your application(s).
- Write a detailed job hunting plan.
   List your goals and how to achieve them. Create a to-do list with a calendar and deadlines, and keep it up-to-date.
- Create an attractive curriculum vitae (cv or resume) and cover letter.
   Send it out in reply to job announcements of interest, and post it online on social media and different job search platforms so that job or head hunters can easily find you.
- Prepare yourself well for (remote) job interviews, as well as assessment tests and exercises.
   Create and practice a good personal elevator pitch, i.e. how to present yourself convincingly in 30 seconds.
   Before each interview, learn more about the company and the open position.
   Practice some mock assessment tests and exercises that are available online.

- Develop a tactful strategy to negotiate the more delicate topics of salary, benefits and work-life balance. Manoeuvre always politely so that you don't have to bring it up yourself.
- Once you obtain a fair offer, take your time, but don't take too long to close the deal.

More practical tips and tricks can be found in Chap. 17 (A Successful Career in the Life Sciences Industry: How to Write your Strongest Resumé and Ace that Interview), Chap. 18 (Skill Building for Career Advancement: Public Speaking and Networking) and Chap. 19 (Training Opportunities for a Career in the Pharmaceutical and Biomedical Industry/Sector).

3.8 Career Perspectives

The life sciences and healthcare sector offers many opportunities for career growth. As the social and economic importance of the sector is still constantly growing, many individuals find it an attractive workplace to progress their professional careers.

This section limits itself to more general aspects of the way individuals can plan and develop their careers and describes possible career paths in the pharmaceutical industry and the broader biomedical sector. As an introduction, some general information is provided on possible career approaches, the way (pharmaceutical) companies are organised and the different management levels.

3.8.1 General Introductory Concepts

3.8.1.1 Career Development Approaches

There are essentially two approaches to develop your career, either as specialist or generalist. Successful companies need both profiles for their daily operations. And it is up to you to find out or to decide which one suits you best. Even the mixed approach might work out best for you.

Specialists have deep knowledge on a subject matter, want to become an expert in their field of interest, are niche players and are perfectly happy with that.

Examples in the pharma industry are the discovery researcher who simply seeks to be successful in designing new drugs, or the pharmacovigilance manager who wants to develop his/her career as an expert in drug-induced liver injury.

The advantages of such an approach are that you will be exposed to less competition, may be better paid and have a lifelong career guaranteed. The downside is that you will have difficulty switching to another position when yours becomes obsolete.

Generalists are competent and skilful in several different fields and can perform multiple tasks. They might have started as a specialist, but progressively want to broaden their knowledge and skill base in order to tackle new challenges and be more widely employable.

Examples in the pharma industry are the international clinical operations manager, responsible for several therapeutic areas and multiple countries, or the general manager of a subsidiary (operating as a mini-company), who switches countries every 3–5 years.

Generalists are more flexible, are perhaps less exposed to burnout and progress more easily to leadership positions. On the other hand, they can be replaced more easily.

3.8.1.2 How (Pharmaceutical) Companies Are Organised

It is good to have a general understanding of how companies are organised, in order to better appreciate your own place in the organisation and to realise better which opportunities you might have to switch positions to develop your career.

Companies can be organised in many different ways, and that is also the case for biopharmaceutical companies. The types of organisational structure most frequently used are hierarchical (most common); functional, divisional or matrix-based; or less hierarchical organisations (team-based, network or flat structures). All have their pros and cons, and again, it will be up to you to find out which one suits you best.

The bigger pharma companies have R & D centres, manufacturing sites and commercial subsidiaries scattered all over the world, so that there is a chance that you can find a job in your own country or nearby. However, you can also choose to go for an international career within a company, either by moving from one centre, plant or subsidiary to another (even in different phases of your career) or by switching to a regional office or the headquarters of the company to accept a position with regional or global responsibility.

3.8.1.3 Management Levels

Companies usually have three major management levels: lower, middle and top management; and this is equally true in the pharmaceutical industry.

The lowest level of activities is in the execution of day-to-day operations. Here you find mainly labourers, technicians, scientists, sales reps and administrative staff.

Lower management includes positions with somewhat more demanding first-line tasks, and line managers responsible for coordinating the frontline activities.

Here you find project, product or process managers, as well as supervisors and leaders of small teams.

Middle management (also known as mid- or B-level management) is responsible for the translation and implementation of the corporate strategy defined by top management to the lower management level.

Here you find heads, leaders, managers or directors of functional teams (e.g. group project or product managers, non-clinical development director, drug project team leader), and the major divisions or departments (e.g. regulatory affairs, quality assurance, pharmacovigilance, marketing, sales, human resources, training and development, information technology and finance managers).

As this constitutes the majority of the company's management team, staff members often start in these positions as associates, and eventually move up to a senior level.

Top management, with alternative names such as senior-, executive-, or C-level managers (also known as the C-suite, the C standing for Chief), are responsible for aligning the corporate strategy, policies and operations with the mission and goals they receive from the Board of Directors.

This is usually a small group of highly experienced and influential professionals representing the major departments in the company, such as the Chief R & D or Chief Technology Officer (CTO), the Chief Operations Officer (COO), the Chief Financial Officer (CFO) and the Chief Marketing Officer (CMO), under the ultimate leadership of the Chief Executive Officer (CEO), the highest-ranking person in a company.

In larger companies, the highest-ranking executive can be the President, combining the functions of CEO and COO/CFO, seconded by a (Senior) Vice President.

In general, the C-suite decides in concert, and the CEO receives instructions from and reports back to the Board of Directors, representing the owners of the company.

3.8.2   Career Management

Career management is a lifelong and time-consuming process of implementing a strategy to achieve your professional dream and goals. It is often described as the combination of career planning and career development (see below). Career management is both important for the employees (on an individual level for continuous job satisfaction) and for the employer (on an organisational level for talent retention). This section focuses on what an individual can do.

3.8.2.1   Career Planning

Career planning is the process of creating an action plan to achieve your career goals. It is a continuous reiterative process composed of essentially four elements:

– Self-assessment, to identify your strengths and weaknesses.
– Research. Explore which possibilities are out there. Find out which jobs and career paths would suit you best in the future to guarantee continuous job satisfaction. Consider all aspects, i.e. job content, competences and skills needed, salary and benefits offered, work-life balance and the need to relocate. Go to job

markets, and contact people who already work in the industry or sector. Think of several career paths, compare them and select one to work on.
- Setting goals. What would you like to achieve in 5, 10 and 20 years from now? Identify career steps that match your current competencies and skills (for the short term), or the ones you want to acquire first (for the mid- and long term).
- Action plan. Create a detailed road map with different actions and their timeline with milestones. Implement it, follow it up and repeat the cycle each time when you want to take your career to the next level.

The company's human resources department may be of help, but their objectives could be different from yours, or they could only offer it to high-potential employees (HIPOs). If needed, go and see an independent career counsellor.

3.8.2.2 Career Development

Career development is all about what you can do to seize future job opportunities that can propel your career forward. Here are a number of examples of possible actions you can take:

- Learn lifelong. Continuous education and training are key. Take extra courses, integrate new skills and be on top of new technological innovations.
- Extend your network, and find a mentor. They might advise, motivate and coach you, or bring you back to reality when you have the tendency to be overly enthusiastic.
- Participate in professional working groups, committees and task forces, both within your current company and also externally (e.g. join a professional association) in order to increase your visibility to other potential employers.
- Attend (international) professional conferences, congresses, seminars, workshops, etc. This is an excellent opportunity to get exposure to others (e.g. when giving a presentation) and to expand your network.
- Keep yourself up-to-date in professional reading.

3.8.3 Career Opportunities

In this section, the focus will be on three aspects in relation to career opportunities: (1) career progression modalities in general, (2) career opportunities in the (bio)-pharmaceutical industry and (3) career opportunities in the wider life sciences sector.

3.8.3.1 Career Progression Modalities in General

During the course of a professional career, there are many possibilities for career advancement.

A number of these modalities will be briefly presented here:

- Job rotation, by assigning newcomers temporarily to other jobs within the company, in order to give them an opportunity to decide where they would fit in best.
- Job redesign, either by enlarging the scope of the job or by adding additional responsibility.
- Career progression up the ladder, either as a specialist without the intention to become a manager (from junior professional to expert professional) or as a manager (from a lower management level to an executive level).
- Lateral or horizontal progression. One possibility is doing the same or a similar job in another location, e.g. general managers heading a subsidiary in a particular country can move several times for a number of years from one country to another, tackling new challenges each time and gaining international experience. Another possibility is to switch (several times) to another department, somewhat similar to job rotation, to learn about other parts of the business before moving to a middle or top management position.
- Special career moves, including taking a break or sabbatical, step up the pace by temporarily accepting a more challenging job or inversely, move to a less demanding job for personal reasons.
- Going international, either by moving to another country (even several ones successively, cfr example above) or by taking up a position with regional or global responsibility in a regional office or at the company's headquarters.
- Going independent, either as consultant or freelancer, or by starting your own company, e.g. as a service provider or full competitor.

Most of the career moves described above can be made within the same company, or by switching to another company or organisation, usually within the same sector, but why not, also by switching to a completely new one.

3.8.3.2 Career Opportunities in the (Bio)Pharmaceutical Industry

There are numerous opportunities for recent or confirmed life sciences graduates to start or continue a professional career in the pharmaceutical industry.

Within one pharma company, all the career progression modalities cited in the previous section are possible, except for going independent. So there is no need to repeat them here.

For a number of decades now, a lot of companies opted for leaner (and meaner) organisations, which resulted in an increased use of service providers. This creates a lot of extra job and career opportunities in this industry.

There are essentially two modes of service provisioning that are widely used in the (bio)pharmaceutical industry:

– *Outsourcing of projects*

Part of the R & D, manufacturing or commercial activities of the business can be subcontracted to a service provider. In the (bio)pharmaceutical industry, these companies are known as contract research organisations (CROs), although their activities surpass the 'research' part of the business. In manufacturing, they are known as contract manufacturing organisations (CMOs). In this mode of operations, the service provider takes over the entire workload of, for instance, the screening of a number of drug candidates, the regulatory non-clinical toxicology test battery, the clinical development of a drug, the clinical quality assurance programme, the submission of marketing authorisation applications, the manufacturing of a drug, the sales promotion of a new drug, etc. For regulatory authorities, however, the marketing authorisation applicant or holder keeps the final responsibility to respect all legal and regulatory rules.

– *Insourcing of staff*

In this service modality, staff members employed by a CRO or other service provider are temporarily insourced in a pharmaceutical company to execute certain tasks. The legal aspects of this type of service provisioning can be tricky in some countries, but are out of the scope of this chapter and book.

The CRO business in the pharma industry is a very important one for extra job and career opportunities. Newcomers in the industry can start in a CRO and gain experience from the approaches and culture of different pharmaceutical companies, before eventually switching to such a company. Inversely, staff members of a pharma company can advance their career by switching to a position higher up the ladder in a CRO.

As much as some pharma companies are called 'big pharma', there are also big full service CROs that occupy a place in the top ten ranking of companies active in this industry, based on their yearly global turnover.

Apart from the research-oriented drug companies, there are also several companies that specialise in generics and/or biosimilars only. Although they don't need to do much research, and the non-clinical and clinical development of these drugs is limited, their commercial activities are important. In total, they offer a fair amount of additional opportunities for jobs and career growth.

There is also the possibility to create your own company, as a service provider or as a competitor to pharma companies, and either start it as a one-person consulting business or opt immediately for a somewhat bigger start-up. In order to be successful in this endeavour, you will need to prepare yourself thoroughly and follow a number of steps:

– Clarify your idea. Know what you want to do.
– Take some extra courses to close your knowledge gap about entrepreneurship. You might even think of getting a master in business administration or MBA.
– Find people and organisations that can help you.
– Do an in-depth market search about your competitors and potential customers.
– Write a business plan.

– Get the financing, legal aspects and staffing done.
– Start promoting your business, and grow it.

It sounds easy on paper, but it can be painstakingly challenging. Therefore, you should be passionate, ambitious, flexible and tenacious.

More detailed information on entrepreneurship and enterprise creation can be found in Chap. 15.

3.8.3.3   Career Opportunities in the Wider Life Sciences Sector

On top of the ones already described above, there are many other job and career opportunities out there in the wider life sciences sector.

For a brief overview of these opportunities, the reader is referred to Sect. 3.2.3. More detailed information on career perspectives in a science and technology park can be found in Chap. 14.

The fact that such a broad sector has only one common ultimate goal, i.e. improving the health of humans (and animals), makes it somewhat easier to enhance your career within this sector by switching from one stakeholder to another. And that is exactly what is happening quite frequently. As an example, you could start your professional career in a CRO, move on to a drug company, switch to a national regulatory agency, get settled at the European Medicines Agency and end your career back in academia.

As a final thought, remember that you should treat your career as a process or project similar to commercialising a drug or a product, with similar phases: launch, growth, maturation, decline and withdrawal (retirement). To be successful, you should pay considerable attention to each of these phases, and prepare them well in advance.

3.9   Conclusion

The (bio)pharmaceutical industry, as well as the wider life sciences sector, offers a plethora of job and career opportunities to young graduates and confirmed professionals in the life sciences.

In order to find your way in this jungle, there is only one piece of advice that stands above all: prepare yourself as best you can. This book is written to help you with that, and this chapter is intended to trigger your curiosity to explore more.

Acknowledgements   I would like to thank Steven Dekens for the graphical support, Maaike Gons and Wouter Eijkelkamp for critically reading part of the manuscript, and Iris Gorter de Vries and Chris van Schravendijk for their critical review of the entire manuscript.

References

ABPI-IPSOS (2021) Pharmaceutical reputation index 2021. https://abpi-ukpharma-reputation-index.ipsos-mori.com. Accessed 26 Jan 2022

BIO-QLS-Informa (2021) Clinical development success rates and contributing factors 2011–2020. https://www.bio.org/ia-reports. Accessed 11 Feb 2022

EFPIA (2021) The pharmaceutical industry in figures: key data 2021. https://www.efpia.eu. Accessed 26 Jan 2022

EUR-Lex (2001) Directive 2001/83/EC of the European Parliament and of the council of 6 November 2001 on the community code relating to medicinal products for human use. Off J Eur Commun L 311:67–128

Fierce Pharma (2021) The top 20 drugs by worldwide sales in 2020. https://www.fiercepharma.com/special-report/top-20-drugs-by-2020-sales. Accessed 31 Jan 2022

Hill RG, Rang HP (2013) Drug discovery and development. In: Technology in transition, 2nd edn. Churchill Livingstone/Elsevier, Edinburgh

IFPMA (2021) The pharmaceutical industry and global health: facts and figures 2021. https://www.ifpma.org. Accessed 26 Jan 2022

Rose KH (2005) Project quality management: why, what and how. J Ross Publishing, Fort Lauderdale, p 41

Rosier JA, Martens MA, Thomas JR (2014) Global new drug development: an introduction. Wiley Blackwell, Chichester

Wouters OJ et al (2020) Estimated research and development investment needed to bring a new medicine to market, 2009-2018. J Am Med Ass 323(9):844–853

Zahid A (2021) 6 reasons why pharmaceutical careers are lucrative. https://www.biospace.com/article/6-reasons-why-a-career-in-pharma-is-lucrative-/. Accessed 26 Jan 2022

Part II
Opportunities Along the Drug/Product Life Cycle

Chapter 4
Career Opportunities in Toxicology

Mark Martens and Miranda Cornet

Abstract In Chap. 4, an overview is given of the career opportunities for toxicologists in the pharmaceutical industry as well as in other industries such as the agrochemical, food, cosmetic and chemical industry. Careers not only in industry are addressed but also in academia, regulatory authorities and consulting and contract research organisations. For each of these sectors, an overview is given of the type of activities where toxicologists are involved. Toxicology is a multidisciplinary science, and a career in toxicology can be pursued starting from a variety of university degrees in the biomedical area. Therefore, attention is paid to the basic education and requirements for a successful career as a toxicologist. Also, the possibilities of postgraduate training are discussed and how they can contribute to becoming an experienced toxicologist and take on career opportunities even beyond the role of toxicologist. To enhance credibility in consulting, legal testimony and defence of toxicology dossiers at national and international authorities, it is essential to be recognised by peers as a qualified toxicologist. This can be done by applying for certification. An overview is given of the most important certifications for toxicologists that are available worldwide.

4.1 Introduction

Toxicology is a multidisciplinary science investigating adverse health effects of chemicals, biologicals and materials in living organisms. These can be medicines (human and veterinary, small molecules and biologicals), medical devices, diagnostics, implants, advanced therapy medicinal products (ATMPs) such as gene and cell therapy, tissue-engineered products, pesticides, biocides, cosmetics, food constituents, food additives, food contact materials, food contaminants, genetically modified organisms, industrial chemicals, building materials, coatings, consumer products,

M. Martens (✉)
Consultant in Preclinical Development and Toxicology, Leuven, Belgium

M. Cornet
UCB Biopharma, Brussels, Belgium

© The Author(s), under exclusive license to Springer Nature Switzerland AG 2023
J. R. Thomas et al. (eds.), *Career Options in the Pharmaceutical and Biomedical Industry*, https://doi.org/10.1007/978-3-031-14911-5_4

natural animal and plant toxins and environmental contaminants. Health effects that are the result of exposure to physical agents such as ionising and non-ionising radiation, sound, vibrations and magnetic and electric fields require specific skills and therefore normally don't belong to the field of expertise of the toxicologist but to experts specialised in each of these physical agents. Toxicology aims to identify and characterise the hazards associated with chemicals, biologicals and materials and to assess the risks for human or animal health taking into account exposure during intended and non-intended contact. The ultimate goal of toxicology is to ensure that there are no health risks associated with the use of medicines or exposure to chemicals, products and materials at home, at work and in the environment.

To assess the safety of products and materials, various aspects of toxicology research have to be considered, and this includes in vivo, in vitro, in chemico and in silico investigations. Toxicological endpoints that are important for health hazard and risk assessment include local tolerance (skin, eyes and respiratory tract irritation and sensitisation), genotoxicity, acute toxicity, short-term and long-term toxicity, carcinogenicity, fertility, embryo-foetal developmental toxicity, pre- and postnatal development toxicity, juvenile development toxicity, neurobehavioural toxicity and immunotoxicity. Pharmacokinetics and metabolism also play an important role in the interpretation of toxicology studies and the assessment of the relevance of experimental toxicity data to human health.

Ecotoxicology and environmental risk assessment concentrates on adverse effects of chemicals and materials on environmental non-target animal species, populations and ecosystems and is also important for the risk management of chemicals, certainly in the agrochemical and biocide industry. Since this is a specific area of expertise requiring different backgrounds and postgraduate training, it is not considered within the scope of this chapter.

Toxicologists occupy positions in a variety of sectors such as academia, government, international organisations, scientific institutes, industry, contract research organisations (CROs), consultancies and non-governmental organisations (NGOs). According to the American Society of Toxicology (SOT 2022), over half of the toxicologists in the United States work in industry, 34% work in academia, and 12% in government.

Apart from the production, evaluation and submission of data for market approval of products, toxicologists can also be involved in other activities such as forensic toxicology, occupational toxicology and clinical toxicology. In forensic toxicology, body fluids and tissues are analysed for the presence of toxic chemicals to help in solving criminal cases. Occupational toxicology deals with the monitoring and risk assessment of exposures of workers to chemicals in the workplace and with the development of occupational exposure limits. In clinical toxicology, various job profiles can be distinguished such as the clinical investigator following up side effects of experimental and marketed drugs, the emergency physician treating acute poisonings, the analytical toxicologist providing support to emergency medicine for the detection and monitoring of acute poisonings and the physician or pharmacist specialised in clinical toxicology information providing support to poison control centres. These disciplines in toxicology will not be further handled in detail in this chapter.

It is the objective of this chapter to give an overview of the different career opportunities in toxicology and the training and skills that are required for a successful career as a toxicologist.

4.2   Basic Skills Required for a Career in Toxicology

To start a successful career in toxicology, a strong basic knowledge in biological, chemical or biomedical sciences at university level is required. Degrees (at least Masters) in biomedical sciences (with options such as pathophysiology, immunology, neurosciences, cancerology or toxicology), biology (with options in molecular and cell biology), biotechnology, biochemistry, pharmacology, physiology, biophysics, pharmaceutical sciences (pharmaceutical care, drug development), medicine, veterinary sciences, chemistry (with option in analytical chemistry) and bioengineering (with options in cellular and genetic engineering, food science, molecular biology) are a good starting point.

Various postgraduate training programmes are offered by universities in Europe that are useful to further expand skills required for a career in toxicology. Examples are courses in toxicology (experimental, regulatory, occupational), pathology, analytical toxicology (bioanalysis), pharmacology, metabolism, pharmacokinetics, immunology, drug development, clinical biology, bioinformatics and biostatistics. An overview of postgraduate training programmes in Europe recognised by EUROTOX for the European Register of Toxicologists (ERT) programme is provided in the table below (EUROTOX 2022):

Topic	Teaching hours	Course provider	Course website
In vitro Testing Methods	22	The European Society of Toxicology In Vitro (ESTIV)	http://www.estiv.org
Principles of Toxicology	Web course	Postgraduate Education of Toxicology, Wageningen, the Netherlands	http://www.toxcourses.nl/courses/general-toxicology/
Molecular and Cellular Toxicology	27		
Target Organ Toxicology and Histopathology	25		
Clinical and Forensic Toxicology	38		
Epidemiology	24		
Toxicity of Environmental Pollutants	25		
Ecotoxicology	26		
	34		

(continued)

Topic	Teaching hours	Course provider	Course website
Genotoxicity and Carcinogenicity			
Target Organ Toxicology and Histopathology	30		
Laboratory Animal Science including 3R	31		
Occupational Toxicology	28		
Immunotoxicology	25		
Reproductive and Developmental Toxicology	25		
Regulatory Toxicology	26		
Risk Assessment of Chemicals	30		
Molecular Toxicology	25		
Food Toxicology	26		
Molecular and Cellular Toxicology	14	EUROTOX-Molecular Toxicology Specialty Section	
Principles of Toxicology	40	Belgian society of Toxicology and Ecotoxicology (BelTox) and Université Catholique de Louvain (UCLouvain), Belgium	https://uclouvain.be/fr/etudier/iufc/programme-toxico.html
Regulatory Toxicology	40		
Occupational Toxicology	40		
Experimental Design and Biostatistics, Target Organ Toxicology and Histopathology, Toxicity of Environmental Pollutants, Exposure Assessment, Epidemiology, Occupational Toxicology, Genotoxicity and Carcinogenicity, Reproductive and Developmental Toxicology, Risk Assessment of Chemicals, Drug Safety Assessment, Regulatory Toxicology, In Silico Toxicology, Immunotoxicology, Analytical Methods in Toxicology	440	Università degli Studi di Milano, Milano, Italy	https://safetyassessment.cdl.unimi.it/en
Principles of Toxicology, Laboratory Animal Science Including 3R, Experimental Design and	598	Medical University of Vienna, Austria	http://www.meduniwien.ac.at/toxicology/php/index.php

(continued)

Topic	Teaching hours	Course provider	Course website
Biostatistics, Molecular and Cellular Toxicology, Absorption, Distribution, Metabolism and Excretion, Target Organ Toxicology and Histopathology, Toxicity of Environmental Pollutants, Exposure Assessment, Epidemiology, Occupational Toxicology, Genotoxicity and Carcinogenicity, Reproductive and Developmental Toxicology, Risk Assessment of Chemicals, Clinical and Forensic Toxicology, Drug Safety Assessment, Regulatory Toxicology, Ecotoxicology, Nanomaterials, In vitro testing methods, In silico toxicology, Immunotoxicology, Neurotoxicology, Analytical methods in toxicology			
Safety Assessment of Cosmetics in the EU	43	Vrije Universiteit Brussel (VUB), Brussels, Belgium	https://www.safetycourse.eu/
Practical Application of Toxicology in Drug Development	37	British Toxicology Society and the American College of Toxicology	http://www.thebts.org/events-2/courseandwebinars/patdd2019/
Assessment of Drug-Induced Liver Injury (DILI): Key Rules and Common Pitfalls. How To Make a Clinical Narrative	11	ACTION COST 17-112 PRO EURO DILI NET and Department of Pharmacology, School of Medicine, University of Malaga, Spain	https://proeurodilinet.eu/1st-working-groups-meeting-2nd-cg-mc-training-school-malaga-14-15-march-2019

The best basis for a career in toxicology is a doctoral programme in one of the many areas of toxicology (e.g. analytical toxicology, forensic toxicology, pharmacokinetics and metabolism, genetic toxicology, reproductive toxicology, neurotoxicology, immunotoxicology, carcinogenicity, in vitro toxicology, occupational toxicology, clinical toxicology, safety pharmacology, pathology) or a related biomedical topic (e.g. pharmacology, bioinformatics, genomics) that can be combined with various postgraduate trainings. Besides the specialisation in a specific topic in toxicology, a doctoral research programme also allows the PhD student to develop skills such as problem definition, data analysis, search and analysis of literature data, performing methodical scientific research, problem-solving and written and verbal communication.

Finally, a career in toxicology means continuous learning not only to be kept abreast of progress in science but also to increase knowledge in other domains of toxicology. Most toxicologists start as a specialist in a particular domain but quickly have to expand their expertise to other areas in toxicology as they move on in their career and increase their responsibilities and oversight in toxicology projects. This is possible not only by postgraduate training but also by training on the job and changing jobs within and between industrial sectors. Changing jobs offers the opportunity to not only learn about other sub-specialities in toxicology but also to be confronted with other chemicals having different toxicological profiles.

4.3   Career Profiles of Toxicologists in Academia

Because toxicology is the science that studies the effects of chemical substances on living organisms, there are many university master degrees in sciences or more particular in life sciences that provide a good basis for a career in toxicology. These include biology, molecular biology, biotechnology, bioengineering, pharmaceutical sciences (drug development, industrial pharmacy, pharmaceutical care), biomedical sciences, medicine, veterinary sciences, chemistry and biochemistry. University degrees with specific undergraduate training in toxicology are pharmaceutical and biomedical sciences. Universities in Europe and around the world also offer postgraduate trainings that can be useful for a career in toxicology. Examples are physiology, cell biology, molecular biology, pharmacology, haematology, clinical biochemistry, histopathology, biostatistics, bioanalysis, pharmacokinetics, drug metabolism, in vitro toxicology, clinical toxicology and epidemiology.

The first step in preparing for an academic career in toxicology consists in obtaining a PhD, potentially complemented by a postdoctoral experience. Most of the time, PhD and postdoctoral topics fit into the overall research programme of the university department. They are highly specialised and focussed on specific aspects of toxicology. Typical examples include, but are not limited to, the development and validation of new in vitro test systems, genotoxicity, immunotoxicity, neurotoxicity, liver toxicity, skin sensitisation and mechanisms of chemical carcinogenesis.

In academia, career paths are possible ultimately leading to head of department and professorship. Besides teaching, the main objective of the academic researcher is to contribute to fundamental science often within the framework of national and international research programmes (e.g. European Research Council (ERC) grants in the EU where collaboration with other universities in Europe is encouraged). The experience profile of toxicologists in academia can be widened by participation in advisory committees of national and international authorities, collaboration with industry or providing laboratory services such as forensic toxicology analysis, clinical toxicology analysis and screening of chemical compounds for specific toxicological or pharmacological properties.

Since postdoctoral career opportunities in academia are limited, many PhDs continue their careers elsewhere. Through project work in collaboration with industry, many scientists find their way to positions of toxicologist in industry or in spin-off biotech companies of the university.

4.4 Career Profiles of Toxicologists in Pharmaceutical Industry

The pharmaceutical industry offers a wide spectrum of career opportunities for toxicologists, spanning the different stages of the drug life cycle from drug discovery to early and late development up to post-approval development. Examples of post-approval development are fixed-dose combinations, different routes of administration, paediatric drug development and new indications. Drug candidates for human and veterinary medicine that are studied by toxicologists are small chemical molecules (new chemical entities, NCEs) and large biological molecules (new biological entities, NBEs) such as monoclonal antibodies, vaccines, peptides and oligonucleotides. NCEs have a low molecular weight, are species independent, are non-immunogenic, are easily metabolised, are short acting and can be given via various routes of administration. NBEs have a high to very high molecular weight, are species specific, are easily degraded, are long acting (except peptides), have complex temporal relationships and are only administered via the parenteral route. Whereas NCEs can show off-target as well as on-target toxicity, effects seen with NBEs are generally on-target or exaggerated pharmacology. Because of these important differences, specific testing approaches in safety assessment are required and ask for a specific experience profile of the toxicologist. Apart from the safety testing of classical pharmaceuticals, toxicologists in the pharmaceutical industry may also be involved in the safety testing of medical devices, implants, diagnostics or advanced therapy medicinal products (ATMP) such as gene or cell therapy, all of which require a specific approach.

Toxicologists are involved at each stage of nonclinical drug development, and at each of these stages, an intensive collaboration with scientists from different disciplines, such as chemical and pharmaceutical development, pharmacology, pharmacokinetics and metabolism, bioanalysis, clinical development and regulatory affairs, is essential.

In drug discovery, activities such as drug design, medicinal chemistry, pharmacology and in vitro metabolism and toxicity screening are often performed in laboratories of pharmaceutical companies. Nowadays, the early safety assessment of lead molecules in discovery focusses as much as possible on animal-free tests.

These consist of reliable in silico and in vitro tools for the screening and selection of lead molecules before moving to short-term in vivo toxicology and pharmacokinetic studies. Examples of in silico and in vitro testing methods that enable the detection of liabilities early in the discovery process with high confidence are genotoxicity and cardiotoxicity, but new methods to detect or predict toxicity in other organ/tissues, such as the liver or the central nervous system, are continuously being developed. Reliable in silico tools are commercially available or have been developed in-house by pharmaceutical companies. The discovery phase is the least regulated phase of the drug life cycle and provides a higher degree of freedom and space to be creative and enhance the discovery of new good drug candidates.

In contrast to discovery, nonclinical safety assessment of new drug candidates in early and late development is heavily regulated and very extensive. Safety assessment in the development phase aims to generate data prior to or in support of clinical development and typically includes short- and long-term toxicology studies in various animal species, in vitro and in vivo genetic toxicology studies, fertility studies, embryo-foetal development toxicity studies, pre- and postnatal development toxicity studies, juvenile development toxicity studies, carcinogenicity studies and studies on specific endpoints such as neurotoxicity and immunotoxicity. In the event adverse effects are found in long-term animal studies such as carcinogenicity, the mode of action and the relevance to man have to be investigated.

In nonclinical drug development, toxicologists play an important role in defining the doses which can be safely administered to human volunteers in clinical trials. They also have to identify all possible parameters that need to be followed up during the clinical trials to monitor any possible toxic effect found in nonclinical safety studies. One of the specificities of the safety assessment of pharmaceuticals is that toxic effects have to be related to systemic (internal) exposure and not to the dose administered as is the case with the safety assessment of industrial chemicals, pesticides and biocides. This requires a close collaboration between the toxicologist and experts in bioanalysis and pharmacokinetics.

Toxicology testing of chemical and biological pharmaceuticals in development must be performed within a framework of national and international guidelines. In an effort to harmonise requirements across the different geographical regions in the world, testing guidelines were developed and issued by the International Council for Harmonisation of Technical Requirements for Pharmaceuticals for Human Use (ICH 2022). Toxicology testing of pharmaceuticals has also to comply with the good laboratory practice (GLP) regulations issued by the Organisation for Economic Co-operation and Development (OECD 2022) to assure the quality and integrity of nonclinical data.

Toxicologists can assume several roles in the nonclinical development department of a pharmaceutical company. They can be involved in the conduct and coordination of exploratory and regulatory toxicology studies performed within the company. The toxicologist is then responsible for the design, conduct, interpretation and reporting of the studies. Over the last decades, however, most of the toxicology testing is delegated to contract research organisations (CROs), which have a lot of expertise in running toxicology studies within a regulatory context.

When studies are performed at CROs, the toxicologist of a pharmaceutical company acts as the sponsor's representative, is involved in the design of the study and monitors the study on behalf of the company. Toxicologists are also responsible for the integration of all available nonclinical safety data in the regulatory submission dossiers.

When sufficient experience is acquired in the safety testing of drug candidates, toxicologists can progress to the role of nonclinical project leader where they take on the responsibility of coordinating all activities related to the safety assessment of a drug candidate such as toxicology, safety pharmacology, pharmacokinetics and metabolism. The nonclinical project leader also represents the nonclinical function in multidisciplinary project teams for a given drug candidate and as such collaborates closely with representatives from several other disciplines such as pharmaceutical and chemical development, clinical development, regulatory affairs, patient safety or market access to progress the drug candidate through the different stages of development up to marketing approval.

Besides work related to molecules under development, the toxicologist in the pharmaceutical industry is also called upon to provide expertise in the risk assessment of drug impurities, packaging leachables and extractables, formulation aids, manufacturing intermediates, and worker's safety in drug manufacturing and conditioning.

Toxicologists employed in the pharmaceutical industry can have a range of different backgrounds including veterinary sciences, medical sciences, biomedical sciences, pharmaceutical sciences, biology, molecular biology, biotechnology, chemistry, biochemistry and bioengineering. Training on the job and working experience can be gained in academia, in laboratories of scientific institutes, in industry and in CROs. Continuous education is a must and can be accomplished by following specialised postgraduate training or continuous education courses in academia and national or international scientific societies. To keep up with progress in science and regulations governing drug development, attending scientific meetings, exchange of experience with peers and taking on new challenges are essential. Only in this way sufficient experience can be gained in toxicology testing approaches and in the safety profile of a wide range of chemical and biological pharmaceuticals. This experience may help in climbing the scientific or managerial career ladder in industry. Toxicologists who are very specialised in a particular field in toxicology, for example, histopathology, and are an authority in their field can choose for a scientific career starting as a scientist and gradually climbing the ladder based on their achievements. After having accumulated sufficient experience in the management of toxicology projects, toxicologists can also choose for managerial responsibilities with a broader oversight of projects such as that of a nonclinical project leader and early or late development leader or can move to higher positions in management.

4.5   Career Profiles of Toxicologists in Industries Other than Pharmaceutical Industry

There are also career opportunities for toxicologists in other industries than the pharmaceutical industry. Examples are the agrochemical, food, cosmetics and chemical industry. In terms of completeness and thoroughness in the safety assessment of chemicals, toxicology research for agrochemicals is most comparable to that of the pharmaceutical industry. The most important differences are that human testing is not allowed and that the testing strategy is strictly defined and thus less flexible. In the safety assessment of pesticides, there is no possibility to assess the relevance of animal toxicology data to man because of the lack of human test data. The only tools available to assess human relevance are comparative in vitro studies using human cells. In contrast to the pharmaceutical industry, this means that the toxicologist in the pesticides industry is the ultimate safety expert who takes decisions on the human safety of the pesticide under development. This requires a vast experience in the conduct and interpretation of the toxicology studies that have to be performed. Although many studies are similar to those performed to assess the safety of drugs, there are some important differences. In nonclinical drug development, also safety pharmacology studies (assessment of effects on the physiology of critical organs/systems such as the cardiovascular system) and the monitoring of drug concentrations in plasma in all toxicology studies (toxicokinetics) are performed. In pesticide safety testing, toxicity is related to the applied (external) dose rather than to systemic (internal) exposure. When toxicities are observed, such as effects on the endocrine system or carcinogenicity, the mode of action must be investigated and its relevance to man established. This requires a thorough understanding of in vitro and in vivo testing tools that need to be applied. Often this type of research is done in collaboration with specialised contract research organisations. Besides the design, conduct or monitoring, interpretation and reporting of toxicology studies, the toxicologist in the agrochemical industry has to produce a report integrating all the toxicology data of the active ingredient and corresponding formulations and present a risk assessment for pesticide residues in crops and exposure of workers and bystanders to pesticides in the field. The toxicologist has also to defend his/her safety assessment at the regulatory authorities during the pesticide registration process. This is the responsibility of senior toxicologists with often a minimum of 10 years of postgraduate experience in the field. In big agrochemical companies, toxicologists work in teams where the product toxicologist can rely on the knowledge and experience of colleagues who are specialised in various fields in toxicology such as reproductive toxicology, histopathology, carcinogenicity and metabolism and pharmacokinetics. Most of the time, young toxicologists start in a speciality close to their training and/or topic of their PhD thesis and gradually acquire also experience in other specialities through teamwork and switching responsibilities. As in the pharmaceutical industry, the toxicologist can choose between a scientific and a managerial career ladder. The best way to acquire experience in a sub-speciality of toxicology is to start working in the laboratory to get a feel for the challenges that must be overcome in experimental work and what it takes to produce reliable test results. Also learning to work under good laboratory practices (GLP) is a must. Nowadays, most of the toxicology work on pesticides is delegated to contract research organisations (CROs) and is monitored by the toxicologist of the agrochemical company.

In the food industry, toxicological expertise is necessary on food ingredients, food packaging materials, food additives, food contaminants, food processing methods and genetically modified foods to ensure that no health problems are associated with the consumption of foods. Often a lot of data can be obtained from other sources, but there are circumstances where new safety research is required such as in the case of the use of new food additives or processing methods. The monitoring and risk assessment of food contaminants such as pesticides, heavy metals, endocrine disruptors and persistent industrial contaminants are important responsibilities of the toxicologist in the food industry. For the safety assessment of genetically modified foods, toxicology data packages are produced that are more tailored towards the specific needs for this type of foods. In such assessment, many other factors are considered, such as characterisation of the introduced DNA, characterisation of the gene insertion site and characterisation of the gene product and its mode of action, digestibility, allergenicity and toxicity. Data on the whole food such as composition, nutritive value and subchronic toxicity using the concept of substantial equivalence are also part of the safety testing package. As is the case with the pesticide and pharmaceutical industry, most of the toxicology tests to be done in the food industry are nowadays performed at CROs. Young scientists with a strong background in food science such as postgraduates and PhDs in bioengineering and with the ambition to specialise in food safety assessment are good candidates to join the food industry.

In the cosmetics industry, the safety assessment of cosmetic preparations and ingredients has undergone a specific evolution in the EU. Animal testing in the safety assessment of cosmetics has been banned for several years now, and new ways to evaluate the safety of products had to be explored. Toxicology testing of cosmetics has therefore moved away from traditional in vivo testing towards animal-free testing using a battery of in vitro and ex vivo tools complemented with in silico assessments and, in some cases, with testing in human volunteers (e.g. skin patch tests for the testing of skin sensitisation). Examples of in vitro/ex vivo test methods include skin permeability testing using human skin samples, skin irritation and corrosion, skin sensitisation, eye irritation and corrosion, phototoxicity, genotoxicity and skin toxicity. Toxicologists working in the cosmetics industry have to be experts in the application of animal-free testing methods and need to have a thorough experience in the conduct and interpretation of these tests in terms of human safety. Also, a good knowledge of the toxicology of raw materials and formulation aides is essential in the safety evaluation of cosmetic products. Toxicologists in the cosmetics industry need also to be able to prepare the dossiers for submission to the authorities in accordance with EU regulations. Specific challenges are the safety assessment of nanoparticles and packaging requirements. Careers of toxicologists in the cosmetics industry are comparable to those of the pharmaceutical and food industry.

In the chemical industry, there are several career opportunities for toxicologists. To put chemicals on the EU market, industry must comply with the REACH regulations. Registration, Evaluation, Authorisation and Restriction of Chemicals (REACH 2022) requires that, according to the tonnage that is planned to be placed annually on the EU market, a number of toxicology tests have to be conducted to assess human safety. These tests range from a basic package of toxicology tests such as acute toxicity, skin and eye irritation, skin sensitisation and genotoxicity up to a complete set of tests including short- and long-term toxicity, reproductive toxicity, embryo-foetal toxicity and carcinogenicity. These tests must be performed according to GLP and OECD test guidelines as is the case with pesticides and biocides. The toxicologist in the chemical industry designs the studies to be conducted within the context of chemical safety regulations and most of the time places and monitors these tests at CROs. The results of these studies are used to comply with EU regulations on the classification, labelling and packaging (CLP) of chemical substances and chemical products. In addition to the toxicology data, typical elements of a REACH chemical safety report are the risk assessment of chemical manufacturing processes, the use by professionals and the use by the general population. It also involves the identification of maximum exposure levels for workers and the general population based on all existing toxicology, epidemiology and occupational medicine data. A REACH dossier is reviewed by the European Chemicals Agency (ECHA 2022) and also by EU member states which requires the toxicologist to defend the dossier at the level of regulatory authorities. A toxicologist in the chemical industry is also called upon for hazard communication to the workers in manufacturing facilities in collaboration with occupational medicine services when new manufacturing processes are introduced or when new data have become available on chemicals used in manufacturing. As toxicology studies have to be designed, placed and monitored in CROs, a good start of a toxicology career in the chemical industry is to take on responsibilities in toxicological testing either in laboratories of academia, scientific institutes, the chemical industry or at CROs and then move to jobs with more product and project responsibilities. Careers of toxicologists in the chemical industry are comparable to those of the agrochemical industry and allow also to move to positions with more oversight such as product stewardship and regulatory affairs.

4.6   Career Profiles of Toxicologists in Regulatory Organisations

National and international regulatory organisations have responsibilities in product safety assessment. According to the sector considered, this can be medicines, foods, cosmetics, pesticides, biocides or chemicals. The type of work of a toxicologist in these organisations may vary from experimental work in national and international scientific institutes connected to these organisations to the evaluation of toxicology data submitted by industry within a regulatory context. Another important task of a toxicologist in regulatory organisations is to help in the development and implementation of testing guidelines and product safety regulations. Often toxicologists active at the national level represent their country in product safety programmes of international organisations. Examples of regulatory organisations in the EU are the European Medicines Agency (EMA 2022), the European Food Safety Authority (EFSA 2022) and the European Chemicals Agency (ECHA 2022). Examples of international non-regulatory organisations providing guidance on product safety assessment to national and international regulatory authorities are the Organisation for Economic Co-operation and Development (OECD 2022), the International Council for Harmonisation of Technical Requirements for Pharmaceuticals for Human Use (ICH 2022), the Joint FAO/WHO Meeting on Pesticide Residues (JMPR 2022), the Joint FAO/WHO Expert Committee on Food Additives (JECFA 2022) and the International Agency for Research on Cancer (IARC 2022). The toxicologist of a national regulatory agency brings the expertise from the national to the international level and gets engaged in the evaluation of toxicology data with their colleagues from other countries to come to a common position. To be efficient in such interactions, a strong background in product safety evaluation is required combined with a thorough understanding of the regulatory context. As it is impossible to have experience in every aspect of toxicology from the beginning, most of the young toxicologists in national authorities start in a sub-speciality of toxicology often close to their postgraduate training and/or PhD topic and further develop their expertise through evaluation of dossiers and interaction with peers of other countries. Toxicologists working at the level of international organisations are most of the time senior scientists with a past career at the national level and who are responsible for the coordination of international projects in close collaboration with their peers at the national level. Career opportunities in regulatory authorities may differ among countries but can be scientific as well as regulatory. Scientific career ladders can be offered in the scientific institutes of national authorities and start from scientist up to head of department and often follow academic career profiles with possibilities to teach at universities. A regulatory career is more focussed on the development and implementation of regulations relating to product safety and is comparable to administrative career profiles which vary from country to country.

4.7 Career Profiles of Toxicologists in Contract Research Organisations

Since most of the experimental work is now delegated by industry and some authorities to contract research organisations (CROs), they have become the places with most experience in the conduct of toxicology studies. Various types of studies are performed by CROs and they can range from routine standard regulatory toxicology tests to investigative studies comprising targeted in vitro and in vivo studies using specialised animal models such as transgenic mice. The big advantage of these laboratories is that they have a high study throughput of a great variety of tests, which allows them not only to gain a lot of experience in the conduct of these tests but also to build extensive databases of historical control data which are very important for the reliable interpretation of toxicology data and to manage genetic drifts in laboratory animals. Because of the high throughput of standard studies, it is also more cost-effective to apply good laboratory practices (GLP) to its fullest extent. According to the type of work, CROs can be subdivided into toxicology, bioanalytical and pharmacokinetic (ADME), pharmacologic (pharmacologic screening and safety pharmacology) and investigative toxicology laboratories. CROs in toxicology also offer regulatory support to their clients besides toxicology testing. This can go as far as to the compiling and submission of regulatory dossiers to national and international authorities.

After having finished university postgraduate training and/or a PhD, the CRO is a good working environment to pick up practical experience and acquire new expertise by additional training not only in the design and conduct of toxicology studies (e.g. animal laboratory science, bioanalysis, pharmacokinetics, clinical pathology, histopathology, reproductive toxicology, embryo-foetal development toxicology, early postnatal development toxicology, juvenile development toxicology, genetic toxicology, in vitro toxicology) but also in the reporting of these studies according to regulatory guidelines and in the management of multidisciplinary study teams as a study director or project manager. As CROs provide services in the compilation of regulatory dossiers for medicines, pesticides and chemicals, experience in regulatory toxicology can be acquired as well. Important for CROs is also effective client support from the agreement on the quotation for a study up to the finalisation of the study report. It is thus possible to accumulate experience in different aspects of toxicology including the interpretation and integration of toxicology data and risk assessment. Career opportunities for toxicologists exist within the CRO, starting from laboratory test specialist to study director/regulatory toxicologist, senior scientist, group leader, technical section head, head of department and even director. A versatile career at a CRO is also very attractive for toxicologists as it offers opportunities to prepare for a further career in the chemical, agrochemical and pharmaceutical industry.

4.8 Career Profiles of Toxicologists in Consulting Companies

There are many companies who don't have a toxicologist to take care of the safety testing and regulatory compliance of their products. If they want to bring new products to the marketplace or want to ensure continued product registration, they have to rely on the support of consulting companies that are specialised in the regulatory environment of their clients. Toxicology consultants are then given the mandate to identify, design, commission and monitor the studies that are needed to ensure regulatory compliance. They also take care of the interpretation and integration of the toxicology data, perform the risk assessment and compile the registration dossiers for the relevant regulatory authorities. Most consulting companies provide toxicological and regulatory expertise to specific industry sectors such as pharmaceuticals, agrochemicals, foods, cosmetics and chemicals. Toxicologists who are employed by consulting companies are most of the time senior scientists who acquired experience in toxicology either in academia, national and international authorities, scientific institutes or industry. Also junior scientists with a biomedical background can be employed by consulting companies. Most of the time, they get involved in the compilation of toxicology data for regulatory dossiers (e.g. IUCLID database) and gradually acquire more insight and expertise in toxicology through training on the job. As most consulting companies have no laboratories (apart from toxicology CROs) and as experience in the conduct of laboratory tests and the interpretation of toxicology data is an asset, it is best to start a career elsewhere before joining consulting companies. Career ladders in large consultancy organisations may vary but are most of the time comparable to those in industry and scientific institutes.

4.9   Certification

For a successful career in toxicology, it is important to be able to demonstrate that you are qualified for the job and that you are recognised by peers as an experienced toxicologist. This can be done by publishing work in the scientific literature and actively participating in international scientific meetings, which is essential for a career in academia. For toxicologists employed in other sectors than academia (industry, consulting, CROs, regulatory authorities), publication of scientific work is not obvious because of reasons of confidentiality, proprietary rights and commercial sensitivity of data. In such case, it is possible to apply for a certification as a professional and qualified toxicologist. Certification enhances credibility in consulting, legal testimony, defence of toxicology dossiers at national and international authorities and application for a position in the private sector. It provides a worldwide recognised standard for competence and current knowledge in toxicology. Here we describe three certification systems: the European Register of Toxicologists (ERT) in Europe, Diplomate American Board of Toxicology (DABT) and Fellow of the Academy of Toxicological Sciences (FATS) in the United States.

ERT
ERT certification is organised by the Federation of European Toxicologists and Societies of Toxicology (EUROTOX 2022) and has been established in 1994. It constitutes a register of toxicologists who excel by high standards of education,

skills, experience and professional standing. The intention of ERT certification is to foster competence in practice and science and to provide to the public an authoritative source of information on toxicological competencies. Individuals who apply for registration and are found to comply with the certification requirements defined by EUROTOX and by the national society of toxicology where the application is filed are qualified to use the title "ERT" (European Registered Toxicologist) with their name.

Registration is performed in two steps. First, the candidate applies for ERT at the registration board of the national society of toxicology. This board evaluates the application according to a process described in the ERT Guidelines for Registration and admits successful applicants to the national register. Second, upon request of the national register, EUROTOX registers these individuals in the EUROTOX ERT register and issues a certificate as European Registered Toxicologist (ERT).

Requirements for registration are (1) an academic degree (e.g. BSc, MSc, MD, DVM, PhD or equivalent); (2) basic competence in the essential areas of toxicology through attendance of appropriate courses and recognised qualifications, or by demonstration of specific practical experience and on-the-job training; (3) at least 5 years of relevant toxicological experience; (4) documentation of the practical experience, evidenced by published works, confidential reports or assessments; and (5) current professional engagement in the practice of toxicology.

Certification is granted for a period of 5 years. After this period, the candidate must apply for recertification with submission of a new dossier containing: (1) updated CV; (2) description of professional activities; (3) certificates of continued education; (4) attendance of scientific meetings, membership of scientific societies and membership of scientific advisory bodies; and (5) publications in the scientific literature.

DABT

Certification as Diplomate American Board of Toxicology (DABT) is organised by the American Board of Toxicology (ABT 2022). ABT was established in Washington, DC, in 1979 and the first exam for certification was given in 1980. The vision of ABT is to establish a globally recognised credential in toxicology representative of competency and commitment to human health and environmental sciences. Its mission is to identify, maintain and evolve a standard for professional competency in the field of toxicology.

Certification is performed in two steps. First, eligibility is assessed based on education and experience. Eligibility is accepted for a doctoral degree in an appropriate scientific field and at least 3 years of full-time experience in toxicology, or a master's degree in an appropriate field and at least 7 years of full-time postbaccalaureate experience in toxicology or a bachelor's degree in an appropriate field and at least 10 years of full-time experience in toxicology. In each case, the applicant must have active involvement in the practice of toxicology within the year immediately prior to application. Second, once eligibility is accepted, the applicant is invited to take an exam. Examination is based on a practice analysis study of the knowledge required for general toxicology and consists of 200 questions. The disciplines in toxicology considered are (1) design, execution and interpretation of toxicology studies, (2) descriptive toxicology (environmental, clinical, nonclinical, forensic), (3) mechanistic toxicology, (4) risk assessment (hazard identification, exposure assessment, dose response assessment, risk characterisation and management), and (5) applied toxicology (public, environmental and occupational health). Candidates who pass the exam successfully receive DABT certification for a period of 5 years. After this period, diplomates can apply for recertification. To be eligible for recertification, proof must be delivered of active practice (employment as a toxicologist), continuing education (100 credits over a 5-year period) and maintenance of expert knowledge.

FATS

Certification as a Fellow of the Academy of Toxicological Sciences (FATS) has been organised by the Academy of Toxicological Sciences (ATS 2022) in the United States since 1981. The vision of ATS is to be recognised as the leading international organisation that certifies toxicologists by peer review of education, professional experience, leadership, demonstrated achievement and scientific expertise. Its mission is to establish a process by which practicing toxicologists are certified based on peer review of the following focus areas: (1) education, both formal and continuing; (2) professional practice of toxicology as evidenced by scholarly publications and non-published technical reports and integrated analyses, editorial services to scientific journals, participation on external and internal toxicology-related committees, professional society membership(s), scientific presentations, attendance of scientific meetings and teaching responsibilities; and (3) professional recognition reflected by career advancement, elected and/or appointed service with national and international professional/ technical committees and review bodies, invited presentations and professional honours and awards.

ATS not only certifies toxicologists by peer review of their professional achievement but also imposes a code of ethics that assures that ATS Fellows, who participate in research and testing, are involved in the determination of hazard, risk and risk-benefit, and who make regulatory decisions that impact public health and the environment, exercise sound scientific judgment, free of bias and based on the scientific data.

4.10 Conclusion

Over the last decades, the consciousness about good health and the awareness of the impact of human activities on the environment has increased worldwide. As a result, the role of toxicology in understanding the potential harmful effects of chemical substances and products on living organisms and in ensuring that they are safe for human use has become increasingly important. This has contributed to today's wide and growing variety of career opportunities in toxicology. As detailed in this chapter, toxicologists are employed in various industry sectors such as pharmaceuticals, foods, chemicals, pesticides, biocides and cosmetics but can also pursue a career in contract research organisations, regulatory authorities and consulting companies. They can also choose for a career in academia, where besides teaching, they have an important role to play in basic research on molecular, biochemical and cellular processes leading to harmful effects in living organisms. Whatever option chosen, careers in toxicology require a strong scientific basis in the biomedical field and continuous training to be kept abreast of the progress in science but also to further expand expertise in toxicology. For a successful career in toxicology, good problem-solving skills, flexibility, continuous learning, an open mind for new ideas, team spirit, good communication skills and leadership are essential. In summary, toxicology is an exciting multidisciplinary science providing a plethora of interesting career possibilities that contribute to the well-being of current and future generations.

Acknowledgements The authors are grateful for the advice given by Prof. Dr. Dominique Lison (UCLouvain), Prof. Dr. Peter Hoet (KULeuven), Prof. Dr. Steven Van Cruchten (UAntwerpen), Prof. Dr. Frank Martens (UAntwerpen), Prof. Dr. Jana Asselman (UGent), Prof. Dr. Joery De Kock (VUB), Dr. Birgit Peter (Charles River Laboratories), Dr. An Van Rompay (Penman Consulting), Dr. Erik Van Miert (Sciensano) and Dr. Steven Verberckmoes (Umicore).

References

ABT (2022). https://www.abtox.org
ATS (2022). https://acadtoxsci.org
ECHA (2022). https://echa.europa.eu
EFSA (2022). https://www.efsa.europa.eu
EMA (2022). https://www.ema.europa.eu
EUROTOX (2022). https://www.eurotox.com/ert
IARC (2022). https://www.iarc.who.int
ICH (2022). https://www.ich.org
JECFA (2022). https://www.fao.org/food-safety/scientific-advice/jecfa
JMPR (2022). https://www.who.int/groups/joint-fao-who-meeting-on-pesticide-residues-(jmpr)
OECD (2022). https://www.oecd.org
REACH (2022). https://ec.europa.eu/growth/sectors/chemicals/reach
SOT (2022). https://www.toxicology.org/

Chapter 5
Job Possibilities in Clinical Research

Benedikt Van Nieuwenhove

Abstract Clinical research is a vital component when developing new therapies for patients as it provides evidence that they are safe and effective. The complexity and regulatory requirements for clinical trials explain why there is a multitude of stakeholders involved and why there are many job opportunities in this field.

This chapter provides an overview of what clinical research is, the different types of studies, and what activities are needed to complete a clinical trial. An overview of stakeholders is provided and for each stakeholder what kind of positions exist. The positions are explained, and the required skills are discussed. Finally, guidance on how to start a career in clinical research is provided.

5.1 Introduction

In this chapter, we are going to zoom in on the clinical development part of drug development: we will be introducing the fascinating world of clinical research and the wide range of job possibilities it offers. The reason why clinical research is fascinating is because it allows everyone involved in a clinical trial to directly contribute to developing new or better therapies for patients. All other aspects of drug development (such as drug discovery, nonclinical development, medical affairs, etc.) are exciting too; however, the difference with clinical development is that you are researching the new drug or product on a human being. Unless you work as a healthcare professional, you will never get closer to a patient than here!

Plus, it even gets better—we mentioned drug development above, but clinical research is not only done in this area: it is also much needed when developing new medical devices (such as pacemakers or health apps), functional food, or in vitro diagnostics. There is even clinical research where no product is involved (e.g., a study comparing two surgical procedures or epidemiological studies). Finally, it is

B. Van Nieuwenhove (✉)
European Centre for Clinical Research Training, Brussels, Belgium
e-mail: Benedikt@eccrt.com

© The Author(s), under exclusive license to Springer Nature Switzerland AG 2023
J. R. Thomas et al. (eds.), *Career Options in the Pharmaceutical and Biomedical Industry*, https://doi.org/10.1007/978-3-031-14911-5_5

worth mentioning that there is also clinical research done with veterinary medicines in animals. This chapter is focusing on clinical research in human beings though.

What is clinical research then? In a clinical trial or study, research on human beings is performed to see if a (new) compound or product is safe and to demonstrate that it is effective (i.e., that it treats the disease for which it is intended). In clinical research with medicinal products, there are typically four phases. *Phase I studies are the studies* where the compound is administrated for the first time to a human being: healthy volunteers are used to test the new compound (for some therapeutic indications, *phase I studies* are done directly in patients). Healthy volunteers are used because the aim is to get the first indication about how safe the compound is and what the effect is on the health of an otherwise healthy person. The very first phase I studies are called "first-in-man studies," but there are multiple phase I studies done before moving to the next phase: there are also studies done to determine the pharmacokinetic profile and the pharmacodynamic activity. Phase I studies are carried out in clinical pharmacology units (CPUs). These can either be academic or private (belonging to a pharma company or a contract research organization or CRO). These studies are also used to determine the dosing of the compound to be used in the next phases of development.

Before phase I studies, there are another type of studies (*phase 0 studies*), where very small amounts of the test drug are administered to a very small group of healthy volunteers or patients. It allows to rapidly screen several potential drugs and to be able to start phase I studies in a more optimal way.

When the phase I studies have successfully been completed, the compound can move to the next stage, *phase II*. This is where the product gets tested for the first time in a population that suffers from the disease for which the product is intended. They are done in a small group of patients and are very selective on who can participate: only patients that suffer from that specific disease but are otherwise healthy. If not, then the results of the safety and efficacy assessments of the new compound could be influenced by other diseases (and their treatment) the participant is suffering from and cause bias. The main objective of phase II studies is to study the safety and continue to determine the optimal dosing. However, you will also start looking how effective the new drug is in treating the disease. This is why these studies are also referred to as proof-of-concept (POC) studies, as it gives a first indication that the compound will work for its intended use.

When the results of the phase II studies are positive, the compound moves to the next stage: *phase III trials* or confirmatory trials. Here the number of patients will be much larger, and the selection of study participants will be less strict, as you precisely want to study the behavior of the new compound in a population that is as close as possible to the patients in the "real world": having other diseases or taking other medication, etc. In addition to safety, the main goal of the phase III studies is to prove the efficacy of the product.

When this efficacy is demonstrated, the developer of the drug can compile a dossier to submit the drug candidate to obtain a marketing authorization, which is granted by a regional (such as the FDA in the USA or EMA in the EU) or national health authority. During the assessment of the marketing authorization application, the regulatory authorities will review all data available from discovery up and until phase III trials.

After obtaining the authorization to market the new drug, the clinical research is not finished: at that time, the post-approval research or post-marketing surveillance studies (PMS) or *phase IV studies* are done. The aim of these studies is to study the new drug in a real-world setting, to compare it with other existing drugs, and to evaluate long-term safety and efficacy.

Clinical research is, after atomic energy, the most regulated industry: this is not a surprise as that research is done with human beings and the participants enrolled in clinical studies need maximal protection. Ensuring that the rights, health, well-being, and privacy of study participants are protected is paramount. Moreover, data collected from study participants should only be done in compliance with data protection regulations. Over the last 60 years, authorities and medical associations have given guidance and developed a regulatory framework to ensure this. The International Council for Harmonisation of Technical Requirements for Pharmaceuticals for Human Use (ICH; www.ich.org) has established a large number of guidance documents, of which many have been adopted into legislation. The most important one for clinical research is the ICH E6 Guideline: Good Clinical Practice. This guideline forms the basis for carrying out clinical research.

The global clinical trials market size was estimated by Grand View Research (https://www.grandviewresearch.com/) at USD 44.3 billion in 2020 and is expected to expand at a compound annual growth rate (CAGR) of 5.7% from 2021 to 2028. However, the market growth was hindered in 2020 because of the COVID-19 pandemic. Nevertheless, the future seems promising for the market due to factors such as globalization of clinical trials, rapid technological evolution, and increasing demand for CROs to conduct research activities. The increasing prevalence of chronic disease and the growing demand for clinical trials in developing countries are also fueling this market's growth. The market is also driven by a rising number of biologics, the need for personalized medicines and orphan drugs, and demand for advanced technologies (Fig. 5.1).

The number of studies being carried out is vast. At the time of writing this book, there are over 400,000 clinical studies entered in the clinical trials database of the American authorities (NIH, clinicaltrials.gov) (Fig. 5.2):

The above introduction makes it clear that a lot of clinical research is being done, which creates a lot of job opportunities in this area: not only within the pharmaceutical industry but also in the investigational sites, regulatory authorities, and the multitude of providers (CROs) delivering clinical research services.

5.2 Life Cycle of a Clinical Trial

To understand the different job possibilities in clinical research, we will first briefly describe how a clinical trial is carried out and who is involved.

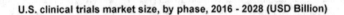

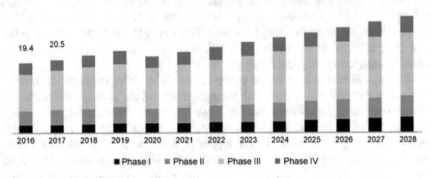

Fig. 5.1 Clinical trial market size in the USA

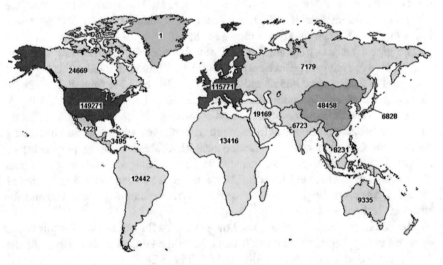

Fig. 5.2 Extract from the clinical trial database. Source: https://ClinicalTrials.gov

As mentioned before, a clinical trial is a study performed on a number of participants (human beings), where researchers want to confirm their research hypothesis: for example, they want to know how a drug works in a specific population or investigate in which subpopulation a specific side effect occurs.

Many stakeholders are involved in carrying out a clinical trial: first of all, there is the study participant (either a healthy volunteer or a patient), there is the investigator (the physician carrying out the research), and his team in the hospital or private practice (study coordinators, study nurses, data managers, etc.). There is also the sponsor: this is the party that takes responsibility over the execution of the study according to the rules (e.g., good clinical practice). This can be a

Fig. 5.3 Life cycle of a clinical trial

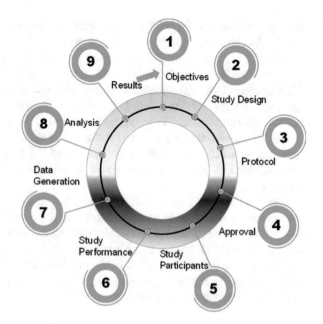

(bio)pharmaceutical or medical device company, but it can also be an academic institution or a nonprofit organization (such as the EORTC, the European Organisation for Research and Treatment of Cancer: https://www.eortc.org/). The sponsor is not always carrying out all trial-related activities themselves: they often use service companies or vendors that work for them. This can be contract research organizations (CROs), central laboratories, courier services, or reading centers, to name just a few. Last but not least, there are also the ethics committees and regulatory authorities that review the study and grant approval to start the trial if all conditions are met. During the trial, they continuously look whether the trial is conducted in accordance with the regulations while respecting the participants' safety, well-being, and rights. The regulatory authorities also review the data resulting from the study at the time an application for a marketing authorization is submitted.

The life cycle of a clinical trial (see Fig. 5.3) starts with defining what the goal of the study is. The sponsor defines the objectives of the trial and describes the primary (and secondary) outcomes to be investigated (e.g., a study on the mortality of the patient group suffering from heart failure with different types of treatment). With these objectives in mind, a study design is prepared: this is a high-level description of what will happen in the study (e.g., what type of patients, what dose of the drug will be used, how long the participants will be treated, etc.).

With the study design, the process of looking how feasible the study starts. Here the sponsor reaches out to the other stakeholders (such as key opinion leaders and authorities) and finds out if the study is justified and realistic (e.g., do those patients with this profile exist). In parallel to that, the full study protocol is prepared. The study protocol is like the manual of the study, describing in detail how the study is going to be carried out and how the data generated from it are going to be analyzed.

Once the study protocol is finalized and the investigational sites that will participate are identified, the process for submitting the clinical trial for approval starts (CTA or clinical trial application). A clinical trial is always reviewed and needs to be approved by an ethics committee. Depending on the type of trial, it is also required that the regulatory authorities grant their approval before the trial can start.

Once approved, the trial can start and study medication (IMP or investigational medicinal product) is delivered to the sites, and the investigators start recruiting study participants after they have agreed to participate (by signing the informed consent).

Once in the study, the participants start the study treatment and undergo all assessments as described in the protocol. From that moment onward, study data is generated and recorded in a database. Verification and validation of the data needs to take place to make sure their quality is in accordance with applicable standards. Once all data is collected and validated in the database, the analysis can start and that analysis results in a clinical study report, which ideally proves the objectives and study hypothesis put forward initially.

5.3 Job Opportunities in Clinical Research

The high number of stakeholders and the level of regulation of clinical research explain its complexity and are the reason why there are so many positions involved. There are well over 50 different positions in this area, ranging from general positions to highly specialized roles, which need a lot of expertise.

These positions do not only exist in a pharmaceutical company. We see the same positions in the medical device industry and in the different types of vendor companies (all together referred to as "the industry"). There are also various positions in the investigational sites as well as in ethics committees and regulatory authorities.

We will be focusing on "starter" positions that are suitable for new graduates and people with limited to no experience.

5.3.1 Positions in Investigational Sites

Depending on your diploma (e.g., as an investigator, you need to be a physician or dentist), you can work in a hospital and coordinate clinical trials there. The most common function is called a "study coordinator." The study coordinator helps the investigator with the organization of the study in the hospital: this starts with making sure that study participants are selected properly (i.e., that they fulfill the study selection criteria), but also making sure that all study assessments are done in accordance with the protocol and with the highest quality standards while protecting the health and well-being of the study participants. The advantage of this position is that you are working directly with study participants which can be very rewarding. As a study coordinator, you work in a hospital (or private practice) mostly in one therapeutic indication, where you work on studies from different sponsors and with different products. This is the main difference with a Clinical Research Associate (CRA) role described below. A CRA covers one (or more) studies and goes to all hospitals participating in a country organized by one (or more) sponsor.

5.3.2 Positions in Ethics Committees and Regulatory Authorities

Ethics committees are in general part of a hospital. They are composed of several members (mostly physicians, but also laypersons, legal representatives, patient representatives, etc.). It is not so common that you see vacancies there for new graduates.

This is different for the regulatory authorities: there are national health authorities, such as the Belgian FAMHP (https://www.famhp.be/en), as well as regional authorities, such as the European Medicines Agency or EMA (https://www.ema.europa.eu/en). A lot of scientists work there as assessors or evaluators for all aspects of drug development, including clinical trial applications, scientific advice, carrying out inspections, and ultimately marketing authorization.

5.3.3 Positions in the Industry

As it becomes clear when reading this book, there are a lot of departments within a pharma company, and most of these departments have tight connections with each other.

The clinical research part or clinical development is part of the R&D group, as it covers the "D" side. This applies to clinical trials up to phase III. Once marketing authorization has been obtained, the further research (phase IV) is often carried out by different groups such as medical affairs, real-world evidence, etc.

Although it is difficult to generalize, as a lot depends on the nature and size of a company, the clinical development group consists generally of four departments: medical or scientific writing, study start-up, clinical operations or project management, and biometrics.

The medical writing group consists of scientists that develop the study synopsis, protocols, informed consent, and clinical study reports and write medical or scientific publications. The position of medical writer does require scientific knowledge, good English writing skills, and experience in the relevant therapeutic area. Quite often PhD graduates can find a role here.

The study start-up groups carry out the feasibility of a trial and selection of the investigational sites participating and prepare for getting approval to start the study. Functions here include "study start-up specialist" and require sound knowledge of the regulatory requirements as well as a good understanding of the epidemiology of the disease studied. Depending on the size of the organization, this department can be integrated in the clinical operations group.

The clinical operations and project management team carry out the study, with positions such as Clinical Research Associates (CRAs), Clinical Trial Assistants (CTAs), and Clinical Project Managers (CPMs).

The CRA is the most common function. Although a CRA is a good starting position, vacancies often require experience. A CRA acts as the link between the sponsor/CRO and the investigational sites: they make sure that the sites carry out the study as described in the protocol and that the rules are respected. The CRA visits the hospitals/investigational sites to make sure that the data generated from the study participant is adequately collected, is of high quality, and guides the site staff with the execution of the trial. Nowadays, with the increased digitalization of clinical research, a lot of these activities can be carried out remotely, but still, the relationships with the site remain very important (hence why almost all vacancies will also require that you speak the local language). More and more, there is also a link between the position of CRA and Medical Science Liaison (MSL) in the medical affairs department. In summary, as a CRA, you need a scientific background, good organizational skills, sense for detail, and strong communication skills.

Clinical Trial Assistants (CTAs) are the back-office support for the CRA and CPM. The CTA is responsible for maintaining the clinical trial documentation in the Trial Master File (TMF), but nowadays, this is often kept electronically. In clinical studies, everything needs to be documented, to demonstrate that the study has been conducted properly. The FDA, the American regulatory authority, claims that if something is not written down, it didn't happen. Needless to say, the CTA plays a key role in this. Although you do not need scientific knowledge to start as a CTA, you very often see that recently graduated masters in life sciences begin their career in clinical research for a short period as a CTA, to get familiar with clinical trial execution and the terminology used. It is therefore a good starter position in preparation to become a CRA. For the CTA position, you need strong administrative skills and have sense for details and be very accurate.

A Clinical Project Manager is the person making sure that the clinical trial runs according to plan (i.e., finishes on time, within budget, and with the required quality). The CPM works with the rest of the clinical operations team (CRAs and CTAs), but also cross-functionally (e.g., with the medical writing or biometrics group). The CPM often works internationally and has to be a good people manager and communicator to keep the team aligned and motivated. Although, in theory, you do not need clinical research experience to be a project manager, there are very few vacancies where that experience is not required. Given the complexity and the international scope of clinical trials nowadays, this is not a surprise. A CPM needs to have excellent planning skills and have knowledge of budget management.

The next department involved in clinical trials is the biometrics department. This department consists of the data management group and the statistics group. Data managers are responsible for delivering a clean database with the data collected during a clinical study. This may sound easy, but a lot of activities come along with this: the data manager needs to interact with the investigational sites, with the CRAs, and the CPMs to have the data collected in a systematic and consistent way. In case of inaccuracies or missing information, they reach out to the sites and CRAs to correct and complete the data where needed. Data needs to be coded to have consistent terminology used across countries where the study is carried out. The function of data manager is a typical starter position, as there is often no, or limited, experience required, although having a life science background will be an asset. You need to have appropriate computer skills and a passion for working with data and have a strong sense for accuracy to be successful in this job.

There are many more positions in clinical research, for example, in pharmacovigilance, medical monitoring, quality assurance, clinical supply management, statistics, etc. Most of these positions require a certain degree of specialization and experience and are therefore beyond the scope of this chapter.

5.4 Clinical Research in a Pharma Company Versus in a CRO

Clinical research is not only done in biopharmaceutical companies. Those companies can also use the services of companies that specialize in executing clinical trial-related activities. These companies are called contract research organizations or CROs, sometimes also called clinical research organizations. Pharma companies outsource a clinical trial or parts thereof to these CROs. There has been an increased outsourcing trend by the pharma industry since the 1980s, and this increase is still ongoing. As shown in Fig. 5.4, the market size of the CROs is estimated to grow to over 90 billion USD by 2026.

The CRO market has been growing remarkably and has resulted in a wide range of different types of CRO companies, ranging from very large, full services companies (such as ICON or IQVIA) with 15,000 to 60,000 employees worldwide to very small, niche CRO players with only a handful of employees.

Why do pharma companies outsource their clinical trials to CROs? The main reason for this is that the clinical research part is the most lengthy and expensive part in the development of a new medicine. With the decreasing drug pipelines and increased complexity to develop new therapies (e.g., cell or gene therapy), the pharma industry is under a lot of pressure to maintain their levels of ROI (return on investment) to compensate for the increasing development costs. A solution for

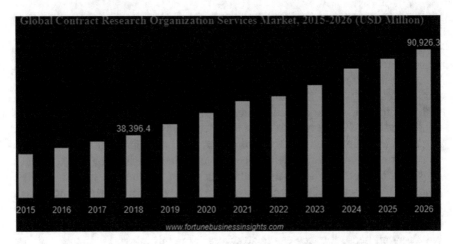

Fig. 5.4 CRO market evolution

this pressure is to outsource the expensive part (the clinical trials) to specialized organizations, who can do it more efficiently and quicker.

5.4.1 Types of Outsourcing

There are CROs for all clinical trial activities: the large CROs can do almost everything (full service), and the smaller ones specialize in either a particular function (e.g., monitoring of a clinical trial), a particular type of trials (e.g., early phase CROs, Phase I Units), or a particular therapeutic indication.

There are many other types of companies that do complementary tasks: central laboratories and reading centers (e.g., that centralize and analyze all blood samples or ECG recordings of all trial participants); clinical supply companies that take care of the packaging, transport, import, and export of study medication; and providers of digital tools used in clinical research, etc.

There are different ways a pharma company can outsource their clinical trials: it can range from outsourcing the full development of a new drug to outsourcing just a single task within a clinical trial:

- Co-development where the CRO is investing in the full development of a new product and only gets compensated if a development milestone has been achieved.
- Full outsourcing: where an entire trial is outsourced to a CRO. The CRO take responsibility of the planning, execution, and reporting of the trial results.
- Functional outsourcing: here a certain function or department will be outsourced (for several trials in the pipeline). For example, a pharma company may decide that all data management activities are outsourced to one or more CROs.

– Insourcing: this is when a pharma company decides to keep trial activities in-house, but "rents" the staff needed for it temporarily from a CRO or in this case also from specialized staffing companies.

It is important to note that despite the outsourcing of a clinical trial, the final responsibility for it remains with the sponsor (the pharma company).

5.4.2 Job Opportunities in a CRO

The same positions as described earlier also exist within a CRO. There are even more job vacancies in CROs than in pharma companies. The main difference is that in a CRO, you might be assigned to several projects from different clients (pharma companies). This allows getting a broader exposure to different types of therapeutic indications and different classes of compounds. The downside is that you "only" provide service and jump from one project to another, without seeing the full picture of the drug development.

CROs tend to hire more junior staff and train them in-house to the required levels of experience. Most clinical research professionals start their career in a CRO.

The insourcing concept deserves special attention: here you will be assigned to a client and work with the client on a project. When the project is over, you are assigned to a new project (eventually from a different client). The advantage is again that you get to know several companies and ways of working in a short period of time. The downside is that you are not part of the staff (the head count) and therefore not involved in all aspects, not really part of the team: often not having access to same level of information and training as the company staff (although a lot of efforts are being made by pharma companies to avoid that).

5.5 Career Development in Clinical Research

Clinical research is in constant evolution. Not only the clinical trial regulations but also in terms of new scientific methodologies that evolve and new technologies that become available and are useful to make clinical research more powerful.

Due to this constant evolution and because of the pressure to perform, companies can seldom afford to hire junior staff members and train them. When you look at clinical research vacancies, the vast majority require experience, sometimes of several years.

This makes it very hard to get these jobs as a young graduate or someone without experience. This is precisely the frustrating part: the industry has a shortage of experienced staff, while a lot of graduates who are talented and motivated cannot find a job because they lack the desired experience.

5.5.1 Required Background

Regardless of whether you have just obtained your master's degree in a life science area, just got your PhD, finished a postdoc, or even had a job before but you want to reorient yourself into clinical research, you will be confronted with the need for experience. Of course, depending on your situation, you might already have some experience which you might want to capitalize on (e.g., research done during your PhD work). It is therefore important that, when you apply for a job, you highlight the relevant experience on your CV and applications. It will distinguish you from other applicants.

It is equally important not to aim too high and to start with something realistic and show ambition to grow.

5.5.2 Clinical Research Competencies

We discussed the starter positions in this chapter. But even for those starter positions, previous experience might be required. As a new graduate, you can apply for these positions, but it remains important to continue to further develop your clinical research competencies and grow your experience to be attractive for the industry.

These competencies are not necessarily the competencies that you have acquired at university. A reference here is the *Clinical Research Competency Framework* that has been developed by the Joint Task Force for Clinical Research Competency (https://mrctcenter.org/clinical-trial-competency/). This was initially developed in 2016 and has been updated in 2020. This framework provides you with the required competencies in eight domains and can be used as a checklist for you to develop yourself.

5.5.3 Ongoing Training and Development

Another way to kick-start your career in clinical research is to do traineeships, where you learn on the job. You can do this on your own, which might be hard given the limited number of traineeship vacancies and lack of mentoring. There is also training organizations such as the European Centre for Clinical Research Training (ECCRT) that have developed starter programs that include traineeships, like the Junior Clinical Researcher STAR Programme at the ECCRT (https://eccrt.com/course_display/junior-clinical-researcher-star-programme/). The advantage of such programs is that they are well structured and provide you with a mentor who will help you tailor the program and traineeships to best fit your interests and talents. They provide all required competencies to start a job and grant a certificate, which opens a lot of doors in the industry.

5.5.4 Where to Look for Vacancies?

There are numerous jobsites, where you can search for clinical research-related jobs. LinkedIn is becoming more and more important as a tool for recruiting talent for companies. It is therefore very important that your LinkedIn profile is up to date and professional. Make use of references and connect with people you know in the industry.

There are specialized recruiting agencies where you can submit your application. They work for the industry in identifying talent, which gives you broad exposure. The downside is that you will only have contact with the actual employer in a later stage and that your application cannot be customized to the need of that employer.

Career fairs can also be very helpful to find out the different possibilities that fit your interest and profile. There you can interact with employers and find out from them what is important to get a job at their organization. This will help you to be better prepared when you apply.

5.6 Conclusion

The area of clinical research is a very exiting one, as it allows life science professionals to apply the latest scientific and technological advancements. It allows to study those advancements for the impact on human beings for the benefit of future patients, which is very rewarding. The number of clinical trials has been increasing systematically over the last decades and has resulted in a wide range of job opportunities. Despite the fact that these jobs require experience, there are possibilities to develop your competencies and acquire experience for you to be successful.

References

www.grandviewresearch.com
Clinicaltrials.gov
Fortunebusinessinsights.com

Chapter 6
How to Get and Develop a Career in a Market Access Role in the Medical Devices' Industry

Vito Palatino

Abstract The medical technology (MedTech) industry includes all the companies that develop, manufacture, and distribute medical devices across the global markets. It is an eminent part of the healthcare sector. It embraces all the medical devices used to simplify the prevention, diagnosis, and treatment of diseases and illnesses. The most known medical technology products are, among others, pacemakers, surgical instruments, imaging instruments, dialysis machines, and implants. The total global medical technology industry's market size is approximating half a trillion US dollars in 2019. Remarkable geography of MedTech industry includes the United States and Western Europe. However, industry outlook proves that Asia and first China are about to play a more notable role in the years to come. Therefore, MedTech companies are playing a critical role in providing medical innovations and satisfying the needs of welfare across the world. However, with limited healthcare budgets and increasing populations, there has been growing pressure on governments, meaning that all medical innovations may find restrictions and major barriers for entry into a specific market. Thus, getting a quick and persistent access to the market has strategically become more important than ever, and its contribution to a company's success is critical. Considering that, all the medical devices' companies, who are willing to successfully launch a new medical technology, should invest their efforts in removing the entry barriers to the market by demonstrating their value. That is the pivotal role of the market access. It is a multi-skills function that requires a strong payer, procurement and policy maker processes knowledge, and business acumen and project management abilities, combined with great communication and negotiation skills.

V. Palatino (✉)
ConvaTec Italia, Rome, Italy

© The Author(s), under exclusive license to Springer Nature Switzerland AG 2023
J. R. Thomas et al. (eds.), *Career Options in the Pharmaceutical and Biomedical Industry*, https://doi.org/10.1007/978-3-031-14911-5_6

6.1   Introduction

In all the healthcare systems around the world, the economic resources are scarce, and the decision-makers are always focused on how to spend them in the most convenient way. The main question every healthcare system must answer, when someone is trying to bring a new medical technology into a market, is: *is it worth it?* However, before considering just the cost control, any government should invest their efforts in finding out how and why purchasing a medical technology and treatments will benefit the healthcare system needs and what are the most valuable solutions for their patients. In that kind of environment, it is not taken for granted that any new medical technology might be launched, adopted, and successfully sold without any effort. Therefore, to effectively introduce a new medical technology in the business and effectively navigate the process, companies must understand the correct local and national market access routes and key stakeholders' expectations and needs, along with the regulatory processes and documentation necessary. This would help to benefit all parties in the healthcare system, including providers, payers, and patients. In a scenario like that, a market access professional can help the firm in accelerating the adoption journey. Being able to effectively demonstrate how a new device will benefit everyone involved is the fastest way to get access to the market and to gain a prompt and consistent adoption of the technology. When setting out to market a medical device, each firm is probably tempted to rely just on sales and marketing department's skills of negotiation and persuasion to get its device into each national health system; but that is not enough, and it is probably the most unsuccessful strategy. *Market access* is the term that encompasses all the business and market requirements that will help to accelerate a medical device's admission into a healthcare system. Among those qualifications, there are health economics evaluation and value dossiers' editing. The aim of market access is to prepare the market and payers in accepting and adopting their technologies and to ensure that all possible barriers are eradicated and the reimbursement price is the most appropriate for the value of the technology.

Thus, this chapter will help you to understand more about that strategic role, what you need to get it, and what will be further room of progression in your career ladder. All the above will be presented in more detail in Sects. 6.2–6.4. After that overview, career perspectives and how taking properly job opportunities in a market access role will be discussed in Sects. 6.5 and 6.6. The chapter ends with some closing remarks (Sect. 6.7) and a bibliography for further reading.

6.2   The Healthcare Market: A Brief Overview

The World Health Organization (WHO) stated in 1998 *"the healthcare sector consists of organized public and private health services (form surgery to health promotion programs to dentistry), the policies and activities of health departments and ministries, health related non-government organizations and community groups, and professional associations.*" Thus, the healthcare fundamental meaning represents every aspect linked to services and devices for taking care of our health. It is not simple defining healthcare with a single word. A broader healthcare outlook considers all goods, services, procurement, and payment processes for achieving and maintaining people's health. It includes, but is not limited to, physician offices, hospitals, labs, radiology centers, physical therapy offices, pharmaceutical and MedTech companies, pharmacies, health insurance companies, group purchasing organizations, pharmacy benefit managers (PBM), corporate healthcare systems, and combinations of insurance-PBM-pharmacy and much more.

Anyone who has worked in the healthcare industry knows that it moves and evolves in a continuous state of limited economic resources; the reasons why it happens depend on:

- *The increase in population's aging and the growing chronic diseases which are raising dramatically the welfare demand, the spending rate, and the request for healthcare solutions*
- *The new health technologies that have a higher price than the standard of care (SoC) but allow the treatment of more disease conditions otherwise not treatable*
- *The slight expansion of each government budget for healthcare that is not enough to satisfy the welfare demand*

A few distinct economical features and elements drive healthcare markets.

- *The governments' involvement in that business sector is rampant. So, policy makers and public payers are playing a crucial role in deciding what technology and healthcare solutions to purchase and how much to pay for them.*
- *The elasticity of healthcare demand (i.e., how much the demand varies as the price increases) depends on several factors as availability of substitute goods, time period, patients' income, who pays, and necessity. For example, insulin is one of the most inelastic goods as whatever the price is, its demand won't change as it is a lifesaving drug. That aspect is a key element of evaluation during the price negotiation process with the governments.*
- *Consumers and manufacturers face inherent uncertainties regarding needs, outcomes, and the costs of services as they do not have the equal amount and quality of information in their hands (i.e., asymmetric information).*
- *The entry barriers and the access to the market of a new healthcare solution depend on stakeholders' engagement, professional licensure, regulation, intellectual property protections, specialized expertise, research and development costs, and natural economies of scale.*

The healthcare market should be considered as a constellation of business industries that provide medical services, manufacture medical equipment or drugs, provide medical insurance, or otherwise facilitate the supplying of healthcare to patients. The healthcare market is segmented by type into *healthcare services, pharmaceutical drugs, medical equipment, biologics,* and *veterinary healthcare.* Healthcare services were the largest segment of the healthcare market, accounting

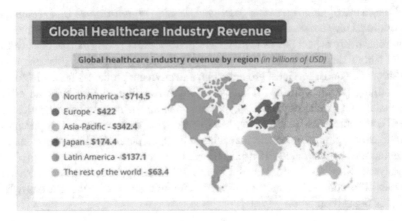

Fig. 6.1 Global healthcare market value in 2018 per region (Smiljanic Stasha, August 2021, PolicyAdvice)

for 79.4% of the total in 2018; going forward, the fastest growing segments in the healthcare market will be biologics and veterinary healthcare, where growth will be at compound annual growth rate (CAGR) of 13.6% and 10.9%, respectively. Pharmaceutical drugs, medical equipment, and then the other segments followed it.

That impressive growth is due to accelerated aging of the population, faster economic growth also in emerging markets (and thus an increasing request of welfare), technological development, and an increase in prevalence of chronic disease. Among the factors that are slowing its growth are the healthcare system reforms across the globe, the increasing stringent government regulations, lower healthcare access, and shortage of skilled professionals. North America is the largest market for healthcare, accounting for 41.9% of the global market in 2018. Asia-Pacific, Western Europe, and then the other regions follow it (Fig. 6.1). The healthcare market is highly fragmented, with many small players. Consider that the top ten companies in the market make up to 7.2% of the total market in 2018.

Healthcare absorbs more than 10% of the gross domestic product (GDP) world-wide. In particular, North America spends up to 18% of its GDP, Western Europe 12%, while emerging markets (Latin America, Asia and Africa) between 5 and 7% of GDP in 2019 (Fig. 6.2). In fact, it is not surprising that the healthcare sector is the US's largest employer.

Between the 1960s and 1990s of the twentieth century, most of the developed countries saw an increasing growth of the healthcare expenditure compared with their GDPs. The increasing healthcare's need became, across the last decades, a direct indicator of the economic development and well-being. However, the gap between the request for welfare and economic resources available arose due to increasing of population's aging, the growing incidence of chronic diseases, the enlargement of the screening and prevention programs' offering, and the raising of the medical devices', services', and drugs' prices and costs due to their innovation. Thus, guaranteeing an equal access to the healthcare system to all the population is

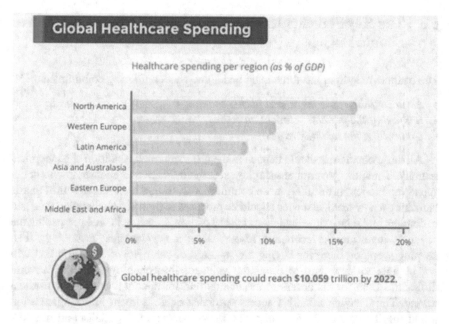

Fig. 6.2 Global healthcare spending by 2019 (Smiljanic Stasha, August 2021, PolicyAdvice)

becoming a massive welfare, social, and political issue that any government and policy maker should promptly address. That is because any healthcare system is running systematically in scarcity of economic resources. Assuming that, global or local corporations are moving across international markets where economic scarcity for healthcare is the normality and where the nonclinical stakeholders are even more influencing into the decisional process. The healthcare industry is facing a fast evolution that push also the MedTech companies to analyze seamlessly the market and the purchasing behaviors to set the right strategy for each scenario. Among those attitudes, the communication toward the stakeholders is playing a pivotal role of that strategy; for example, the large availability of the information for the patients and payers about therapeutic, medical procedures and new devices is leading to a higher awareness than in the past. The increasing usage of the digital communication tools by the patients (social media, blogs, webpages, etc.) has changed the way in which they are interacting with the MedTech corporations, the healthcare providers (HCP), and the payers. Therefore, any company who wants to approach the healthcare market with a new medical technology must carefully consider those critical elements and should count on market access professionals (or department) who are able to interact and negotiate with all stakeholders, both clinical and nonclinical. That is crucial for any MedTech company as the healthcare market is facing several and consistent budget constraints, and moving the decisional power outside the traditional clinician area of influence as it happened just 5 to 7 years ago.

6.3 The Key Stakeholders a Market Access Professional Should Engage

The healthcare system has three main and somewhat contrasting commitments:

- *Assuring the people the widest access to care*
- *Improving the patients' clinical outcomes*
- *Controlling the healthcare costs*

All those conditions should happen in the just mentioned condition of economical scarcity. Thus, the government and key stakeholders have to choose how to better spend the money in fulfilling those commitments. In that scenario, any firm that is launching a new medical device should be prepared to fight in a challenging field and to demonstrate more value than the *standard of care*. In fact, it is vital persuading the payer in investing the economic resources on a new medical technology than keeping spending them for buying the standard of care. However, a firm that will not be able to show and to proof the value of its technology will face several difficulties both for the access to the market and for adoption of the new medical device. Thus, having a market access specialist or department in its organization might fulfill that aim. In fact, market access managers or specialists are the key professionals who will likely be able to target, persuade, and engage all the key stakeholders about the firms' value proposition. To do that, market access professionals should target and then map the necessary stakeholders to engage and to involve; this kind of activity is called *stakeholders' mapping*, and it is an essential stage of a stakeholder's engagement journey. When it is performed correctly, it brings brilliant results. In mapping the stakeholders, market access professional must answer the following questions:

- *Who is/are the main stakeholder(s) to engage?*
- *What is their range of influence?*
- *Who is/are the most influencing stakeholder(s)?*
- *Where can I reach them, and what roles do they have?*
- *When do I have to involve them?*
- *Is their attitude neutral, supportive, or blocker?*
- *How are the different stakeholders linked to each other?*
- *Is there any formal step/process to be followed to engage them?*

The main output of the mapping should be a deep understanding how to cope with both the company's objectives and stakeholder's needs and expectations.

There are numerous and different stakeholders to involve, and their network complexity is rising, above all in those healthcare systems where the welfare governance is delocalized and assigned to local government agencies or institutions.

Therefore, the main stakeholders the market access manager should engage are:

- *Payers*
- *Patients*

- *Clinicians*
- *Policy makers*
- *Health technology assessment (HTA) bodies*
- *Distribution channels*

The *payers, or often payors,* are those who decide how much to pay and how spending, ruling, and investing the economic resources can satisfy the healthcare demand. They are strategic gatekeepers; they decide how to allocate the money and which kind of entrance barriers should be raised for a new technology. The payers include those stakeholders in charge of planning and setting the procurement and tender processes for each medical device's segment, and they are the necessary partners a market access manager must engage. They pay HCP, hospitals, clinics, and pharmacies to deliver clinical procedures and outcomes. Across the globe, the payers can be public and private. An example of public payer is the minister of health and its government delegate (i.e., NHS), public hospitals, and clinics. A typical example of private payer is the healthcare insurances.

The *patients* are playing an increasing role in influencing the access and the adoption of new medical technologies, mainly through their associations; and they represent even more often long-term and chronic patients. They are the end users of a medical device and thus a firm must care about their level of satisfaction and in keeping high the *customers' experience*. They could affect the decisions at both local and national levels as their increasing awareness about the therapeutic options available is changing the relationship between patient and healthcare provider (HCP), putting both at the same level of influence. They want to be informed and be involved into the decisional process in getting the right therapy for caring their disease; and the patient's associations are tapping into the procurement and buying decisions even more frequently. Therefore, the patients (and their associations) are one of the most important stakeholders to consider in the market access strategy because putting them at the center of the care process (i.e., patient-centric approach) ensures a better diagnosis, an effective therapy compliance, and a prompt removal of barriers to the access. Involving the patient means giving them flexibility, freedom of choice, and finally a higher compliance and acceptance of therapy; the ultimate result is helping the healthcare system in raising the bar of their service quality and efficiency.

The *clinicians* are all those who suggest, prescribe, or directly use a medical technology in order to diagnose or treat a disease. They are used to be the most important, often the solely, decision-maker in the past; nowadays, they are part of the stakeholders' scenario and must be engaged by a company in order to give the payer all the clinical data and evidence useful for an accurate evaluation of a new technology. They are necessary because they proof the real clinical (and superior) value of a MedTech innovation, and they will support its adoption.

The *policy makers* represent the political share of the stakeholder's maps. They could have both national and regional influence, and they shape the rules and regulations that govern the healthcare systems. They make their decision after consulting and collect clinical, patient, and health economic data about a new medical technology.

The *health technology assessment (HTA)* is a process that aims to evaluate the impact of a new technology, new drug, or organizational model on the performance improvement of a healthcare service. Every country has national and local HTA bodies which are private or public entities that are arranged in networks across each region. Those organizations perform HTA of a medical device, drug, or organization in order to provide decision-makers with objective information regarding health technologies gathered by an interdisciplinary group through a well-structured analytical approach. HTA can help stakeholders in making decisions about reimbursement, in providing recommendations on medicines and other health technologies that can be financed or reimbursed by the healthcare system.

The *distribution channel* represents the last mile of a market access journey. It is the way a medical technology reaches the patients. It is made of several elements as distributors, wholesalers, pharmacies, hospitals, trade associations, and supply chain. A medical technology could be provided through different distribution models as:

- *Direct distribution (i.e., in hospital distribution)*
- *Indirect distribution (i.e., distribution by private pharmacies and orthopedic shops)*
- *Direct-to-home/home delivery distribution (i.e., distribution at the patient's home)*

The medical devices' distribution is thus the final step of a technology journey that can be critical to satisfy the therapeutic needs of a patient. A failure or a barrier into the channel will mean preventing the access to the technology for several patients, so that a market access professional has to manage and to handle the distribution stakeholders carefully to guarantee free access and a seamless availability of a medical technology. One of the main aspects a market access manager or specialist must take care of is to ensure that the reimbursement price of a technology is profitable enough for both corporate and distribution stakeholders; the reimbursement price is the result of a negotiation process that involves payers, trade association, and distribution channels. If the reimbursement is not appealing for all the rings of the distribution chain, the medical device supply could face a constraint or even a stop in reaching the patients.

Engaging with key stakeholders is crucial for the correct interpretation of their expectations, needs, and concerns. Moreover, by embedding their feedback into a company's strategy and daily business, each corporate is able to address their common issues and develop long-term solutions, so that an open and constructive dialogue is crucial to improve the corporate's ability to create sustainable value and growth.

6.4   The Challenge of Value Demonstration

The healthcare environment has been changing considerably in recent years due to technological innovation, growing cost pressure, as well as increased evidence requirements for approval and coverage. As a result, the launch process needs to consider new strategies to differentiate the innovative technologies and effectively communicate their value to each stakeholder. Such activities include generating real-world evidence to prove their value to regulatory authorities, using value-based pricing approach to get the right reimbursement price by payers, and proposing patient-centric solutions to improve end user satisfaction and adherence as well as increasing the adoption. Moreover, to facilitate approval, access, and adoption, companies should put in place actions to enlarge the overall business opportunity by increasing stakeholder's awareness about their value proposition. As stated above, the healthcare market dynamics is fast changing, is shifting the influencing burden from clinical to nonclinical stakeholders, and is moving the focus from product features to product value. That is due mainly to budget restrictions, increasing needs for health, limit to the access, and the shifting to a more specific and personalized medicine. Thus, it is mandatory for any company to demonstrate that its solutions are not only clinically safer and more effective than the standard of care (SoC), but also more valuable for the healthcare system. It means that a MedTech company must build and effectively communicate a value proposition for the technology in order to justify a higher reimbursement price and its access to the market. The value is the key to proof to the stakeholders how much it is worth to pay and adopt a new medical technology replacing the existing health solutions. The stakeholders are increasingly watching carefully at the value-based medicine when taking their purchasing decisions. That is due mainly to several barriers that in pre- and post-launching phase each company might be able to cope with. Those limitations are:

- *Budget ceiling for medical devices*
- *Payback systems*
- *Therapeutics and diseases' guidelines and recommendations*
- *Costs monitoring*
- *Reference prices*
- *Regional/hospital budgets*

However, defining the value in healthcare is not easy as it is difficult to identify and to measure parameters uniquely accepted by each stakeholder. As Michael Porter stated in a paper published in 2010 on *The New England Journal of Medicine*, "the value in health care is the ratio between the outcomes and costs generated by a new therapeutics solution"; it is like saying that the value is "each health outcomes got per each dollar spent to buy that innovation." The factors that contribute to determining the value of a technology compared to the standard of care could be:

- *Superior clinical outcomes and/or safety*
- *Better patient compliance to the therapy*

- *Faster recovery time*
- *Higher hospital resource savings (i.e., personnel efforts, length of stay, readmission rate in inpatients, etc.)*
- *Higher overall costs saving*

MedTech companies need to be on the same page with this evolving healthcare scenario and stakeholders' value concept. A company's value and evidence-generation process needs to change into an economic modeling system that addresses prompt commercial strategy questions while providing a secure start and a driver to long-term evidence-generation strategies. Definitely, it is important for a company and its market access department, before and after launching a new technology, as well as alongside the entire product life cycle, to build and show how their medical solutions might help the patients and the healthcare system to perform better and to govern the costs.

6.5 The Key Skills and Competences for Getting an Opportunity in a Market Access Role and Its Career Development

The worldwide dynamics in healthcare industry are continuously fast changing, and thus any MedTech corporation should reinvent its business model, its go-to-market strategy, its market approach, and its organizational matrix. The growing need for healthcare, the increasing margin erosion, the pushing on cost control, and the shifting of the influence power from clinical to nonclinical stakeholders are flourishing the importance of value demonstration for each innovative technology launched into the market. For those reasons, having a market access figure into the human resource's "arsenal" is vital to guarantee a bright future to a MedTech firm.

The market access is first a matter of cross-functional strategy with the pivotal aim to proof and communicate the value of the medical technologies, with an absolute patient-centric approach. Market access is one of the winning tools for a company to *jump the gun* of the market evolutions, and it must be involved, with a value-based strategy, from the beginning to the last stage of a medical devices' life cycle (i.e., R & D phase, pre-launch strategy, price setting, and launching phase).

The priorities for a correct market access strategy and thus for a market access professional are:

- *Identify and build the value proposition* by a careful and detailed knowledge of both stakeholders and company needs and expectations
- *Proof the value proposition* through creating tools and *real-world* evidence clear and objective, by mastering HTA and health economics and outcomes research (HEOR)

- *Communicate the value proposition* to the entire internal and external stakeholder landscape to get a prompt and long-lasting access to the market and be properly rewarded for its innovations

Market access is essentially the way MedTech companies guarantee a rapid and consistent access for their innovative technologies, at the right price, across various countries and regions, to reach and to benefit patients and the healthcare services. Therefore, market access is focused on demonstrating the value of these products to gain access and supply the national health service of one or more countries; after that MedTech companies are then reimbursed, likely with a higher price, as the product is prescribed by HCP and used by patients. Market access is a niche department in MedTech firms, yet an ever-expanding one within that industry, with a fast-growing need and interest for strong talent within the sector. Thus, to be part of this appealing world, a market access professional should be able to:

- *Be business oriented*
- *Have a holistic and cross-functional approach to the business*
- *Integrate the market access strategy to the corporate one*
- *Manage projects*
- *Understand and generate real-world evidence (i.e., the clinical evidence gathered during the real clinical practice with the medical device)*
- *Communicate effectively across the internal department and to the external stakeholders*
- *Knock down the barriers among the company silos to effectively execute the market access strategy*
- *Link the R & D pipeline to the strategy*

Even though the skills required for a market access manager are changing over time, the core competencies could be summarized as follows:

- *Deep understanding of the stakeholder needs and decision-making process of the healthcare and business environment*
- *Broad understanding of tender, bidding, and procurement process*
- *Extensive knowledge of reimbursement and funding processes*
- *A strong academic background and an interest in life sciences are required, but it is not always mandatory for an application*
- *Strategic thinking and mindset*
- *Project management abilities*
- *Cross-functional collaboration*
- *High ability in strategy execution, communication, and negotiation*
- *Builds and provides solutions to improve patient experience and satisfaction*
- *Technical skills and/or professional experience and knowledge in value dossier building, pricing and reimbursement, health economics models and analysis, HEOR, and real-word evidence*
- *Informative, persuasive, and influential*
- *Provide data-driven insights*

- *Previous professional experience in medical device's clinical education, sales, and/or marketing*
- *Proficiency in English as usually involved in international projects*

The job title for market access roles may change and is different across the companies, and you should consider that when starting a job research. The keywords to use, for an open market access position research, usually are:

- *Market access*
- *Market access and government affairs*
- *Field stakeholders*
- *External/regional/public affairs*
- *Reimbursement and access*
- *Patient access and advocacy*
- *Market/business development*
- *Key/private account*
- *Value access and pricing*
- *Tendering and value*
- *Health economics, market access, and reimbursement*
- *Regional/national access*

Often the title of *specialist* follows the above one for the people with 3 to 5 years of job experience, while *manager* refers to professionals with at least 5 years of experience in the healthcare business. Lead, leader, and director are titles for people with more than 10 to 15 years of experience, most of them preferably spent in a market access role.

The market access role is hardly a starting point for a career journey because it requires a bit of experience and understanding about the business and the healthcare environments. However, an internship or a stage in a MedTech company's market access department might ease your career in that role. Commonly you can reach this kind of position after some years spent in other positions like:

- *Health economics specialist*
- *Clinical project management*
- *Public/medical/regulatory affairs*
- *Clinical education*
- *Sales and marketing*

However, one of the key competencies required is a deep and full understanding of the business and stakeholders' perspective, so that all the experiences that might enrich that aspect will ease your way to the market access. Often a master or an education got in health economics, HTA, HEOR, or an MBA might facilitate getting a position in market access.

The salary range is quite interesting in the market access field. According to *salary.com*, the wage for a market access manager is about $67,000–90,000 per year, while a market access director could reach an average salary of $165,000 per year, accordingly. As per *Paramount Recruitment* 2019 research in the United Kingdom,

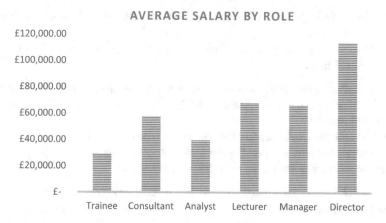

Fig. 6.3 Average salary in market access roles

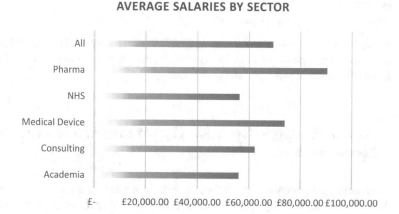

Fig. 6.4 Average salary in market access roles by sectors

the average salary in market access varies from £29,454 for a trainee to $113,737 for a market access director, with the MedTech sector placed as the second-best payer, preceded by pharmaceutical one (see Figs. 6.3 and 6.4). Certainly, the salary range depends on the size of the company and on the complexity of its business.

Being a market access professional means to be seamlessly updated about healthcare policies, procurement regulations, competition, business intelligence, and patient needs. It is a role that requires to be always a step forward and to envision the future evolutions of the healthcare market. Thus, the preparation and a continuous learning are paramount aspects that any successful market access expert should own.

Once you have jumped into a market access role, after some years spent in that, you might consider different options to develop your career. In fact, being in a market access position will offer you multiple choices that will boost your professional development.

For instance, if you prefer continuing your experience in market access, you might be appointed as:

- *A market access manager and then director/vice president with a team to manage a broader territory (i.e., Global, EMEA, Asia-Pacific, or rest of the world) or larger business*
- *An advisor for market access in a consultancy firm*
- *Business/commercial development manager and then director for the same region where you started or for a larger geography*

However, due to the strategic importance of the market access professional and his/her transferable skills, you might aspire also to other business roles such as:

- *Sales director*
- *Business unit manager/director*
- *General manager*
- *Strategic accounts manager/director*

Of course, those lists above are just an example of what you might do within a market access career pathway, but there are many other opportunities that will allow you to be successful in your professional journey.

6.6   How to Effectively Get a Job Opportunity in a Market Access Position

Finding a new job opportunity starts from a specific need: you are willing to get a brand-new, more interesting, and ambitious career. To do that, the first step is to understand what you are looking for. So, ask yourself which direction you want to take and what is the vision about your future moves in your career ladder. The second step is to prepare your best business card, writing your *resume*. In fact, striving for a new job position is a true competition between you and other candidates, and editing a great resume is the pivotal stage to reach the best ranking in that race. A resume is a fluid, tailored, and customized document that must speak about you and your professional background, but above all, it must be your first sales aid to persuade the recruiter to select your profile among hundreds or even thousands. A single resume does not fit for all the job postings; you should customize it according to the job description and use it to show and to proof the recruiter how your profile fits with the position requirements. Thus, update, change, and adapt it every time you make a new job application.

The key features of a well-done resume should include:

- *Personal details*
- *Work experiences (highlighting the most recent one)*

- *Educations, qualifications, and certifications*
- *Skills, interests, and referees (only if requested)*

It should not include:

- *Why you have left each job written on your resume (but be prepared to answer these questions in your interviewer)*
- *Current salary details*
- *Inexact information*

Some general tips about a resume are the following:

- *Keep it in a length of two to three pages*
- *Ensure that the resume is clear, structured, concise, and relevant*
- *Use bullet points instead of long sentences*
- *Check up for typos, grammar, spelling, and formatting errors*
- *Be sure it makes sense and easy to read*

The resume is your best marketing tool. So, it must be your reference for the recruiter and it should be the landmark to follow during further interview stages.

The third move is writing a tailored *cover letter*. While a resume tells a potential employer about your skills, experience, and education in a condensed way, a cover letter is a document you send, with your resume, which provides additional information about skills and experiences related to the job you are applying for. It especially explains details of your resume in more depth and the reason why an employer should recruit you; it is the first impression a hiring manager has of you. Recruiters use cover letters to slim the applicant pool and choose the group of interviewees they want to talk to.

The key features of a good cover letter should include:

- *Customized heading and recipient details*
- *The most interesting and relative experiences and skills you can offer for the open position*
- *A length of one to two pages*
- *Information about your past and present experiences and how they could impact your ability to succeed at the new position*
- *Explanation about your motivation for working with them and why it will fulfill your career goals, passions, or interests*
- *A respectful call to action such as "I look forward to hearing from you about this opportunity"*

It should not include:

- *The same detailed information of your resume*
- *All the skills and competencies you have got alongside your job experiences*

Like the resume, you should write a customized cover letter per each job application you make. Valid supports in writing both your resume and cover letter are on the web where you could find several models and examples that may help you in writing correctly those two fundamental documents.

Once you have applied for a market access job position and your profile and resume seem to be interesting for the recruiter, it is time to get prepared for the interview. The *preparation* is key and it is the most important aspect to successfully face an interview. Even if you are confident, and you know your stuff, it is still important to prepare for your interview.

First, you should collect plenty of reading materials, tools, and advice on the interview process. After that, you should get information on who will be interviewing you, background information on the company and role, and any feedback from previous interviews (if applicable).

You might find a lot of information on the company's website, LinkedIn pages, and social media channels. You should invest time finding out about the company culture, reading on case studies, and looking at any examples of their work you can find online. Be sure to be informed on the latest directions within the market access role and any relevant industry updates or news; there are several sources to use for it on the web. Usually, you may be asked to write an exercise about the market access role, and a presentation to highlight the interviewee's knowledge and presentation skills or a task to discuss a project you have worked on previously. Give everything a thorough read to double-check for any spelling and grammatical errors.

The interview process takes at least two stages, but often a third or a fourth appointment could be necessary.

Second, questioning plays a pivotal role in a successful job interview. You will answer general questions about your experiences, the reason why you are looking for a new opportunity, and your knowledge on the company. You should answer specific question related to the market access role, such as projects executed and your contribution to the results, how much you are independent in learning and running tasks and activities, or how you are able in engaging customers and stakeholders. Definitely, an interview with a recruiter or an associate of a company has a two-way main purpose: discover how much your professional and cultural background fit with the company and how much the company and its culture and mission are a good fit for you. To do that, it is a good idea if you prepare and ask some key questions to the recruiter or to the interviewer during the meeting.

Some examples of these could be the following:

- *What are the soft skills you are looking for in that position?*
- *How do you link your cultural beliefs to the business strategy execution?*
- *Who is/was covering that position so far? Why do you have that vacancy?*
- *What would be the career progression? What are the development opportunities for that role?*
- *What is the organization structure? How is the team composed?*
- *What is the next 5- to 10-year strategy of the company?*
- *Could you tell me more about you? (i.e., interviewer's background, experience, and reason why she/he is working there).*

Finally, it is crucial for a successful job interview that you fully understand if that job description fits with you and your professional background. Above all, you should check if it matches with your career aspiration because a good job position and a competitive salary are quite important, but the most critical aspect for your life-work balance is working with passion and loving what you do every day.

6.7 Conclusions

Alongside the chapter, my main purpose has been to give you an overview on what a market access role represents in reality, the framework in which it moves, and what are the challenges and opportunities you may face in doing that. What you have read and (hopefully) learned is mainly based on my over 17 years of experience in the healthcare industry, so it is a direct witness of what I have learned and experienced in the MedTech and healthcare business. As you may have read, the market access role in a company is a critical one because the only way to get access and to be rewarded for a medical innovation is to proof its superior value; and that will be necessary anytime someone needs to launch and commercialize a new medical device in any market. That happens as the spending capacity and the willingness to pay of governments and payers are even thinner, so that they carefully evaluate if a new technology is worth to be purchased or not. The market access is already an asset in pharmaceutical companies, but it is becoming even more important and necessary in the MedTech industry. Nowadays, researching, developing, and launching a new medical technology into any market without the support and the help of a market access department is clearly a ruinous strategy because any payer around the world will ask himself those key questions: *Do we really need that technology? Is it worth purchasing it and even pay more for it? How will it affect my healthcare service? Does it satisfy the patient needs?* A market access expert will just help a company to answer those questions, by creating, demonstrating, and communicating the superior value of its innovation to the payers. Becoming a market access manager is probably not the first role you will apply for or cover in your career pathway, but it will be for sure a great step to success for your career development as it requires several hard and soft skills to understand the business, engage the stakeholders, and successfully realize your projects. It is a 360° role that interacts with several departments and that should be involved from the early development to the post-marketing stages of a medical technology product's life cycle. Again, it is a strategic role that could help you raising the bar of your professional background, and maybe help you to accelerate your career ladder, facilitating you way to a top position that is even more interesting across the MedTech industry.

Bibliography

Business Wire (2019) The $11.9 Trillion Global Healthcare Market: Key Opportunities & Strategies (2014–2022) - ResearchAndMarkets.com https://www.businesswire.com/news/home/201 90625005862/en/The-11.9-Trillion-Global-Healthcare-Market-Key-Opportunities-Strategies-2014-2022%2D%2D-ResearchAndMarkets.com

Chong E (2018) Accelerating market access for a maturing medtech industry in APAC. IQVIA White paper

Clifton D (2019) HEOR and Market Access 2019 salary and workforce insight survey. https://www.pararecruit.com/salary-surveys/heor-and-market-access-salary-survey-2019

Data G, Mariani P (2015) Market access nel settore healthcare. Strategie, attori, attività e processi. Franco Angeli Edizioni

Gallo A (2020) Harvard business review. https://hbr.org/2014/12/how-to-write-a-resume-that-stands-out

Guinness L, Wiseman V (2011) Introduction to health economics, 2nd edn. McGraw-Hill Education

Page Personel UK web page (2021) Write a great CV. https://www.pagepersonnel.co.uk/advice/career-advice/looking-job/write-great-cv

Porter ME (2010) What is value in health care? N Engl J Med 363:2477–2248

Porter ME, Teisberg E (2006) Redefining health care: creating value-based competition on results. Harvard Business Review Press

Roche (2018) Stakeholder engagement. https://www.roche.com/sustainability/approach/stakeholder_engagement.htm

Salary.com (2022). https://www.salary.com/research/salary/recruiting/market-access-manager-salary

Salvatore C, Boscolo P, Tarricone R (2013) Planning and control of medical device investments by Italian public health authorities: a means to improve the decision-making process. J Med Mark 13(3):135–141

Shaw E (2021) Interviewing within market access: the essential guide. https://www.carrotrecruitment.co.uk/blog/interviewing-within-market-access

Smiljanic S (2021) The State of Healthcare Industry – Statistics for 2021. https://policyadvice.net/insurance/insights/healthcare-statistics/

Stewart C (2021) Medical technology industry - Statistics & Facts. https://www.statista.com/topics/1702/medical-technology-industry/#dossierKeyfigures

Talent.com (2022). https://www.talent.com/salary?job=director+market+access

Tarricone R (2020) Un'introduzione alle valutazioni economiche e al technology assessment in sanità. SDA Bocconi

Tarricone R et al (2017) Key recommendations from the MedtecHTA project. Health Econ 26 (Suppl. 1):145–152

Tarricone R et al (2021) Establishing a national HTA program for medical devices in Italy: overhauling a fragmented system to ensure value and equal access to new medical technologies. Health Policy 125(5):602–608

World Health Organization (1998) Health promotion glossary. Division of Health Promotion, Education and Communications (HPR) Health Education and Health Promotion Unit (HEP)

Chapter 7
Job Opportunities in Pharmaceutical Marketing

Vicky van den Nieuwenhuyzen

Abstract Pharmaceutical marketing is the set of promotional activities that ensures that medicines reach patients by first identifying the customer's needs and desires and then meeting them in the best possible way. This process is crucial during the commercialisation phase of the drug. The pharmaceutical market is very different from the traditional consumer market in several ways, including the highly regulated environment. In this chapter, we explain the main activities of marketing professionals, the required qualifications and skills, as well as the career opportunities.

7.1   The Importance of Commercialising a Medicine

Many years of intensive research and development precede the commercialisation of a drug. Of the original thousands of drug candidates, only a few make it to the finish line. For years, investments are made in studies that will or will not show the added value of a medicine. These investments are substantial, sometimes running into billions of euros. During the commercialisation phase of a drug, the aim is to recoup all investments, ideally even more, in order to cover expenditure on drugs that have never seen the light of day. More than 20% of revenues on average are often reinvested in research and development.

The commercialisation phase starts with obtaining a good market authorisation. A good price and reimbursement must also be negotiated with the various national health authorities (market access). These elements are essential for the success of the medicine, but are not sufficient to take the medicine to patients. First of all, all stakeholders, such as specialists, general practitioners and pharmacists, must be informed of the existence of the medicine. It is the role of the marketing, medical affairs and sales departments to explain the proper use of the medicine to all concerned. Information plays a crucial role in pharmaceutical innovation. After all, as long as healthcare professionals (HCPs) are not informed about the existence and

V. van den Nieuwenhuyzen (✉)
Servier Benelux, Brussels, Belgium
e-mail: vicky.vandennieuwenhuyzen@servier.com

© The Author(s), under exclusive license to Springer Nature Switzerland AG 2023   137
J. R. Thomas et al. (eds.), *Career Options in the Pharmaceutical and Biomedical Industry*, https://doi.org/10.1007/978-3-031-14911-5_7

use of new medicines, there can be no innovation. Marketing, medical affairs and sales ensure that HCPs receive all the necessary information about their medicines, so that they can make the right choice when choosing a treatment according to the individual patient.

Of course, one of the most important goals during the commercialisation phase is to get the sales up in order to be able to invest in research and development again. But informing HCPs is just as important. Marketing, medical affairs and sales actually ensure that the HCPs are educated about the correct use of their medicine.

Medical affairs, marketing and sales work hand in hand here, but each from a different angle. These three departments work in a complementary way and the best results are achieved when these departments are coordinated. Depending on your own interests, you may be more or less interested in one department or another, but you can also progress from one department to another.

7.2   What Is Pharmaceutical Marketing?

Marketing is present in our daily lives. You come into contact with it both at home and at work; through TV, radio or word-of-mouth advertising; through the well-known press advertisements, banners and so on; but also through, for example, an interview in which an artist announces his new record or the presence of a minister at the opening of a museum.

People usually associate marketing with the profit sector. But marketing also comes into play in the non-profit sector. Think of open days in hospitals, recruitment campaigns for defence, awareness-raising campaigns of climate organisations, brochures for religious organisations, petitions for human rights, etc. In this context, too, marketing is necessary to achieve a good result and fulfil the mission of these various non-profit organisations.

There are different definitions of marketing. Philip Kotler, a well-known American professor of international marketing, described marketing as delivering customer satisfaction in a profitable way. You can also describe marketing as the set of promotional activities that ensure that the product reaches customers by first identifying the customer's needs and desires and then meeting them in the best possible way.

However, the pharmaceutical market is very different from the traditional consumer market in several respects. Let us take the example of a prescription medicine. Although patients are the end user of the medicine, they are not the ones to decide. It is a doctor who decides which medicine to prescribe. The medicine is not only bought by patients, as the social security system also contributes to this purchase. Compared to the consumer market, customers (read patients) are more loyal to their brand. Finally, the pharmaceutical market is also highly regulated compared to the consumer market. For example, direct communication to patients about prescription drugs is prohibited in most countries.

It is one of the reasons why marketing professionals in the pharmaceutical market tend to have a life sciences background and not necessarily a master's degree in marketing management. Marketing in the pharmaceutical sector is very different from the consumer market in many respects. One reason is that the focus lies more on patients than on the product, and therefore in-depth scientific knowledge is required to understand the patient's world. Depending on the size of the company, we find different positions within a marketing department: project manager, product manager or brand manager, digital officer, competitive intelligence officer, business analyst or data manager, etc. The smaller the company, the more often the different functions are combined in one person, often under the name of product manager.

Every marketing process consists of a number of successive steps:

– A detailed analysis of the strengths and weaknesses of your product and the opportunities and threats of the market (= SWOT analysis)
– Defining a clear objective
– Developing a marketing strategy
– Developing an action plan
– Implementing, evaluating and adjusting the action plan where necessary

---

What does this all mean concretely?

7.2.1   Insights, Insights, Insights

The first step in the marketing process is a thorough analysis of the drug and its therapeutic area. A *thorough knowledge of the medicine* is an absolute requirement. For this, the product manager can rely on the scientific file compiled by the *medical affairs* people. Understanding, demonstrating and articulating the added value of the drug relative to potential competitors throughout the product life cycle is one of the main activities of medical affairs. This requires a non-commercial, evidence-based strategy and communication with academics and HCPs. Medical affairs provides objective, clinical and scientific information about the importance of the medicine for patients and the actual uses of the medicine. They must maximise the value of the medicine by ensuring that medical insights are understood and used throughout the organisation, to provide a competitive advantage. At the same time, they must protect the credibility and interests of patients and other stakeholders by ensuring scientific rigour, ethical communication and adherence to guidelines. The information they provide is intended both for internal stakeholders within the company and externally for potential prescribers in the healthcare sector.

In addition, marketing and medical affairs should collect as much information as possible that may be important in determining the positioning of the medicine and drawing up the communication plan. Marketing will focus more on the business-related aspects, while medical affairs is more scientifically oriented.

- It is important to know what impact *demographic, environmental, sociocultural, technological, economic or political-legal factors* have on the positioning of your medicine. For example: What age group is your medicine intended for and how large is this group? Is your medicine seasonal? What is your price and/or reimbursement compared to the market?
- It is not only in the consumer world that people speak of *influencers*. The opinion of key opinion leaders, medical journalists or scientific associations can have a significant impact on the perception of your medicine. For example: What is the place of your medicine in the guidelines produced by an internationally recognised scientific association?
- Next, the various *target groups* that may prescribe and/or recommend your medicine must be identified. Who can prescribe and/or recommend your medicine? What is the potential of the different target groups? What are their needs and wishes?
- The most important step is probably mapping out the *patient journey*. What are the different patient profiles that can benefit from your medicine? When and where are they diagnosed? Who is monitoring them? What are the pain points during their patient journey? What are their specific needs, necessities or wishes?
- Finally, the *other players* on the market should also be examined. Who are the main direct and indirect competitors? How strong is their presence in the market and what is their image among HCPs and patients?

In order to find out all this information, marketing uses a mix of quantitative and qualitative analyses. The qualitative analyses help to understand the market, while the quantitative analyses help to measure the market. It is the sum of these analyses that ensures that marketing obtains accurate, relevant information. You can use internal data (e.g. sales figures), data purchased from external healthcare data science companies (e.g. IQVIA), image studies commissioned from HCPs or patients, feedback from sales or by visiting specialists or organising advisory boards. Depending on the company, this can be followed up by the product manager himself, or in cooperation with *a business analyst (competitive intelligence)*. In any case, these tasks require the necessary analytical skills, whereby you must be able to approach all data in a critical, objective manner, make connections and draw conclusions.

7.2.2   Thinking Strategy

On the basis of these analyses, marketing will develop *a strategy* with corresponding brand positioning. Brand positioning describes the specific place a brand occupies in the minds of healthcare professionals and how the brand differentiates itself from other competitors. Marketing and medical affairs will decide together which main properties will be focused on and which image to convey about the medicine so the HCP remembers it. This involves defining a so-called unique selling proposition

(USP), coming up with a good name, a catchy logo and a simple but unique slogan. This image will be communicated to the HCP throughout the marketing mix. The marketing strategies for an innovative drug which is being launched or a natural product that is already well advanced in its life cycle require a different approach.

During the determination of the strategic imperatives, marketing will also consider patient targeting and HCP targeting. Not all patients within one indication are the same, and market analyses may have shown that the medicine better meets the needs of one group of patients versus another group. In terms of HCPs also, targeting can help to define priorities. Depending on your medicine, you may have to inform certain specific specialists and not all general practitioners. And even within the segment of specialists, there may be differences in interests or areas of expertise that cause you to adapt your message according to the HCP targeting.

To define the right strategic imperatives, the product manager must be sufficiently business-oriented, but also patient-oriented. After all, this sector is not just about sales, but focuses on patients and their needs.

7.2.3 Designing and Developing Omnichannel Campaigns

An important task of marketing is to develop a fully fledged omnichannel campaign. The well-thought-out and well-defined brand positioning still has to reach the HCPs. For this purpose, the product manager has a range of communication channels (online and offline) at his disposal, which he has to coordinate. The goal is to get the right content through the right channel to the HCP at the right time. Therefore, a product manager should be able to bring several projects to a successful conclusion at the same time. He must have excellent communication skills, both oral and written. Moreover, he must be a hero in multitasking and proactive work and have strong organisational skills.

The most important communication channel in the pharmaceutical industry has always been *the medical representative or key account manager (sales). During the visit of a medical representative* to specialists, general practitioners or pharmacists, the brand positioning is explained, and the practical use of the medicine is well illustrated with the help of clinical studies. Marketing prepares the entire strategy for the sales department with accompanying visual aids, brochures, leave behinds, patient advisories, emails and so on. During the preparation of such a sales campaign, all the skills of a product manager come into play: in-depth product knowledge, analytical skills, strategic insight, but also his creative talent in developing documents that appeal to HCPs and/or patients. After months of preparation, the icing on the cake comes when the product manager can present his campaign to the medical representatives at so-called cycle meetings. In this context, it is important that the product manager is able to give an engaging and convincing presentation to motivate and inspire salespeople with his elaborate strategy and action plan.

Another important channel of communication is *congresses*, which are a permanent part of the ongoing education of HCPs. Most of these scientific events can take place, thanks to the financial support of pharmaceutical companies. In return, pharmaceutical companies are allowed to be present with a promotional stand in the exhibitors' hall where leaflets, publications, videos and so on about the medicine are made available. Depending on the national or regional character of the congress, marketing and sales, respectively, follow up these sponsorships. Marketing takes care of the design of all stands. Together with medical affairs, marketing is also responsible for organising symposia at some congresses. During such symposia, experts are invited to give a presentation on their work, scientific news or a clinical case related to the therapeutic field of the drug. Medical affairs will mainly have input in the drafting of the programme. Posters and invitation must also be developed. This is the responsibility of the marketing team.

Press advertising is also part of the marketing mix. It is complementary to the other communication channels and provides a reminder of the name, logo and slogan. Marketing is responsible for designing the press page and publishing press ads.

For some years now, *digital media* have occupied an important place in the media mix. The digital world is also catching up with the pharmaceutical industry, which by nature is rather conservative. The COVID pandemic certainly contributed to this. Moreover, there are also more and more digital natives who graduate to HCP and consult a multitude of (digital) sources. Finally, these digital media also offer additional opportunities to interact with HCPs.

As a result of this digital evolution, marketing teams are also investing more and more time and energy in developing online communication channels, e.g. virtual meetings, websites, opt-in programmes, newsletters, approved emails, podcasts, social media presence, etc. The digital transformation within the pharmaceutical industry is in full swing and requires new skills. Many teams are now reinforced by *digital officers* who support the teams in developing omnichannel campaigns.

The digital officer or digital marketing manager is responsible for providing best in-class support to brand marketing teams in designing and executing programmatic, social media and digital marketing campaigns overall. The digital officer works hand-in-hand with local brand teams and external agency partners to define, audit and drive best digital marketing campaign executions aligned with brand business goals and objectives communicated by product managers or brand managers. This includes supporting campaign strategic planning, design, execution and measurement.

In addition, a digital officer contributes to the development of promotional teams' skills in digital media and channels (acculturation/training) and leads to the digital transformation of the teams by bringing value with digital inputs. The digital officer has to ensure a consistent environment/infrastructure with all IT tools (e.g. VEEVA CRM (Customer Relationship Management), Google Analytics, Power BI) and uses data/digital analytics to contribute to the elaboration of the strategy. In other words, a digital officer must be able to work well cross-functionally, as he has to coordinate digital projects with marketing, medical affairs and sales teams.

7.2.4   *Drug Promotion Regulation*

All communication on medicines is highly regulated compared to, for example, the traditional consumer market. The pharmaceutical industry is committed to making its medicines available within a global ethical framework and in compliance with all national and international regulations and laws. This means that particular attention is paid to providing accurate, correct, objective and scientifically based information to the various stakeholders. The promotional material must not be misleading in any way and must mention both the benefits and the risks of the medicinal product, so that the correct use of the medicinal product can be ensured. Moreover, it also seeks to ensure the greatest possible transparency in the relations between the pharmaceutical industry and HCPs. In accordance with (inter)national legislation, nothing is offered to HCPs that could in any way influence their prescribing behaviour.

As a product manager, you must therefore not only be creative and have good scientific knowledge. You must also be familiar with the ethical framework in which to work and familiarise yourself with the many regulatory internal and external procedures.

In this context, many companies have a *person Responsible for Information and Publicity (RIP)* who checks, before publication, that all advertising made by the company conforms to the laws and regulations concerning medicinal products advertising. The person responsible for information is a doctor or a pharmacist approved by the Ministry of Public Health. This person often also ensures the follow-up of compliance rules within the company with regard to samples, contracts, GDPR, internal procedures and so on. He assists the various internal departments with training and checks.

7.2.5   *A Full Range of Tasks*

Besides all marketing activities, a product manager is also responsible for budget management and forecasts. A product manager is allocated a considerable *budget* to carry out all the analyses and to steer action plans in the right direction. Often he has to defend this budget once a year to his hierarchy and make sure that the budget planning is respected. The product manager must also forecast the future market demand for the drug. *Forecasts* are often prepared using statistical models (e.g. by extrapolating historical sales data) or based on certain assumptions and hypotheses (e.g. the possible impact of the launch of a competitor). Based on the forecast, the supply chain can order or manufacture the necessary raw materials to meet the expected future demand for the medicine.

At first glance, marketing seems to play a role only from the moment the medicine comes on the market. This is probably also its main area of action. However, through regular contacts with HCP and thorough market knowledge, marketing is also well positioned to provide background information to other internal stakeholders (R & D,

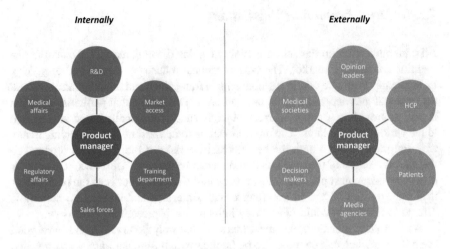

Fig. 7.1 The cross-functional role of a product manager

market access, etc.). Some strategic recommendations may help in the development of the drug, e.g. to identify the right populations where the needs are greatest, to formulate the right reimbursement criteria and so on. A junior profile will initially focus on implementing the action plans, but as experience grows, his role in these strategic considerations can grow more and more.

In other words, a product manager "manages" really all aspects of his medicine. Therefore, he is also the central contact for many departments (Fig. 7.1). Internally, he advises on reimbursement strategies to market access, looks for information or research opportunities in R & D, determines the value of the drug together with medical affairs, translates this into campaigns for sales and has to make sure that the various internal stakeholders are all on the same wavelength. Externally, through all his marketing activities, he comes into contact with scientific associations, opinion leaders, policy makers, journalists and so on.

7.3   Qualifications and Skills

You do not need to have studied marketing to get started in pharmaceutical marketing. In this particular market, a degree in life sciences is more appropriate. An additional education in marketing, digital communication or market research is a plus that can help differentiate you from other candidates. Often, the necessary time is invested in internal training when you start working in a pharmaceutical company. These trainings then include not only a scientific course on the medicines but also a course on marketing and/or sales.

However, you can also distinguish yourself from other candidates by experience in other departments. If you have any sales experience as a medical representative or key account manager, this is definitely a plus in order to then work in a marketing department. After all, one of the most important core activities of marketing is to prepare campaigns for medical representatives. But you can also start in a marketing department after an experience in R & D or medical affairs. Both are useful experiences.

It is also important that you have the following skills:

- Excellent interpersonal and communications skills to efficiently and productively communicate, both orally and in writing
- Strong tactical and analytical skills to identify and understand complex issues and then developing appropriate cross-functional solutions
- Patient-oriented mindset to develop well-adapted patient solutions
- Planning and organizational skills, including ability to follow tasks/assignments through to completion
- Good team player and proven ability to work with cross-functional teams
- A creative and curious mindset and a strong focus and drive
- Entrepreneurial, leadership, eager to learn, positive energy, service mindset and a results-oriented, can-do attitude
- Ability to adapt quickly and cope with changing situations in a world that is moving fast

7.4   Career Opportunities

As previously discussed, you can find several positions within a marketing department. A junior profile can start as a *project manager* or *junior product manager* under the supervision of a *senior product manager* or *brand manager*. A brand manager is responsible for several products within one range or therapeutic area. Often, they start on a national level and can then grow to an international level to develop more corporate strategies.

Some positions within a marketing team are focused on particular missions, such as a *business analyst* (see Sect. 7.2.1) or a *digital officer* (see Sect. 7.2.3). They often support several product managers or business units working in different therapeutic areas. In other words, on the one hand, they are focused on one part of the entire marketing mix, but on the other, they have the opportunity to be active in different therapeutic areas for drugs that may be at different stages of their life cycle.

Depending on the company and the therapeutic areas, a product manager or brand manager may report to a marketing manager or a business unit manager. A *marketing manager or marketing director* is responsible for all product managers and marketing activities of the company. In addition to the marketing manager, there is a sales manager who leads the team of medical representatives. A *business unit manager*, on the other hand, is responsible for marketing and sales, but only within the therapeutic domain of his business unit.

7.5   Conclusion

In short, a product manager is like a mini CEO of his product. He is responsible for every aspect of his product. In this capacity, he plays a central role in the life cycle of the drug and interacts with all departments involved in the drug, from R & D to sales. Through these cross-functional collaborations, the product manager can gather a lot of knowledge. This unique position also allows the product manager to discover where his interests lie if he wants to develop further. Perhaps a bright future in medical affairs awaits him, or he prefers the sales techniques of the sales team, or decides to grow further in the exciting and varied world of pharmaceutical marketing.

Chapter 8
Working in Medical Affairs and Clinical Operations: Life-Changing Careers

Drago Vuina, Amal Chalfoun, Ana Ines Chiesa, Laura Salvi, Giusi Lastoria, and Arianna Gattoni

Abstract Innovation represents the driving force of every technologically advanced sector, but in the pharmaceutical field, it acquires particular importance since it concerns the health and quality of life of patients. Research and development (R&D) sector and departments are a real human and technological asset for pharmaceutical companies, and together with innovation, they are the engine of their growth. It is also an important sector that welcomes many young graduates, offering them various professional roles.

In addition to the know research and development department, there are many pharmaceutical companies such as the Danish Novo Nordisk, which presented three other scientific and core departments, which express the most medical, clinical, and regulatory roles and functions. At Novo Nordisk, Italy, for example, these three souls are located within a single large department called Clinical Medical and Regulatory (CMR).

Medical affairs experts, who work in this department, are the medical face of the company; their experience outside scientific and clinical aspects allows to facilitate the flow of information between the scientific community and the organization. Within the company, they act as a link between research and business, both at local (country) and European or worldwide level (global teams). Clinical operations is the department that deals with the management of clinical trials and therefore follows the development of a drug from phase I to phase IV. Within this department, there are various professionals who work in teams to bring new drugs and therapies to the market. In Novo Nordisk, the regulatory department is responsible for collecting all the necessary and fundamental information for development. It deals

D. Vuina
CVP - Novo Nordisk Italy, Rome, Italy
e-mail: drv@novonordisk.com

A. Chalfoun · L. Salvi · G. Lastoria (✉)
Clinical, Medical and Regulatory Department, Novo Nordisk Italy, Rome, Italy
e-mail: amcf@novonordisk.com; zlrs@novonordisk.com; giul@novonordisk.com

A. I. Chiesa · A. Gattoni
P&O, Communication and Sustainability – Novo Nordisk Italy, Rome, Italy
e-mail: aaic@novonordisk.com; ngat@novonordisk.com

with the registration and marketing of pharmaceutical products and managing the preparation of the entire drug registration dossier to obtain the first authorization for drug placing on the market and for the authorization of the future and next indication. Starting a career at Novo Nordisk is more than getting a job. It is an opportunity to improve the lives of millions of people living with a serious chronic disease.

8.1   Research and Development

Scientific and technological research, innovation, and the constant challenge in reaching and bringing to the market safe and effective treatments and cures to improve the lives of people suffering especially from chronic diseases (e.g., diabetes, obesity, hemophilia, growth disorders) is something that cannot be achieved without people. People always represent a wealth and a fundamental point for the success and effectiveness of anything, regardless of their work, from where they live, and their point of view. We mean the people who work together to achieve these common goals and who believe in what they do, day by day: we can therefore refer to clinicians, patients, caregivers, patient associations and scientific societies, patient family, nurses and other healthcare professionals, researchers, pharmaceutical companies, etc.

For example, Leonard Thompson—the first person with diabetes to be treated with insulin—was injected with insulin extracted from the pancreases of cattle (IDF International Diabetes Federation 2019). Since then, the management of this chronic pathology has changed dramatically. The therapeutic options available today have come a long way since 1922, when the first insulin injection was administered. However, they may well be considered antiquated 100 years from now. Innovation is never a single event; it is a collection of small discoveries and breakthroughs that bring about transformation. And this takes time. For example, in 1889, German researchers Oskar Minkowski and Joseph von Mering first discovered that dogs developed symptoms of diabetes when their pancreas gland had been removed. Yet it was not until 1921 that insulin was discovered—on a different continent entirely (Vecchio et al. 2018). The process of developing a medicine takes time (on average 10–15 years) and significant financial resources (Fig. 8.1) (Karamanou et al. 2016). A collaborative process, research and development (R&D) involves a broad range of stakeholders, patients, hospitals, healthcare professionals, health authorities, and the pharmaceutical industry (Vecchio et al. 2018; Karamanou et al. 2016). While the result of the R&D process may be an innovative new medicine, the process itself also yields a deeper understanding of diabetes and, consequently, improvements in the care of those living with diabetes (Van Norman 2016; Novo Nordisk 2014).

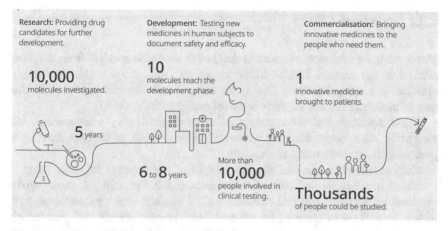

Research: Providing drug candidates for further development.

Development: Testing new medicines in human subjects to document safety and efficacy.

Commercialisation: Bringing innovative medicines to the people who need them.

10,000 molecules investigated.

10 molecules reach the development phase.

1 innovative medicine brought to patients.

5 years

6 to **8** years

More than **10,000** people involved in clinical testing.

Thousands of people could be studied.

Fig. 8.1 Research & Development

8.2   The Roles of Medical Affairs and Clinical Operations in the Constantly Evolving Scientific and Health Scenario

At Novo Nordisk, Italy, the functions of medical, clinical, and regulatory are located within a single large department called Clinical Medical and Regulatory "CMR." These three functions belong to the three departments specifically named:

– Medical affairs
– Clinical operations
– Regulatory and safety

The CMR department work in close contact with each other and with other company departments, including marketing and sales, with the common and greatest goal to discover, spread, educate, communicate, and ensure and monitor the clinical benefit in real life, better treatments for people living with a serious chronic disease, like people with diabetes, obesity, diseases related to growth disorders, and blood coagulation disorders. Novo Nordisk is a dynamic company and these three departments perfectly embody the dynamism of the company and its DNA.

The CMR department in its three souls works first of all in close synergy with the other internal departments (Marketing, Market Access, Sales) and, as regards external relations, collaborates, supports, and interacts with various interlocutors.

Moreover, the CMR department works in close collaboration with clinicians, that is, the medical specialists in the specific therapeutic area where the company develop drugs investing in research and various clinical and scientific activities.

It also works in addition with national scientific societies, patient associations, investigators involved in company clinical trials, payers, pharmacist, nurses, key opinion leaders (KOL), universities, and biotech companies worldwide, depending on the specific activities involving the various functions of the three departments.

8.2.1   Medical Affairs

The continuous evolution of scientific and health scenarios requires from the pharmaceutical and medical devices' industries a significant change in processes, organization, and company roles. One of the central and strategic functions in this transformation of the last 10 years is that of medical affairs (MA).

Within a pharmaceutical company, medical affairs (MA) plays a key strategic and supportive role, representing the real-world clinical needs of patients, healthcare professionals, and other decision-makers.

Medical affairs is essential for the success of a company. Its main value is contained in scientific and clinical competence and in the ability to build strong relationships with the scientific community. The Medical affairs professional deals with a drug at every stage of its life cycle (pre-launch, launch, and post-launch phases) supporting its appropriate use and working and interacting with internal and external interlocutors for the various scientific and clinical activities, during the phase before the marketing of the drug and then in the post-marketing phase. Medical affairs intervenes in numerous development activities including those of strategic vision, clinical research, and understanding and interpretation of scientific data, up to the generation of scientific publications. In addition, it collaborates in the definition of market research and training within the company, for example, of the drug's scientific representatives (Fig. 8.2).

The numerous activities of medical affairs are declined both in the offices (medical advisor (MA)) and in those of the territory (regional medical advisor (RMA) or medical science liaison (MSL)).

The MA is required to represent the medical-scientific reference of the therapeutic area for the company and the national scientific community, through the production and dissemination of medical scientific knowledge. Another focus area for medical advisor in the office is planning Novo Nordisk's presence at national congresses and

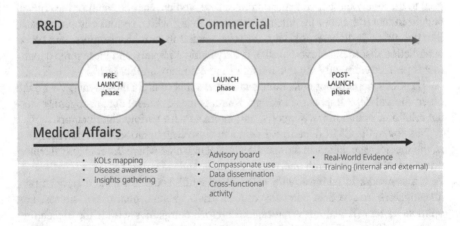

Fig. 8.2 The strategic role of the MA during the drug life cycle

symposia, providing guidance on investigator sponsored studies, and being the main drivers for producing and publishing abstracts, scientific papers, and posters at congresses and scientific journals.

Likewise, the RMA is a professional located in the area whose main responsibility is that of promoting peer collaboration relationships with opinion leaders by providing medical and scientific support.

Its main function is therefore to facilitate the exchange of scientific information between the medical community and the pharmaceutical company.

Within the medical affairs in Novo Nordisk, the various activities are reflected and are placed within five well-defined focus areas, which have the following objectives:

- Evidence generation: Support evidence generation and real word-evidence dissemination and interpretation, and drive consistent scientific communication across phases in clinical trial programs
- KOL and association engagement: Structured engagement processes with national and global key opinion leaders and associations
- Publication planning: Make Novo Nordisk a national and world leader in ethical scientific publication practice
- Medical education: Continuously disseminate science to physicians in a compliant manner
- Medical guidance: Scientific and process alignment across Novo Nordisk

Why is real-world evidence (RWE) important?

One of the most important focus areas, in which medical affairs works, is the real-word evidence area.

Novo Nordisk invests and supports various activities that fall under the RWE umbrella, with the aim of adding scientific knowledge and clinical data to what is traditionally collected by randomized clinical trials (RCTs) that are part of drug development programs (pre-registration phase 3 studies). RWE is playing an increasingly important role in decision-making related to regulatory, reimbursement, and access of new medicines. It is predicted that its use and importance will only increase in the future. External stakeholders are shaping the RWE environment, and FDA (HMA/EMA) and EMA (Makady et al. 2020) have published guidance documents on use of RWE in decision-making in order to speed up the process of bringing innovative products to patients in need. This increased focus on RWE within the regulatory environment is likely to also pave the way for more use of RWE among other stakeholders. RWE supplements evidence from RCTs by providing an understanding of the real value of a treatment by supplementing clinical efficacy with clinical effectiveness. Real-world studies can, thus, be used to address different questions and endpoints than RCTs. Furthermore, with real-world data (RWD) being more accessible, the cost of conducting a real-world study is also lower than conducting a RCT. The potential of RWE is expanding to the drug development phase. RWE is often considered a post-launch tool; however, new ways of leveraging RWD and RWE are in the drug discovery and development phase. In these early stages, real-world insights can provide an understanding of the

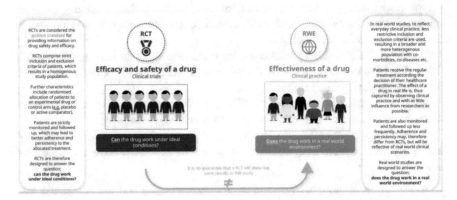

Fig. 8.3 RWE vs. RCT

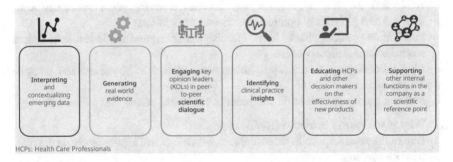

Fig. 8.4 How medical affairs acts to advance patient care

holistic environment of a disease area, incl. disease characteristics (burden of disease, unmet needs), and the characteristics of the real patient population, treatment pathways, and patient experiences. Such early insights can be used to design smarter and more patient-centric clinical trials with the right populations, subgroups, comparators, and value-based endpoints relevant for stakeholders, which can reduce the risk of expensive trials not showing anticipated results (Fig. 8.3).

The Job request of medical affairs professional is experiencing significant growth, especially in the last 10 years, during which the investments in research and development specifically for the treatment of chronic disease and for those companies that have a rich and varied pipeline have the need to expand the scientific knowledge toward the scientific community. It is easy to predict that in the next few years, the demand will continue to increase. The MA/RMA figures are based on a valid scientific and clinical preparation, as well as soft skills, in order to guarantee an equal comparison with opinion leaders. It is therefore indispensable and essential for the MA/RMA to develop both technical and management skills, such as those of negotiation, consultancy, project management, and problem-solving (Fig. 8.4).

In Novo Nordisk, each therapeutic area, i.e., diabetes, obesity, and the biopharma (hemophilia and growth disorders), is characterized by a well-structured medical affairs department, which comprises office and territorial roles (MAs and RMAs). Medical advisors report to a medical manager who works in office (diabetes medical manager, obesity medical manager, and biopharma medical manager), while the local RMA reports to another medical manager who instead works on the territory.

All medical managers of the different therapeutic areas report to a single medical director, who is the CMR director, who heads the entire CMR department.

Possible roles within medical affairs:

1. Medical affairs entry-level roles

   - Regional medical advisor (RMA)
   - Medical advisor

For both the roles, a scientific master's degree is the minimum requirement. A PhD could be a plus as well as postgraduate courses in the pharmaceutical management field. In terms of skills, the ability to work in group, the intellectual curiosity, and a patient-centric approach could accelerate the learning curve for both these roles. For the RMA role, it is crucial that the ideal candidate is willing to travel frequently.

2. Medical affairs career development roles

   - Medical manager
   - Medical director

8.2.2 Clinical Operations

The clinical operations department has the aim to drive clinical operation expertise and innovation to ensure an efficient, world-class, patient-centric, clinical trial execution.

Clinical operations (CO or ClinOps) is the department that deals with the management of clinical trials and therefore follows the development of a drug from phase I to phase IV. Within this department, there are various professionals who work in teams to bring new drugs and therapies to the market.

The clinical operations can be located within a pharmaceutical company or within a CRO (contract research organization). In recent years, most pharmaceutical companies have removed the clinical operations (CO) department from their workforce to outsource it to CROs.

Within Novo Nordisk, clinical operations fall within the CMR department and there are several roles that this department holds. All roles included in the CO department focus on the management of clinical trials. In particular, clinical studies must be conducted in accordance with the study protocol, GCP (good clinical practice), and current regulations.

In the complex world of clinical research, there is a key connecting figure between the sponsor (generally a pharmaceutical company) and the investigator center or site (doctors, patients, and nurses). This is the role of the clinical operations department and specifically this is the role of the clinical research associate (CRA), the first professional figure which characterizes the CO department also in Novo Nordisk, defined by the GCP as the "person delegated by the sponsor to organize, follow and control the progress of the clinical study at the experimental centers."

A clinical research associate (CRA), also known as a clinical monitor, has the role of overseeing the conduct and progress of a clinical trial. A clinical study can be conducted in a hospital, in a private clinic, or even in a doctor's office. The main tasks of the CRA are to manage initially the setup of the trial, through the selection of the most suitable centers and through staff training, and in the subsequent phases, to monitor the progress of the trial, ensuring the integrity of the data collected, with respect to the rights, safety, and well-being of the subjects participating in the study.

Specifically, a CRA must ensure that the physician and his staff correctly comply with the standards of good clinical practice and the study protocol; verify that all documentation relating to the use of the drug has been correctly completed; verify the compilation of informed consents for each study subject; ensure that adverse events, whether serious or not, are reported correctly and promptly; verify the completeness and accuracy of data relating to medical records; and ensure the review and archiving of regulatory documents.

We can talk about home-based and office-based CRAs, depending on whether the work is done from home or from the office, and in most cases, a willingness to travel for 50–70% of the time is required in order to perform all the necessary visits to the various centers participating in the studies.

The work of a CRA is extremely important for pharmaceutical companies, which are currently trying to reduce the development time required to receive approval for placing their products on the market as much as possible. Proper monitoring is therefore the first mechanism to help reduce these times, which is why the demand for competent and expert CRAs is constantly growing, so much so that demand is now often greater than supply.

In addition to the CRA, other key roles in Novo Nordisk within clinical operations are:

- Clinical trial assistant (CTA): multifaceted figure who has the task of supporting the team in the management of the clinical trial; he/she plays an more administrative role.
- Lead CRA: leads the group of CRAs that run a clinical trial.
- Head of clinical operations, who heads the clinical operations department.

Possible roles within clinical operations:

- Clinical operations entry-level roles

  - Clinical research associate (CRA)
  - Clinical trial assistant (CTA)

These professionals have a scientific master's degree (Biology, Biotechnology, Pharmacy and Chemistry, and Pharmaceutical Technologies, just to mention few of the most common one). It is frequent that they have already some professional experience in clinical operations consultancy firms.

These are the principal skills required to work in clinical operations:

- High attention to detail and precision
- Excellent organizational and time management skills
- Problem-solving skills
- Excellent communication skills, as you interface with different roles
- Knowledge of English (it is essential since all the documents of the study are in English, and we often collaborate with teams also present in other countries)
- Knowledge of the processes that regulate clinical research, of GCP, and of the regulations in force

- Clinical operations career development roles:

  - Lead CRA
  - Head of ClinOps

To progress in this area, it is required to have project management and leadership skills.

8.2.3 Regulatory and Safety

The regulatory and safety department has multiple responsibilities, multiple areas of expertise, and a connection point between different company dimensions, in constant transformation and with a much more dynamic nature than one might think at the start: a world to be discovered and explored.

For a pharmaceutical company, adhering to the rules and regulations in force is a crucial aspect to ensure the quality, safety, and effectiveness of its products. This is specifically dealt with by the regulatory department which plays a fundamental role in terms of R&D and product compliance.

In Novo Nordisk, the regulatory department is responsible for collecting all the necessary and fundamental information for the development of a drug in safety both in the pre-registration phase and in the post-marketing phase. It deals with the registration and marketing of pharmaceutical products, managing to prepare the entire registration dossier that it is necessary to produce and submit to the national regulatory agencies (e.g., AIFA for Italy) to obtain the authorization for the marketing of the drug. The regulatory is therefore a fundamental department, which supports all the other departments in product development to achieve greater success.

Very often, it is also part of the department within which clinical operations and medical affairs are also located; it is thus, for example, in Novo Nordisk, within which in addition to carrying out the regulated functions and also dealing with pharmacovigilance and product safety.

Over time, the regulatory function within companies has evolved and expanded. The regulatory function, differently from the past, no longer coincides with a simple administrative activity but has taken on a strong scientific as well as a strategic connotation. It is constantly in contact and interaction with all the other functions.

The regulatory department actually interfaces with the most varied business areas: from quality to pharmacovigilance, from research and development to marketing, all across the total supply chain. Creating a constructive and fluid dialogue with the various players in the pharmaceutical company is essential to make processes more streamlined and effective.

To minimize errors, and speed up registration times and consequent marketing of the drug, it is very important to be able to count on the support of the regulatory department right from the product development phase. Crucial is also the guidance that the regulatory affairs department can provide to the technical R&D functions in interacting with regulatory bodies.

The role of regulatory affairs in companies such Novo Nordisk remains crucial as well as in many other companies even following the launch of the product on the market. Should there be any changes to be made to the original project, it is the responsibility of the regulatory function to support the various departments in the implementation of product compliance.

Within the CMR in Novo Nordisk, the regulatory department also deals with pharmacovigilance (PV) activities. Monitoring drug safety is an important activity that provides fundamental information at every moment of its life cycle.

In the regulatory department in Novo Nordisk, the pharmacovigilance activities are accountable and guided by the regulatory and safety manager who reports directly to the medical director in charge of the entire CMR structure.

The regulatory and safety manager manages all aspects concerning the set of activities aimed at identifying, evaluating, understanding, and preventing adverse effects or any other problem related to the use of medicines, so that the relationship between benefits and risks is favorable for the population to which the pharmaceutical product is intended. His/her duties include ensuring that all information relating to product safety reaches the attention of health personnel, through the preparation of periodic safety update reports, the management of communications to and from the Ministry of Health, and the dissemination of information notes and updates to doctors who prescribe drugs (Fig. 8.5).

Typically, entering the world of regulatory business requires a degree in a science subject, especially those more related to pharmaceutical development, such as chemistry and pharmacy. The master's degree is not always necessary, but it can be a nice advantage and a good way to specialize in regulatory affairs, especially if the course of study was more general. Furthermore, as the world of regulatory affairs is constantly progressing, periodic refresher and training courses on regulatory changes are also recommended. For this purpose, there are also many online courses, which allow you to save time without having to give up updating. Internships and internships can be a good way to enter this world, especially in large companies, more used to managing new graduates with no experience and more willing to offer this type of positions, advertised on the net and on social networks. It is also possible

Fig. 8.5 Regulatory and
PV strategic work areas

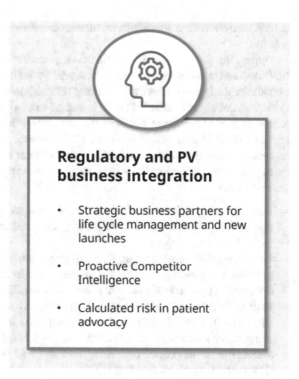

to get to regulatory affairs from related, perhaps more technical, sectors, for example, quality assurance, i.e., to start a career as regulatory affairs specialist, it is required a high level of attention to details and intellectual curiosity.

8.2.4 Life-Changing Careers

A career in the CMR (Clinical Medical and Regulatory) department is a great opportunity for working in one of the most diverse teams within a pharmaceutical organization, in terms of background and support provided to the line of business. In fact, CMR is involved in interactions with doctors, developing and implementing regulatory strategies, providing medical education, and collecting data to support efficacy and new product development.

As already mentioned, a solid, scientific university background is a must have, and a master's degree or a PhD could further enrich the technical knowledge. But it is also crucial to have the willingness to collaborate across all the functions of the company.

With these premises and having these objectives, in Novo Nordisk, for example, there is a graduate program, a program of 2-year, that can be understood as a global career journey with a minimum of three rotations with at least one international rotation.

During the program, you will gain a deep understanding of our company, our business, and our company values. You will be included in and drive global and national projects, as well as build a strong international network of professional and dedicated colleagues. This initiative is aimed to students (early career programs), with the scope of attracting highly qualified people—this includes bachelor students, pre- and postgraduate master students, PhD students, and postdocs in life sciences, as well as medical doctors in the early stages of their careers.

In particular, Novo Nordisk offers some graduate program tracks, among which are as follows:

- Manufacturing technology: This has been designed to develop the next generation of key project managers, specialists, and product owners within the field of
  technology and innovation.
- Pharmaceutical development: This 2-year graduate program will give you comprehensive knowledge of the key departments in the drug development value
  chain, from the early clinical trial phase to the regulatory approval process as well
  as drug safety surveillance. You will get to know the drug development process
  from multiple stakeholder angles, enabling you to find the niche where your
  competencies and interests coincide. We have two different tracks within pharmaceutical development: regulatory, medical and safety, and trial management
  (Novo Nordisk; Novo Nordisk Italy).

This is why it is possible to state that, in every situation, in every job and for each individual, change is constant—change in lifestyle, change in technology, and change all over. This is particularly true for a pharmaceutical company like Novo Nordisk, which has a focus in driving change in every single therapeutic area (diabetes, obesity, rareD). The pharmaceutical environment is truly a dynamic industry, where success in clinical trials could have a direct impact on patients' quality of life. That's why Novo Nordisk continuously pushes to improve the way its employees work and the lives of the patients we serve, creating innovative solutions that fit the way people want to live. To accomplish this, it embraces a spirit of open-mindedness and experimentation, striving for excellence without fixating on perfection.

8.2.5   Conclusion

Working in a pharmaceutical company requires to always keep up with the times and follow internal and external rhythms. This is especially true for multinational companies. For graduates who come from medical and scientific faculties and who often have no idea of the roles and skills and the job prospects that a company can offer (being very focused on research or on the academic profession), the functions of medical affairs and clinical operations but also of regulatory and safety can represent a great opportunity.

The main roles described in the medical affairs and clinical operations department are characterized by great dynamism and versatility. The medical advisor, regional medical advisor, and clinical research associate figures, together with the managerial roles of these departments as further growth opportunities, have the task to support and guide the core activities of the company from a scientific and clinical point of view. This happens interacting with different interlocutors (external and internal) at all levels and at different moments in the life cycle of drugs and for different reasons (information, education and communication scope, publication support, study coordination, and so on).

The key roles of these two departments can be considered the scientific and medical face of the pharmaceutical industry, representing on the one hand the point of connection between the scientific community and society itself, and on the other hand, the pivot that maintains the internal company balance between the marketing/business area and research.

Finally, it can be said that these are strategic and core roles and function within a pharmaceutical company, thanks to a mix of scientific and clinical knowledge and communication skills and relationships with the outside world, able to supervise and guide all stages of production and dissemination of a service/product and supporting its proper use.

References

HMA/EMA Task Force on Big Data

IDF International Diabetes Federation (2019). http://diabetesatlas.org/resources/-atlas.html

Karamanou M, Protogerou A, Tsoucalas G, Androutsos G, Poulakou-Rebelakou E (2016) Milestones in the history of diabetes mellitus: the main contributors. World J Diabetes 7(1):1

Makady et al (2020) What is real-world data? A review of definitions based on literature and stakeholder interviews Pharmavoice Whitepaper, Real World Evidence comes of age

Novo Nordisk. Assessing the value of diabetes clinical research (2014)

Novo Nordisk | driving change to defeat diabetes. www.novonordisk.com

Novo Nordisk Italy. www.novonordisk.it

Van Norman GA (2016) Drugs, devices, and the FDA: part 1: an overview of approval processes for drugs. JACC: Basic Transl Sci 1(3):170–179

Vecchio I, Tornali C, Bragazzi NL, Martini M (2018) The discovery of insulin: an important milestone in the history of medicine. Front Endocrinol (Lausanne) 9:613

Chapter 9
The Role of Medical Science Liaison

Roberta Manfroni

Abstract Building a pharmaceutical professional career can be extremely challenging, especially if the existing roles within the pharmaceutical companies are not fully known or understood. Among these, the medical science liaison (MSL) role, acting as part of the medical affairs department, has been consolidated for some years, but it is still evolving.

This chapter provides a comprehensive overview of the main characteristics and responsibilities of the MSL and explains how this role can contribute to the implementation of the company's strategy. Key areas discussed include history, different definition of the role, MSL typical activities, as well as some tips for those who are about to define their professional objectives.

The aim of this chapter is to provide the reader with key elements necessary to imagine himself acting as a medical science liaison within the medical affairs department and to evaluate whether it may meet personal characteristics and interests.

9.1 Introduction

The medical science liaison (MSL) is a field-based scientific professional reporting into the medical affairs department. We can begin this journey by asking ourselves what the initial conditions for the development of this figure were. The idea came in 1967 at the Upjohn Company where the development of increasingly sophisticated drugs required to build a team with a strong scientific background to facilitate the scientific exchange with the stakeholders (Gupta and Nayak 2013).

At the beginning, the company selected the first of those who later became MSLs among the sales representatives who demonstrated to have the strongest scientific knowledge (https://medicalaffairsspecialist.org/what-is-an-msl). Then this role slowly acquired its own identity, but only in the last few years, we are witnessing an exponential growth in demand of these professionals from the pharmaceutical

R. Manfroni (✉)
Medical Science Liaison, GW Pharma Italy S.R.L, Milan, Italy

© The Author(s), under exclusive license to Springer Nature Switzerland AG 2023 161
J. R. Thomas et al. (eds.), *Career Options in the Pharmaceutical and Biomedical Industry*, https://doi.org/10.1007/978-3-031-14911-5_9

industry. As evidence of this, we can mention what was reported by the MSL Society: "according to a 2018 global MSL Society survey, 68% of managers plan to expand the size of their MSL teams within the next two years." (https://www.themsls.org/what-is-an-msl/).

Together with the increasing complexity of marketed products, there had been other important changes in healthcare systems. In fact, pharmaceutical decision-makers shifted from prescribing physicians to pharmacy and therapeutics committees. Consequently, the MSLs elevated the quality of relationship, starting to work with both key opinion leaders (KOLs) and decision-makers to focus not on product sales, but on advancing standards of care and on optimizing patient outcome (Morgan et al. 2000). According to Pharma Market Network, "Key Opinion Leaders are physicians who influence their peers' medical practice, including but not limited to prescribing behaviour." (https://www.pharma-mkting.com/glossary/?name_directory_startswith=K)

Recently, some companies began to refer to KOLs as key external experts (KEE) or therapy area experts (TAE) to better emphasize their expertise in a specific field.

Anyway, it is important to point out that there is a big difference between companies in the way the role is conceived. In fact, there is currently no standard definition of it. If we make a quick research on the web, we will find different interpretations, some of them focusing more on communication skills required to create strong business relationship with the stakeholders, while other ones concentrate more on specific scientific skills of the MSL.

I personally believe that the meaning of the "mission" for an MSL simply lies in the name: a professional working in the *medical* department, with a deep *scientific* background and knowledge, acting to create *liaison* between the company and the relevant external stakeholders.

In addition, as we will see later, this role really depends on the life cycle of the products; therefore, in a same company, we can assist to a temporary increase or decrease of MSLs demand at different times.

Apart from the different definitions, it is clear that, despite being born from a commercial department, the MSL nowadays is a non-promotional role, independent of sales representatives and marketing colleagues (Koot et al. 2019), although in a context of cross-functional collaboration. Nevertheless, it is questionable whether the stakeholders are aware of this difference. Between June 2019 and January 2020, three Spanish Scientific Societies invited their members to participate in a survey developed by the MSL task force of AMIFE (Asociación de Medicina de la Industria Farmacéutica Española) to address the knowledge of the MSL role. Interestingly, more than 70% of HCPs (healthcare professionals) knew the MSL role and were able to differentiate the MSL role from others in marketing/sales departments. Another encouraging result emerging from the same survey is that the KOLs agreed on the importance to create partnership with the MSLs in developing scientific projects (de Castillo et al. 2021).

9.2 How Do I Become a Medical Science Liaison?

At this point, perhaps you are curious to know how you can start a career in this field. Indeed, there is not only one way to start working in the medical affairs department. With regard to education, you will need to prove to have a high scientific education in life sciences, for example, a PharmD, PhD, medical, or relevant scientific degree, but the minimum requirements are set by the companies that might decide to require a specific education or knowledge in a distinctive therapeutic area.

In most cases, a minimum experience in the role is required, but there are also opportunities for entry-level candidates. In the last case, the educational aspects need to be particularly strong. An experience as a researcher or a previous career as a clinician could be positively considered by recruiters.

There are also some specializing courses or Master programs useful to understand the role and to get ready for the interview, even if they are not mandatory.

Another possibility to become MSL goes through the promotion from other roles within the company. Essentially, in my experience, the background of MSLs I used to work with can be divided into two groups:

- Sales representatives who showed a particular aspiration and suitable skills to be part of the medical affairs department
- Clinical research associates or other roles within the clinical operations department

The first group may be compared to the case of the first MSLs selected at the Upjohn Company. Sometimes, I heard about companies that tend not to hire people from sales department, even if they are a minority. In my opinion, a previous experience in a field role can certainly ease territory management. This means, for example, ability to reach and approach the stakeholder for the first time, being able to move around different departments of hospitals. In fact, even if it may seem obvious, it is not immediate to get used to field life!

A clinical research associate (CRA, also called "monitor") is a professional who oversees all aspects of clinical trial conduct (http://www.clinicalresearchassociatecra.com/cra/). In fact, he/she is responsible for monitoring clinical studies at investigational sites according to all applicable regulatory requirements. The CRA can be a pharmaceutical company's employee or employed in specific companies, called contract research organizations (CRO), that provide research services to pharmaceutical companies.

The progressive transition from an in-house model of clinical development department to an outsourced one may also have contributed to the increase of MSL demand as an essential contact point between the sponsor, the CRO, and the KOLs in the management of sponsored clinical trials (https://themsljournal.com/article/msl-and-cra-a-responsibility-model-for-the-efficiency-of-clinical-research-and-clinical-trials/).

In some way, the MSL could be seen as a "natural evolution" for CRA's career. Some argue that the roles are quite similar, but there are important and significant differences I would like to explore with you.

In general, the CRA role is more technical compared to the MSL role in which communication skills are crucial and prevail. The CRA manages all aspects of a sponsored clinical study. When he/she plans a monitoring visit at an investigational site (hospital), he/she usually spends the whole day there, meeting the entire team involved into the study: the pharmacist for study drug check, the clinical engineer for equipment testing, the principal investigator (PI), and sub-investigators to perform site trainings and review study documentation. In addition, the CRA organizes and verifies material shipment at/from the site and focuses on the most important activities of a monitor: source data verification and electronic case report form (eCRF) review. All these activities don't require a continuous presence of site staff during the visit. Therefore, as it is often the case, the PI provides the CRA with a space for his permanence and makes himself available when necessary.

In contrast, the MSL works closely with the stakeholders on different medical projects, not only clinical studies: he/she goes to a hospital specifically to meet a stakeholder or diverse stakeholders involved in different projects at the same site.

9.3   Who Are the Stakeholders?

We commonly refer to the stakeholders to indicate people with whom the MSL interacts. It is important to note that the MSL works very much with the internal stakeholders (i.e., colleagues of the same company) that are, indeed, more diversified than the external ones (Fig. 9.1). This makes sense if we think about the peculiar role of the MSL as a "bridge" between external healthcare environment and the company from a strategic point of view. As a result, he/she has to liaise with different internal departments, even if most of his/her time is spent on field.

With regard to the external stakeholders, the MSL is a reactive role. This is true in the context of scientific therapeutic exchange, where interaction is based on an unsolicited request on a specific topic requested by the stakeholder. Note that the communications of the MSL must be non-promotional, scientific, and balanced. In addition, the MSL, in contrast to the sales representative colleagues, can respond to unsolicited off-label requests, that means for unapproved indications or pre-approval information.

On the other hand, the MSL may ask the stakeholder for an introduction meeting or engage him in some medical projects, such as involvement of a KOL in a sponsored clinical trial. These types of activities are, by definition, proactive. Anyway, it is the choice of the companies to establish the level and borders of proactive interactions of the medical affairs personnel.

Fig. 9.1 Graphic representation of MSL internal and external stakeholders

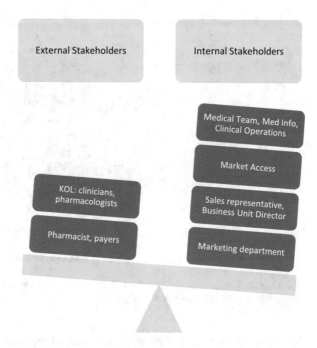

9.4   What Are the Activities Carried Out by the Medical Science Liaison?

To become familiar with the MSL activities, first of all it has to be highlighted that they can be extremely variable between different companies, but also within the same company at different times. In fact, the role needs to be very versatile as it is a key strategic function.

The difference between the activities of sales representatives and medical science liaisons is not just about being promotional or not.

If we focus on the development of a new drug and its launch on the market, it is interesting to note, for example, that work effort of the two figures changes a lot over time. Based on my experience, I tried to graphically represent this aspect in Fig. 9.2. The MSL gradually reduces his activity over the product life cycle, whereas the sales representative starts and exponentially increases his activity from launch on the market onward.

The MSL starts to work on launching a drug long before the launch date. This is even more true if the company works in a new or complex therapeutic area. One of the most important strategic tasks to be conducted is the so-called KOL identification and mapping. In fact, it is crucial to identify and to foster collaboration with the external experts who are, as already anticipated, people with expertise in the therapeutic area of interest for the company. Based on medical needs identified by the medical affairs department, the "KOL identification" will allow the medical affairs personnel to engage the proper KOL to fill in scientific gaps. In other words,

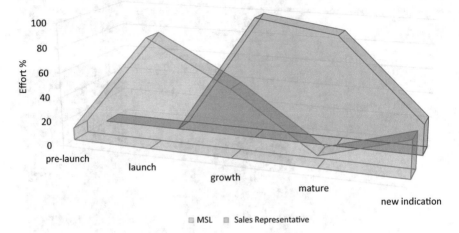

Fig. 9.2 Graphical representation of the different work efforts between MSL (blue) and sales representative (red) in launching of a new drug

the MSL, by interacting with the KOL, tries to understand his area of scientific interest and whether the company can partner with him. In addition, "KOL mapping" will allow to establish the level of recognition between peers (international, national, or local) and the network through which the KOLs interact.

After launch, MSL activities will slowly decrease, even if he/she can reactivate his/her effort if new indications are foreseen to be available. In fact, the MSL can present, upon request, information about clinical development programs and often takes part to the pre-feasibility process for phase 3 clinical trials. In this case, the MSL, but in general the medical affairs personnel, will work closely with the clinical department (internally, or with outsourced CRO) to identify the best researchers to run a sponsored clinical trial. This type of studies is often international, so managed at global level. This facilitates a cross-country collaboration and MSL involvement in international activities.

An important task of the MSL is to support clinicians who want to carry out an independent study on a company's drug. These studies are called investigator-initiated trials (IIT), or investigator sponsored trials (IST). While maintaining complete independence on the study protocol design, the MSL is the main contact point to liaise between the company and researchers if any kind of support (e.g., financial, drug supply) is requested by the clinician. Each company will set up a specific procedure to evaluate if it is possible to support clinicians.

Within the context of therapeutic exchange with external experts, it is not unusual that the KOL asks the MSL to conduct a hospital meeting within his department, even before the launch of a new drug. Based on specific needs identified by the KOL, the MSL will present data on different topics, such as disease aspects, unmet needs, and pharmacological and clinical data of a specific drug.

In some way, the MSL can be considered the arm of the medical lead on field. In fact, he/she is one of the most important resources for the company for insights gathering. By collecting and processing insights from field, the company is able to understand healthcare environment with its changes and can adapt its strategy to new dynamics. For the great contribution that he/she can bring, the MSL often takes part in cross-functional meetings with sales, marketing, and market access departments to discuss, for example, brand plan implementation at local level.

The MSL continuously collaborates with key roles within the medical affairs department (e.g., medical lead, medical advisor) for implementation of medical projects, such as national or local advisory boards.

Being an MSL requires the highest level of scientific/medical knowledge. This means that some of the time has to be dedicated to self-study, including literature update. A very useful way permitting both to keep up to date and gathering insights is participation at congresses/symposia. At the end of these events, a scientific report is usually drafted and shared within the medical affairs department. In many companies, the MSLs also support the medical presence at international congresses.

With regard to the internal stakeholders, the MSL is always available to provide the commercial field force with internal scientific training, especially for colleagues who share the same territories with the MSL.

Finally, depending on the companies' structure, the MSL interacts with global functions and can participate in cross-country working groups and activities, such as journal clubs.

As I mentioned at the beginning, depending on life cycles of products and company assets, the MSL can be more focused on specific activities. Not only activities, but also MSLs number can vary over time in the same company to meet the needs of a specific moment. Based on MSL team size and where they are located, the extent of territories to be covered can be established. Anyway, an MSL usually manages big areas, more than one region. This should be considered, since time spent for travel is generally considerable; it is also requested to be available for overnight staying and, sometimes, flexibility to work during the weekend since some congresses cover partially Saturdays or Sundays.

As you might have noticed, the figure of the MSL is involved in many activities, but I would also like to highlight that the role has much more to do with quality than quantity.

9.5   Planning of MSL Activities

Since the MSL is a reactive role, there is obviously a certain degree of flexibility and uncertainty in defining in advance the percentage work effort to be dedicated to the various activities. Anyway, some companies may hypothesize it in order to guide the MSL in planning and reporting of weekly activities. In Fig. 9.3 you can find an example of how an MSL plan looks like.

MSL Plan

1. Field activities/virtual interactions ~ 65%
   - Therapeutic info exchange
   - Reactive hospital meetings (HM)
   - Clinical trial related activities (IIT, sponsored clinical trials)
   - Congresses/educational events participation
   - Advisory board

2. Internal activities (home office) ~ 25%
   - Home study, trainings, and scientific update
   - Field medical project planning
   - Administrative tasks (e.g., expense report)

3. Internal meetings ~ 10%
   - Medical meetings
   - Journal Club
   - Training to colleagues
   - Company meetings

Fig. 9.3 Example of an MSL plan

In addition, depending on the company's structure and pipeline, the MSLs can be responsible for more than one product; consequently, another aspect that can be considered in defining an MSL plan is the different percentage work effort on different products.

9.6 Hard and Soft Skills Required

Recruiters for jobs require both hard and soft skills from the candidates. They are, respectively, technical competencies required to play a specific role (such as a particular degree, number of languages needed, or the wealth of experience) and behavioral aspects that have more to do with personality.

To establish long-term peer-to-peer scientific relationship with the KOLs, the MSL needs a strong scientific background. As I already anticipated, talking about hard skills, the companies set a minimum level of education needed; in general a master's degree in life science is required. An advanced degree, such as a PharmD, MD, or PhD, in research is a plus.

In addition, considering the increasing involvement of the MSL in global activities, such as working groups, best practices sharing and journal clubs, an advanced English level is needed. Therefore, if you want to apply for a medical science liaison position, bear in mind that a part of the intake interview is usually held in English.

Regarding soft skills, as you may imagine after reading the previous paragraphs, managing many activities in large areas requires an excellent organizational ability. It is essential to set priorities to plan weekly activities, optimizing traveling time and field colleagues' requests. As anticipated, the MSL will spend most of the time on field, and, sometimes, overlapping internal urgent activities to be managed occurs. This requires a high level of flexibility and availability to change plans quickly.

The MSL is characterized by having strong presentation skills, and speaks clearly and in a credible way, focusing on the main concepts and bearing in mind he/she is in a non-promotional role. He/she is also a skillful communicator, with persuasion ability to lead the discussion and very good listening skills. To gather useful insights from interactions with the healthcare professionals, the MSL should be provided with so-called business acumen, that is, the ability to identify the best opportunities for the company. In fact, he/she usually receives many requests from the field, and it is not always possible to fulfill all of them. Therefore, he/she has to be able to evaluate and report the most profitable ones from a strategic point of view.

Finally, remember that one of the missions of the MSL is to act as a "liaison" between the company and the healthcare environment. This requires both a good attitude to build and maintain strong professional relationships with the healthcare professionals (networking skill) and proactively contributing to a continued internal info exchange (teamworking skill).

I tried to cover the most important hard and soft skills to be considered as a valuable medical scientific liaison, but, of course, any other personal skill will help you in your daily work.

9.7 Future Perspective

The pharmaceutical and healthcare environments are constantly evolving. In addition, we live in a complex and uncertain world. The last 2 years have significantly affected our life and way of working, especially if we think about the field roles' need to interact with clinicians who have been on the front line in dealing with the pandemic (COVID-19). Social distancing has forced us to find new ways to communicate with the stakeholders and led to rapid development of digital interactions. Some companies have been wondering what we learned from the pandemic time; therefore, it is possible that the MSL engagement with healthcare professionals will evolve in some way. Obviously, virtual interactions have *pro* and *cons*, so they will unlikely completely replace face-to-face interactions. In my opinion, it is possible that they will coexist and the MSL will learn how to make the best of them, maintaining openness to both possibilities according to the different scenarios he/she will face.

9.8 Conclusion

In this chapter, the role of the medical scientific liaison was explored. It is a function that is acquiring increasing strategical importance in the pharmaceutical companies.

Starting from the origin of this role, I provided you with information on "field life" of an MSL, the various internal and external stakeholders with whom he/she interacts, the most important activities he/she is responsible for, and main skills required by interviewers. With regard to the last point, an experience abroad will be considered very positively by recruiters (this is true for any kind of role you are applying for).

It is important to remember that the MSL will act differently depending on the companies' structure and size, whether they are big pharma or mid-size pharma or start-up. Each company will establish characteristics, activities, number, and general profile of its MSL team.

As general tips, applicable for different roles, I would also like to tell you to maintain an attitude of openness to different opportunities that will arise (I did not even know of the existence of this figure during my university studies and now I love it!). It is not easy to be hired from the beginning in the desired role, but remember that you could start and then change department and roles within the pharmaceutical company if you prove to have the right skills that fit with the role. In this case, a new role always requires a change of mentality and demands patience, so give yourself time to take on new responsibilities.

Finally, it is also important to take care of building your working network with colleagues and recruiters and make yourself available on the professional network platform.

I hope that this journey within the role of the medical scientific liaison will help you to have a clearer picture of how this figure can contribute to the company's success. I have just to say "good luck!" to you.

References

de Castillo G et al (2021) The medical science liaison role in Spain: a survey about the. Opinion of HealthCare Professionals

Gupta SK, Nayak RP (2013) An insight into the emerging role of regional medical advisor in the pharmaceutical industry. Perspect Clin Res 4:186–190

https://medicalaffairsspecialist.org/what-is-an-msl visited on 09 Jan 2022

https://www.themsls.org/what-is-an-msl/ visited on 15 Jan 2022

https://www.pharma-mkting.com/glossary/?name_directory_startswith=K visited on 29 Jan 2022

http://www.clinicalresearchassociatecra.com/cra/ visited on 22 Jan 2022

https://themsljournal.com/article/msl-and-cra-a-responsibility-model-for-the-efficiency-of-clinical-research-and-clinical-trials/ visited on 24 Jan 2022

Koot D et al (2019) Medical science liaisons (MSL) in Africa: a perspective. Pan Afr Med J 33:313

Morgan KD, Domann DE, Collins GE, Massey KL, Moss RJ (2000) History and evolution of field-based medical programs. Drug Inf J 34:1049–1052

Chapter 10
Career Development for Physicians in the Biopharmaceutical Industry

Anke Van den broeck and Ann Dhoore

Abstract Although the pharmaceutical industry is in need of physicians and can offer them great career opportunities, only few physicians make the switch due to insufficient information. In this chapter, we address the most common questions with regard to this unknown career path and give more clarity on what can be expected in the short and long term.

10.1 Introduction

Being a doctor does not limit you to working in immediate patient care. The opportunities after medicine studies are much more varied than many are aware of. One of these opportunities is a career in the pharmaceutical industry. Although physicians are highly valued profiles for a large variety of roles within the pharmaceutical industry, only very few doctors take the step (Erikson et al. 2009).

One of the reasons is the lack of information. It is fair to say that working in the pharmaceutical industry is very different from working in individual patient care and as the medical curriculum barely includes information beyond a clinical career, physicians who consider the switch are confronted with many questions on which it is often very difficult to receive a clear answer.

Therefore, we would like to answer the following questions in this chapter:

1. Why would a physician choose a career within the pharmaceutical industry?
2. What to expect as a physician working in the pharmaceutical industry?

A. Van den broeck (✉)
Amgen Belgium & Luxemburg, Brussels, Belgium

AstraZeneca BeLux, Groot-Bijgaarden, Belgium
e-mail: anke.vandenbroeck@astrazeneca.com

A. Dhoore
Amgen Belgium & Luxemburg, Brussels, Belgium

Grimbergen, Belgium

3. When do I take the step and what do I need?
4. How do I develop my career, and what are key factors for success?

10.2 Why Would a Physician Choose a Career Within the Pharmaceutical Industry?

The pharmaceutical industry plays a pivotal role in providing healthcare for patients and developing medicines and equipment for use. It is a key asset to the European economy and is growing year over year leading to a growth in employment rates and therefore an increased need for highly educated profiles (Data center: Pharmaindustry-R&D 2022).

- As a doctor, you have *unique qualifications* to work in the pharma sector:

    The medicine curriculum is unique as it combines scientific knowledge and clinical experience. This wide knowledge of the human body, diseases, and therapeutic approaches is an important asset as it allows you to be(come) an expert in many domains. Moreover, during your internships, you have learned to solve complex and challenging problems, to make decisions, and to closely monitor their impact.

    As a doctor, it is crucial to work with high ethical standards where the patient is in a central position. You collaborate with people from diverse professional and personal backgrounds, whereby it is also crucial that you adapt your communication style according to your stakeholder.

    Finally, it is crucial for the pharmaceutical industry to have a good relationship with the medical community, whereby you can interact with your colleagues as a physician.

    This mix of scientific and soft skills, combined with an interest in scientific innovation and a high ethical standard, is very important in the pharma industry. In some countries, some responsibilities within the pharma industry are therefore legally linked to having obtained a medical diploma.

- The pharmaceutical industry can be a *unique employer.*

    Although a clinical career is considered the most obvious option during medicine studies, it does not give job satisfaction to everyone. For some, it is already obvious during their basic medical training, others experience this during their specialization (advanced master's degree) or even much later in their career.

A better work-life balance and flexibility are one of the reasons (Lahiry and Gattu 2020) for doctors to make the switch, but there are many more drivers (Sweiti et al. 2019):

1. The pharmaceutical industry has a significant effect on healthcare at population level, so beyond individual patient level. As a co-worker of a pharmaceutical company, you can contribute to bring benefit to society and make a greater difference for the patients in general. You can focus on those domains with a

high medical need where you as a clinical doctor are confronted with a lack of therapeutic possibilities.

2. It is an innovative, dynamic, and fast-paced environment that is intellectually stimulating and is based on intense collaboration between different roles, including an intense collaboration with the medical community. One example of the continuous change is how clinical development has evolved over the last decades and continues to transform (IQVIA report: The changing landscape of Research and Development 2019).

3. Talent development is a crucial pillar of the pharmaceutical industry. If you are interested in management skills, in strategy development, or in other personal development, it is certainly an environment where you can develop leadership and other professional and soft skills (see below). Personal development is however never a one-way direction: the company will invest in you, but of course expects you to work professionally and ensure good return on investment.

4. Career planning and adapting your objectives to your individual needs, interests, and stage of life are possible. It is important to realize that when you make the switch towards the pharma industry, a world of opportunities will open up for you. This can address the need for flexibility and work-life balance, but it also requires flexibility from you. We will discuss later on how you drive your career development. In addition, pharmaceutical companies tend to offer competitive and performance-based salaries.

The pharmaceutical industry has a wide range of opportunities for physicians:

- On the one hand, there are *various departments* in which you can work as a doctor, such as:

  – Clinical research/drug discovery
  – Clinical drug development
  – Medical affairs
  – Clinical pharmacology
  – Pharmacovigilance/safety
  – Sales and marketing department
      In these departments, there are also several positions that can be considered, and this list is not exhaustive. Many of these departments are described elsewhere in this book. A distinction can be made between an entry job—the first job within the industry—and jobs that you perform later in your career.

- On the other hand, there is also a *wide range of companies and disease areas*. A same role can be very different because of the portfolio that falls within the responsibilities, but also because of the type of organization. A distinction is often made between big pharma and smaller pharmaceutical companies or start-ups:

  – *Big pharma* is a term used to describe global pharmaceutical companies (many having their central offices in the USA) that have growing influence over the practice of medicine worldwide. The big pharma companies have a broad range of products in many disease areas and offer clearly defined positions with extensive responsibilities in a solid framework. Some also make a

distinction between a pharmaceutical company, with products on a chemical basis and a biotech company with medicines on a biological basis, but nowadays many biotech companies do much broader activities and vice versa.
- *Smaller pharmaceutical companies* often focus on specific therapeutic areas and niche markets. Roles in small pharma companies could be more combined roles, with responsibilitles for fewer products. Since healthcare is a very dynamic, innovative industry, there are also many start-ups, such as spin-offs from research organizations.

10.3   What to Expect as a Physician Working in the Pharmaceutical Industry?

The pharmaceutical industry and clinical practice are very different. One of the most notable differences is that direct patient contact is no longer part of the daily routine of physicians in the pharmaceutical industry. Some companies do offer options for physicians to practice clinical medicine part-time or fulfill their academic duties, but this is rather limited and might be particularly helpful for physicians during their transitional period. Instead of direct patient contact, in the pharma industry, you contribute to the development of therapeutics for thousands of patients at a time, thereby having a medical impact on a larger scale.

This also has an impact on individual recognition: instead of direct patient-doctor gratitude, projects in pharma are often long-term efforts and some projects have a more indirect impact. For example, you may create high-quality educational materials that can be used by others.

High quality is also not always a guarantee for high success rates, for example, during reimbursement discussions where many other factors besides the quality of the reimbursement dossier play a role.

Projects and deliverables are also seldom the responsibility of one individual but rather team efforts. Teams often consist of people with different roles, but also with different backgrounds, working together in partnership without a hierarchical ladder. The decision-making process can therefore be very different from what a doctor is used to in clinical practice.

As a result, the working day naturally looks completely different, with scientific study being part of the core activities, and—depending on the position—a large part of the day being spent on meetings. Back-to-back meetings are common, but in general, the days are easier to plan and there is a higher degree of flexibility. The components of a working day are of course highly dependent of your role and can therefore vary during your career. When you develop, for example, into a people manager position, your activities will be influenced by the needs of your team.

As in any other industry, priorities and tactics in the pharmaceutical industry are set according to the objectives, and performance is measured using key performance indicators.

And finally, as in any other innovative industry, setbacks are part of the dynamic environment. The overall likelihood of approval for products from Phase 1 was 7.9% in 2011–2020, and this does not even include the reimbursement procedure (Bowden et al. 2021). As a consequence, every physician in the pharma industry will be confronted with changes, from a minimal change in product portfolio to major reorganizations during his career. Also independent from the development success rate, acquisitions and mergers are relatively common in the pharma sector. This should nevertheless not be an area of concern as in every change there is a new opportunity.

Despite the major differences between pharma and clinical practice, it is also important to highlight the similarities. The most striking similarity is that physicians in both fields are dedicated to improving the lives of patients. *A physician is still a physician in the pharmaceutical industry* (Weihrauh 2000). To achieve this, both disciplines require strong scientific knowledge and knowledge of clinical practice and patient pathways. Strong knowledge requires continuous education and learning, but equally strong collaboration with the medical community. Therefore, physicians in the pharmaceutical industry continue to collaborate with experts in academia across different fields, for example, as part of their involvement in clinical trials.

10.4   When Do I Take the Step and What Do I Need?

When a physician considers to switch to the pharmaceutical industry, the most frequently asked questions are the following:

- When is the best timing?
- Is additional training/education needed?
- How do I get started?

The best timing to switch is determined by (1) your personal conviction about the switch and (2) the right preparation.

• With the information above, we have tried to fill part of the information gap, but in order to have an even better picture, we recommend you talk to several people who have made the switch. Physicians that work in the pharma are an important source of information on the differences between the career paths and on expectation management. As mentioned, everyone has his/her own story, and all these different perspectives will help you to find out better what to expect.

There are examples of doctors returning to their original job because the role within the industry was not what they had imagined, so it is not impossible, but we believe this can be avoided by better information.

Only late in my career, after the completion of my Advanced Master in Specialist Medicine and my PhD, I made the switch. Some people ask me if I consider my Master in Surgery as a waste of time, but I needed this time to feel that a clinical career was not my best option: I needed my PhD to experience a nonclinical career and I needed to finish my education to experience the impact of being accountable for the patient. Moreover, I still benefit from the skills that I acquired during my training. In retrospect, I did take a risk because I was not well informed, and therefore I stress the importance of understanding the different aspects of a career in the pharma industry.

- The right preparation is linked to the frequently asked question whether additional training is needed, such as a PhD, a business school, a specialty, and a training in pharmacology. It is important to make a distinction between what is and is not necessary for a certain role. Each role has a specific job description including requirements on competences that one has to meet. In addition, in the model of LifeLongLearning (see below), personal growth never stops and competences can also be acquired during your career.

For an entry-level job in pharma, a scientific background is a standard requirement. A Master in Medicine degree is therefore sufficient. We personally consider additional clinical experience to be of great value, and therefore we would be in favor of starting an Advanced Master in Family Medicine or a Advanced Master in Specialist Medicine. As mentioned, a good understanding of clinical practice is necessary in the pharmaceutical sector, and this clinical experience can hardly be acquired afterward through additional training. Moreover, you build up a clinical network, which can be very useful afterward in the collaboration with the medical community. Some job descriptions also require experience within the pharma industry or at least with clinical trials, so clinical experience with trial execution can address this requirement.

How much clinical experience is needed, so whether or not you need to finish this additional master, and which discipline you would choose, is individually very different.

The Pharmaceutical Medicine Specialty training is a separate education developed to become a pharmaceutical physician. It offers a broad preparation for a role in the pharma industry (Setia 2018). In the UK, it is one of the fastest-growing medical specialties, but this specialty is currently only recognized in a small number of European countries (UK, Switzerland, and Ireland), and is therefore not required.

Other common additional degrees, such as a PhD or a business school, can certainly provide additional competences and skills—such as presentation skills or business acumen—but these can also be acquired later, so they are not strictly necessary.

In addition, it is important to mention that technical competences are only one part of the story. As mentioned, collaboration is crucial within the pharmaceutical industry. An evaluation of your soft skills, such as communication, positive attitude, critical thinking, teamwork, ethical behavior, etc., will certainly be part of the assessment when you apply for a certain job. To guide you, these are also often mentioned in the job description.

To conclude, you should not worry about the best timing, as the timing to switch to pharma is only important for your own decision-making process and does not affect your career opportunities. A career within the pharmaceutical industry is dynamic and many factors play a role, as explained in more details in the next section.

When you are convinced that a career in the pharmaceutical industry is right for you, a wealth of possibilities opens up: different functions and/or different companies. Therefore, take your time to understand the specifics of the role and the values of the company, and use recruitment agencies, but also people in the field to guide you. LinkedIn is a good way to make connections, and there is certainly a great willingness to share information.

10.5 How Do I Develop My Career, and What Are Key Factors for Success?

Working life on average spans between 35 and 45 years which is the majority of our adult life. And we all prefer to do so in a way which fulfills our aspirations. These aspirations are however very individual and are influenced by different variables including our *personal situation in life*. In a very traditional way, career development is seen as a way to acquire increasing responsibilities and authority. It is however our view that in order to have a long-lasting and fulfilling working situation, one should take into account that careers can and will have a less linear evolution.

People can maybe move out of a role or a company and move in again, and they may stop working for a while and resume work again or work as employee or as independent consultant, move between working regimes which can be very different from the classical full time or 50–90% etc.

Most of us work to have an income which allows us to lead the life we aspire. Having a good compensation and benefits package is important. However, based on our experience, the most motivated and engaged employees are those who find that there is a *good alignment between the mission, vision, and values (M/V/V) of the company and of their supervisor(s) and their own values*. This alignment is, for instance, measured by the Great Place To Work (GPTW)$^{©}$ index. This is all the more relevant in those sectors where the "War for Talent" is high, as is the case for the biopharmaceutical industry. So before joining a company, we would advise candidate employees to make an analysis of the M/V/V: most companies will clearly describe them on their website. And set up meetings with current and (even better) former employees of the company: what do/did they like in their company, what are the challenges, etc. A well-informed start is already the good beginning of a hopefully motivating "career."

10.5.1 You Drive Your Career Development

As mentioned, there is no "one-size-fits-all" model for career development. As a result, *you will be expected to drive your own development*. Having a good collaboration with your supervisor is key, but in this world of "remote" working, it is sometimes easier to have *a network of advisors*, with some of whom you can have face-to-face meetings. This can be somebody from the human resources department of the company or a formal or informal mentor.

While it is important to be very clear about your career aspirations and training needs, it is also important to bear in mind *certain assumptions of your employer*:

- ROI (return on investment): while you can dream about having a steep evolution in your career, most companies have a (often unwritten) rule that you need to have "performed" in a certain role before moving to another one. A timeline of *18 to 24 months* of being in the same role is often seen as a minimum, but this can of course depend on the opportunities (see below).
- Successful performance: you cannot expect from a company to move you into another role, and especially not if this role will entail having more responsibilities, if you are not delivering up to standards in your current role.
- Manage your boss: very often a manager does not like to see one of the team members leave, especially not when this is a high-performing individual. It is good to have this in mind, when expressing your ambitions, and ensure that you will not leave a void once leaving the team or the role.

10.5.2 CMO Model

One of the models used in career development, is the so-called CMO model: *C = Competences, M = Motivation and O = Opportunities* (Fig. 10.1)

10.5.2.1 Competences or Skills

As a medical doctor, you have already acquired an important amount of *knowledge*. This knowledge is however mostly focused on the immediate treatment of and interaction with patients. Working for a biopharmaceutical company requires an additional set of *competences or skills*. Some of these are needed to be successful in every role that you will have, and others are linked to the role that you want to evolve into. Below you will find a short description of some of the most common competences.

1. Business Acumen

   Depending on *the life cycle of the company, the business model will be different*. A start-up company with a limited number of molecules will have

Fig. 10.1 CMO model

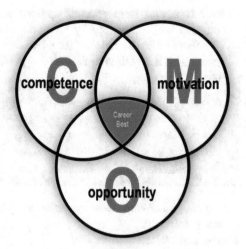

different challenges than what a well-established company with products in different stages of their life cycle (pre-launch, launch, on the market, post patent, etc.) will experience. Most companies will inform their collaborators on a regular basis about the financial results and expectations. It is key to acquire an in-depth understanding of these numbers, and the business challenges and opportunities of your company. The good news is that most (if not all) companies will offer a good training about this in the course of your career. In addition to this, working for a biopharma company requires adhering to strict rules and standard operating procedures (SOP). Every new starter will have to complete a whole set of trainings, such as a "Code of Conduct." These trainings will give a first glance at all the different aspects of working within a biopharmaceutical company.

2. Cross-functional collaboration

Irrespective of the role you will be in, you will be required to work with many different people. And in general, a biopharmaceutical company has very *different types of personalities*, unlike the academic or scientific world where you might find a larger concentration of certain typologies of people. It is important, and very often eye-opening (and fun), to have an assessment of your own personality. This can be done by an assessor accredited by companies such as Insights® and MBTI®, but you can also use an online (and free) tool such as 16 personalities (http://www.16personalities.com). Cross-functional collaboration is almost always easier and more successful when you understand what your colleague needs or why (s)he reacts in a certain way.

3. Therapeutic Knowledge

As a medical doctor, you will be expected to be the subject matter expert of the therapeutic area in which you will operate. Sometimes you will join the company having indeed already specialized in a certain field (such as oncology, diabetes, neurology, etc.), but very often in the course of a career, you will move into different therapeutic domains. Also, disease management is in constant evolution, so it is key to keep yourself updated on these evolutions. And while your company will most probably give you access to a lot of information, and you will (hopefully) be able to attend national and international congresses and seminars, it is key to invest sufficient (personal) time on this.

> *We once recruited a young talent who told us that her hobby was reading professional literature. While we thought that this might be a sign of being somebody who is really narrow-minded (which she wasn't at all), she was very rapidly recognized both locally and internationally to be the real Subject Matter Expert.*

Being passionate about what you are working for will quickly be recognized and appreciated.

4. Stakeholder Management

Another important competence when working for a biopharmaceutical company is managing internal and external stakeholders.

- Internal stakeholders: members of your team, the commercial team, colleagues from headquarters, health economics team, clinical development, etc.
- External stakeholders: government authorities, regulatory bodies, healthcare professionals including prescribers, etc.

In order to be able to represent your company in the best way, it is key to develop your competences on how to speak with stakeholders and *create solid networks* on which you can rely and with whom you can collaborate in the most optimal way. Certain people have a natural ability to create such relationships, but even than it is important to know the boundaries of what can be done and what is not compliant.

Pre-corona most of the stakeholder management was done in a face-to-face setting, which for many people is easier than *in the virtual setting*. After 2 years of Covid, we have seen certain people thrive in this newly developed competence and become role model and advisor to their peers.

5. Presentation Skills

Unless you have been a PhD student, or have followed a special degree in Business Management and may have been required to make presentations to diverse audiences, you may not have had a real opportunity to acquire experience in making professional presentations. And while this is a crucial competence, for certain people, presenting in front of large audiences may be a real challenge. And having to do so virtually is not necessarily easier, We would even argue to the contrary. But the good news is that this is again a competence which can be learned. There are lots of trainings available to help you making snappy presentations which capture and keep the attention of your audience. And you can even get trained on using your voice in the best possible way, and using appropriate body language.

6. Other competences

Above you will find just a few of the more general competences which are needed to be successful in a pharmaceutical company. Depending on the role you aspire to move into, you may need to focus on developing other skills. Some of these skills can be acquired during (rotational) assignments, certain can be learned throughout company offered programs, and yet other ones will require classroom training. On the different ways of learning, see Sect. 10.5.2.4. Some of the examples include (but are not limited to): people management, digital capabilities, health economics, financial analysis, and marketing and sales.

10.5.2.2 Motivation

At the age of 18, when starting higher education, many of us do/did not have a precise idea of what we would like to do in life.

By studying general medicine or any other scientific degree, related to the human body, your ambition probably was to do something concretely with the knowledge you acquired, but as you have read in the other chapters, there are so many different ways in which you can apply your knowledge. And once you have decided to join a biopharma company, you will find that there are so many opportunities which you can pursue. It is therefore crucial to make a good analysis of what it is that really makes your eyes shine. This is very much linked to your *core talents and your personality traits*.

A core talents analysis will help you discover your character (personality or "who you are"), your talents (potential or "what you could be with training and/or practice"), and your motivation (desire, or "what you yourself want") in a very detailed and nuanced way. Exploring more in depth those personality traits will help you discover the things, jobs, projects etc. that give you most of your energy.

Example: if you really like to see the big picture, take risks and experiment new things, then don't go into a role which has a lot of repetition and needs a great sense for detail. Or another example: you like to be involved in a task which needs a lot of attention, is quite predictable, and you can do on your own, and you are excited when the end result matches your expectation, you might probably be less happy in a role with more ambiguity and unpredictability. In the latter case, you were probably happy as a child to make complex puzzles, or endlessly build things with Lego.

So to phrase one of the coaches on core talents if your core talent is to become an apple, try to be the juiciest, most brilliant apple, and do not try to be a pear.

The above seems to be common sense, but we have seen too many people aspiring roles which did not fit their personality or talents. This may be linked to the perception that only certain roles will give you the highest prestige, power, and income.

So some of the things you may ask yourself are as follows:

- Do I like to manage people, and do I get excited to help them grow and work through others? Don't I mind being available for others even at less appropriate moments? Then you will probably be happy being or to become a *people manager*.
- Do I prefer to do things on my own, and do I always check the work of others, because I feel that I can and will do it better? Do I like to work at my own pace, and prefer not to be "bothered" too much by others? Then you will most probably thrive in a career as *individual contributor*.
- The good news is that both roles (People Manager and Individual Contributor) can have the same ranking and prestige.
- Am I interested in other cultures and healthcare systems, and do I like to travel (even though this has become less relevant due to the Covid pandemic and its restrictions)? Then you maybe want to move into a *global role*, become a *regional leader*, or aspire a role at *headquarters level.*
- Do I really want to become the expert in one domain, or do I like to move between different therapeutic domains?
- Etc.

10.5.2.3 Opportunities

Most companies have a whole array of developmental opportunities, and this is definitely also the case within the biopharmaceutical industry. Below you will find a brief overview of some of the steps you can take in your career. And our expectation is that—as career development is becoming much more flexible—those opportunities will only increase in the future.

Type	What is it	Advantages	Potential downsides
On-the-job training (OJT)	An OJT is a temporary assignment in another (type of) role. Very often this will be for the replacement of a person who is out for a certain period. But it can also be to launch a new project	Full focus on a new role Provides the opportunity to experience another role without committing to it on a more permanent basis	Uncertainty about the sustainability Duration may be too short to make good assessment Disappointment when going back to former role
Rotational assignment/ new starters program/ MBA class	Some companies recruit starters in their company by ways of a rotational program. This means that selected people can experience very different	Opportunity to experience a wide variety of roles within a pharma company Often combined with experience in other	Requires a lot of flexibility from the participant Duration of each of the assignments may be too short to have a really good impression of

(continued)

Type	What is it	Advantages	Potential downsides
	roles, some of which may even be abroad	affiliates or even other countries	what the role entails In most cases, the ROI is mainly for the participant, less so for the company High investment from the company, no guarantee on longer-term commitment from the participant
Stretch assignments	One of the most common ways to develop new competences is to take on a stretch assignment Examples: • Taking on the role of your supervisor in her/his absence • Taking additional responsibilities in a certain project • Reimbursement: besides writing the medical part, also work on the economic and marketing aspects of the product	You continue to do your own job, and can always fall back on it Opportunity to gain additional competences and experience new challenges	Often these stretch or additional assignments come on top of the normal workload, so this requires extra time investment from the participant without always being rewarded (from a monetary standpoint) for it It requires good time management and being able to juggle with sometimes competing priorities
Lateral move or promotion within the company	Most companies post the open positions on their internal website. If this is not the case, it is good to inquire with your HR department how you can get informed about them It is always good to be informed about the recruitment process (internal and external), who will be involved, what are the requirements	Moving into the next position within your own company has the advantage that you already know a lot of the procedures	Moving into your next position requires a certain flexibility: you give up what you know, and hopefully will be happy in the new role but there is no guarantee Moving back to an old role (sometimes lower level) can be possible if the role has not yet been backfilled, but will require sufficient maturity to not experience this as a "failure"
Moving into another company	There is of course the possibility to move into a role with another company	It can be very meaningful to experience the culture, procedures, etc. from another company Certain roles are not available within your own company so if you aspire one of those roles,	You leave behind something you know to move to the unknown. . . . And may regret this. But every new challenge represents a new opportunity Make sure to really understand what's

(continued)

Type	What is it	Advantages	Potential downsides
		you may need to move out	behind a certain role title—these can be misleading and may not cover your aspirations or expectations

10.5.2.4 70-20-10 Model

Learning does not and cannot stop once you have left the university, and many new competences will only be acquired once you have left the school environment. That's why we talk about LifeLongLearning.

But the differences with how you learned as a young adult and how you will continue to learn once you have started working in a professional environment are quite substantial.

You will still need to have a certain amount of "teacher-led" training, whether or not in a virtual environment, but this will only represent a minority of your learning activities.

In addition to this, it is always advised to do a lot of self-study. Most business schools provide excellent materials, and there are also lots of materials available on a whole variety of topics. You just have to "Google" a certain topic to get access to these materials. Many of them are for free, but if you want to go more in depth, the companies or schools will most probably require a subscription fee. Most pharma companies have negotiated company-wide licenses to such materials, so it is always good to first inquire what training and study materials are available within your company.

The 70-20-10 model (see picture below) states that by far the most effective training is acquired by on-the-job experiences. Once you have started in a certain area, function, or role, there is still so much that you will need to find out about it, and what is expected from you. On average, this takes about 3 to 6 months, but depending on the complexity of the role, it can even take up to 1 year. This is why many companies have a policy that you have to remain at least 24 months in a certain role, in order to have sufficient ROI.

And finally, another good way to learn is by listening to peers, getting advice from them, etc. The most meaningful learning activities are often those which happen during the meetings with peers from inside or outside the company, sharing best practices, but also mistakes to be avoided. It is quite impressive to see how much energy is wasted by "reinventing the wheel," whereas it can be so easy to "steel with pride." And this requires working on your networks and making sure that you keep your eyes and ears open for what is happening across the company or within your therapeutic domain. Often Best Sharing Practice (BSP) sessions are organized by the company, but you may want to set up your own networks or select certain seminars or congresses (virtual or in person) to attend (Fig. 10.2).

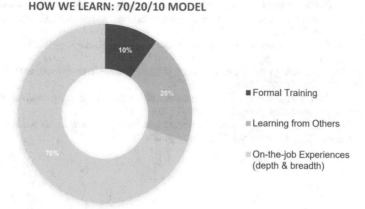

Fig. 10.2 Learning model

10.6   Conclusion

It is impossible to describe the perfect recipe for career development.

Working for a biopharma company is very exciting for a physician as you can have impact on the lives of many patients and as it can provide you many different career opportunities.

As mentioned above, there are so many variables and there is certainly not a "one-size-fits-all model," neither for the decision to make the switch, nor for the development of your career. In this chapter, we have nevertheless tried to give you many elements to consider in this journey.

There may however also be moments when you will have to face more difficult situations. The development of a pipeline product may be stopped; a very promising drug may not receive FDA or EMA approval, or may not be reimbursed at local level; your company may be acquired which may change your role; your role may be stopped due to restructuring; etc.

It is always good to understand the reasons behind those decisions, but it is just as important to move on and look ahead as new opportunities will always arise.

References

Bowden R, Chancellor D, Chaudhuri SE et al (2021) Clinical development success rates and contributing factors 2011–2020 report. https://qlstechnologies.com/research/. Accessed 2 Mar 2022

Data center: Pharmaindustry-R&D (2022). https://www.efpia.eu/publications/data-center. Accessed 2 Mar 2022

Erikson C et al (2009) Oncology workforce: results of the ASCO 2007 program directors survey. J Oncol Pract 5:62–65

IQVIA report: The changing landscape of Research and Development (2019). https://www.iqvia.com/insights/the-iqvia-institute/reports/the-changing-landscape-of-research-and-development. Accessed 2 Mar 2022

Lahiry S, Gattu S (2020) Real-world perspective on career of pharmaceutical physicians in India: a working report (2018). Perspect Clin Res 11:150–157

Setia S et al (2018) Evolving role of pharmaceutical physicians in medical evidence and education. Adv Med Educ Pract 9:777–790

Sweiti H et al (2019) Physicians in the pharmaceutical industry: their roles, motivations, and perspectives. Drug Discov Today 24(9):1865–1870

Weihrauh TR (2000) Career opportunities for female and male physicians in the pharmaceutical industry. Med Klin (Munich) 95(6):322–326

Part III
Opportunities in Supportive Functions

Chapter 11
Job and Career Opportunities in Regulatory Affairs/Science

Ann Emmerechts and Josse R. Thomas

Abstract This chapter focuses on job and career opportunities in Regulatory Affairs/Science in the biopharmaceutical industry, with some additional information on possible options in related industries and regulatory authorities.

As an introduction, the terms 'Regulatory Science' and 'Regulatory Affairs' are clarified.

The core of the chapter is dedicated to regulatory functions in the biopharmaceutical industry, with topics such as the purpose of Regulatory Affairs/Science, the international context, roles and responsibilities of Regulatory Affairs/Science professionals and job opportunities.

Then follows a brief description of regulatory functions within regulatory authorities.

The next part is devoted to requirements for a successful career in Regulatory Affairs/Science, with topics such as wanted qualifications, personal skills and experience.

The chapter ends with some reflections on career perspectives and closes with a short conclusion.

The development and commercialisation of medicines, medical devices, in vitro diagnostics, digital health products, food supplements and other healthcare products, services or solutions is highly regulated.

It is not surprising then that this broad biomedical sector offers a wealth of job and career opportunities for regulatory professionals, within essentially three fields of stakeholders:

A. Emmerechts (✉)
Head of Regulatory Science Benelux and Switzerland/Austria clusters, GRS Europe/Canada, Bristol-Myers Squibb, Braine-l'Alleud, Belgium
e-mail: ann.emmerechts@bms.com

J. R. Thomas
PharmaCS, Merchtem, Belgium

– The regulatory authorities (e.g. medicines agencies, notified bodies, international organisations), with the mission to regulate this sector.
– The pharmaceutical, biomedical and healthcare industry (e.g. pharma, biotech, medtech), which has to comply with these regulations.
– Academia, where research is done to support the regulatory decision-making.

Collaboration between these three stakeholders is important and more and more encouraged.

This chapter will focus on opportunities for regulatory professionals within the biopharmaceutical industry, but will also briefly touch upon opportunities within the other fields of interest.

11.1 Regulatory Science Versus Regulatory Affairs

Several definitions are in use of 'Regulatory Science' and 'Regulatory Affairs'. As this can be confusing for the outsider, this is an attempt to bring some clarity.

Regulatory science is defined by the US Food and Drug Administration (FDA) as *the science of developing new tools, standards and approaches to evaluate the efficacy, safety, quality and performance of all FDA-regulated products* (FDA 2022). The FDA conducts and supports regulatory science research that *facilitates evaluation or development of FDA-regulated products, and supports regulatory decision-making and policy development.* The recent report Advancing Regulatory Science at FDA: Focus Areas of Regulatory Science (FARS) identified areas that need continuous research investment to move regulatory science into the twenty-first century (FDA 2021).

According to the European Medicines Agency (EMA), *regulatory science refers to the range of scientific disciplines that are applied to the quality, safety and efficacy assessment of medicinal products and that inform regulatory decision-making throughout the lifecycle of a medicine* (EMA 2022). In March 2020, the EMA published its Regulatory Science Strategy to 2025 (EMA 2020), complemented in December 2021 with a list of Regulatory Science Research Needs (RSRN) *to close gaps and improve medicine development and evaluation to enable access to innovative medicines for patients.*

Thus, the term regulatory science is more used in a proactive way, i.e. to shape and optimise regulations according to scientific underpinnings, concerns and progress.

In contrast, the term Regulatory Affairs is more used in a reactive way, i.e. how to comply with the existing regulations, and how to implement the current regulatory principles during the whole drug or product life cycle.

Both disciplines have their place in the regulatory landscape, can be considered complementary and influence one another mutually. Depending on the function within academia, health authorities or industry, the focus can be rather on Regulatory Science or Regulatory Affairs.

Additional reading on this topic can be found in Regulatory Affairs Vs Regulatory Sciences (Punia 2013), Regulatory Science and Regulatory Affairs (Molins 2017) and Regulatory Science: Europe Is Flying Blind (Johner 2020).

In this overview we will further mostly use the terminology 'Regulatory Affairs'.

11.2 Regulatory Functions Within the Pharmaceutical Industry

11.2.1 The Purpose of Regulatory Affairs

The core business of the Regulatory Affairs department in the pharmaceutical industry is to drive the regulatory vision providing high-quality strategic leadership, and to manage regulatory processes in line with business and R&D objectives.

Overall, the primary goal is to ensure timely registration of new products and line extensions and as such obtain marketing authorisations for medicinal products, mainly addressing a high unmet medical need (but also other products in area's where the medical need is less prominent), and manage the life cycle of the medicinal product, by submitting variations and product updates.

The type of medicinal products varies from small molecules over biologicals to ATMPs (advanced therapy medicinal products such as cell, tissue and gene therapy), combined or not with a medical device, new (innovative) products, but also generics and biosimilars.

11.2.2 The International Context

Depending on the region or country, one deals with different health authorities, such as the FDA (USA), the EMA (EU) and the Pharmaceuticals and Medical Devices Agency (PMDA, Japan), being the three largest pharmaceutical markets in the world. However, smaller countries also have important health agencies, such as the Medicines and Healthcare products Regulatory Agency (MHRA, UK), Swissmedic (Switzerland), Health Canada (Canada) and all the EU member states working closely with the EMA.

The role of the agencies can be categorised as:

1. Support of the development of medicines via scientific, legal and regulatory advice.
2. Evaluation of clinical trial applications.
3. Evaluation of the data in support of a request for marketing authorisation.
4. Making recommendations for granting marketing authorisation.
5. Safety monitoring of medicines/medical devices on the market (pharmacovigilance/ materiovigilance).

6. Watching over the quality, safety and efficacy by carrying out inspections and controls to verify compliance with legislation and the different good practice guidelines, i.e. GLP, GCP, GVP, GMP, and GDP.

11.2.3 Roles and Responsibilities of Regulatory Affairs Professionals

To achieve timely registration of high-quality, effective and safe medicines, it is important as a regulatory professional to be on top of the pharmaceutical legislation and the development of procedural and scientific guidance for development and evidence generation on the quality, safety and efficacy of the medicine, and to explore innovative regulatory procedures and practices such as accelerated assessment for bringing products to the patient addressing high unmet medical needs.

Effective and consistent communications with health authorities/agencies, a primary external stakeholder, is key and owned by the Regulatory Affairs function. As science and the ecosystems constantly evolve, both the industry and health agencies continuously monitor and set out the priorities. In the EU for instance, these health agencies developed *The European medicines agencies network strategy to 2025* which sets out how the network will continue to enable the supply of safe and effective medicines, in the face of developments in science, medicine, digital technologies, globalisation and emerging health threats (EMA and HMA 2020).

In addition to marketing authorisations, it is also the responsibility of the Regulatory Affairs manager to submit clinical trial applications to the local competent authorities to obtain the necessary approvals to start clinical trials in a country, in accordance with local legislation, i.e. in the EU the newly implemented Clinical Trials Regulation (CTR).

The implementation of early access programmes such as compassionate use programmes, in line with company policies and practices as well as local legislation, to provide access for patients to non-approved medicines, also belongs to the tasks of the Regulatory Affairs department.

Within a company the Regulatory Affairs function overall acts as a key partner to all the corporate departments along the drug/product life cycle, e.g. discovery research, pharmaceutical development and manufacturing (chemistry, manufacturing and controls, CMC), non-clinical development, clinical development, value, access and pricing, medical affairs and marketing. Just to mention but a few examples of its key roles:

- In pharmaceutical development and manufacturing (CMC): support the operational teams with expert knowledge about the myriad of guidelines on product and process quality.
- In non-clinical development: timely inform the team on the necessary preclinical studies before the start of the different clinical development phases.

– In clinical development: strategic input in preparing the clinical development plan (e.g. protocol, which studies in which countries, which comparators to use); owning the interactions with health authorities (e.g. applying for technical or scientific advice, or preparing the end-of-phase 2 (EOP2) meeting with the FDA); getting approval to start any clinical trial anywhere (e.g. an Investigational New Drug (IND) application in the USA, or a clinical trial application (CTA) in the EU).

Also at the local level, the regulatory department partners with the medical affairs, value, access and pricing and marketing departments, supporting local market activities such as promotion of the product, pricing and reimbursement processes, as well as with the pharmacovigilance and GDP functions in the management of the life of the medicinal product, and with the clinical operations function in the start-up and monitoring of clinical trials in the country.

It is also the gatekeeper to ensure that the products on the market meet the criteria as defined in the marketing authorisation dossier, and meet all rules and regulations regarding promotional and non-promotional activities.

Inspections and audits are supported by Regulatory Affairs and therefore interact closely with the quality assurance department in preparing internal or external audits and inspections, all across the product life cycle.

A good internal collaboration with all the stakeholders mentioned above is of paramount importance.

Pharmaceutical companies organise their Regulatory Affairs function in different ways.

One way is according to geographical territory, either responsible for one single country, or a particular region (e.g. the European Union, or Asia-Pacific), or worldwide.

Other common ways are according to the type of products handled (e.g. small molecules, biologicals or ATMPs), the therapeutic class of products or the development phase (e.g. pre-approval vs. post-approval).

This often leads to a more complex matrix organisation, whereby functional, divisional and hierarchical structures are combined, and team members can report to different managers.

At corporate level, Regulatory Affairs is gaining momentum to become more implicated in top management decision-making. Therefore, Regulatory Affairs roles can be found within regulatory *strategy,* regulatory *CMC*, regulatory *operations* and regulatory *policy*. More specifically:

• *Regulatory strategy* provides regulatory expertise and scientific/regulatory input into drug development programmes early on and into all regulatory procedures. They are the primary contact with the health agencies and ensure the implementation and execution of the regulatory strategy in the respective country/region, taking into account the country-specific regulations, legislation and dynamics.
• *Regulatory CMC is* responsible for the development and implementation of the global CMC regulatory strategy through all development phases to registration and post-approval lifecycle stages. They provide strategic regulatory expertise

and guidance for the development and review of technical protocols and reports (e.g. assay development, validation, stability, product development).

- *Regulatory operations* manages procedural activities and operational tasks such as:

  - Responsibility for dossier format and content: planning, generating highly complex electronic submissions (publishing the eCTD, i.e. the electronic common technical document which is the format agreed and accepted by major health authorities for the submission of registration dossiers) and delivering a broad variety of regulatory documentation (prepared by scientific and medical writers) to regulatory authorities.
  - Archiving activities in complex regulatory information management systems.
  - Labelling activities: ensuring end-to-end labelling processes from label content development (creation of the CCDS—Company Core Data Sheet) to health authority-approved labelling (prescriber's information/SmPC, package leaflet, pack texts) to implementation of approved labelling in the market via artwork management.

All this while using advanced automation tools and streamlined processes and applying technical guidelines globally.

- *Regulatory policy and intelligence* shapes and builds the regulatory ecosystem for innovative drug development by providing key regulatory policy insights and updates on the latest health authority thinking.

  This department informs the company of global regulatory developments, responds to influence and integrate regulatory policies and engages internal and external stakeholders to drive strategic policies supporting global regulatory science and drug development functions.

  It interacts with trade associations and health authorities on policy matters and engages in proactive policy topics, such as real-world data, digital health, rare diseases, paediatrics, diversity in clinical trials and patient-focused drug development, as well as engages with patient advocacy organisations, medical societies and key industry stakeholders.

It is clear that the job in Regulatory Affairs over the years evolved from a more administrative (tick-the-box-function) to a strategic partner. It is important to understand the end-to-end development process of a medicinal product and interdependencies. Science and technology is evolving very rapidly, and Regulatory Affairs/ Science is in the driving seat for all these evolutions. The relationship between health authorities and company is crucial and must be seen as a partnership, fostering communication with high transparency.

11.2.4   Job Opportunities

In the pharmaceutical and biomedical industry, a wide variety of job opportunities exist, essentially in all the functions of Regulatory Affairs described above.

At entry level, one might start as a Regulatory Affairs specialist, coordinator or analyst, and later on move up to Regulatory Affairs manager. In these functions, one might be the (or one of the) expert(s in a team) responsible for a country or a region, for a particular development phase, or for CMC for instance.

After a number of years spent as specialist, one might want to take up a leadership role, and become a team, project or department leader or director. And again, this will be possible in the broad variety of Regulatory Affairs functions mentioned above.

In the more decision-making roles at corporate level, e.g. in regulatory strategy or policy, extensive experience in Regulatory Affairs will be required, before being able to take up a senior management position.

Within the biopharmaceutical industry, job opportunities can be found in:

– Large to midsize biopharma companies in the roles as described above.
– Start-ups where one is no expert in one area and needs to look 'over the fence' to work very closely and even do the job of the other departments in the company. There the role is more of a coordinating nature where the outsourcing to Contract Research Organisations (CROs), and managing those CROs is an important part of the job.
– Companies specialised in generics and biosimilars.

A large number of jobs are also available in CROs: in this setting one works for (bio)-pharmaceutical companies who outsource certain activities. These functions are mainly in very specialised domains focussing on one aspect of Regulatory Affairs.

Similar opportunities also exist in the medtech industry, developing and commercialising medical devices, in vitro diagnostics and digital health applications. This is a rapidly evolving sector, as more and more of these devices and solutions (whether or not combined with medicinal products) are being developed, each with their own legislation. In this area, the development of combination products, e.g. drug-eluting coronary stents or precision medicines with a companion diagnostic, requires compliance with several regulations (e.g. for drugs and medical devices, or for drugs and in vitro diagnostics), and hence a lot more expert regulatory advice.

And finally, the multiple national, regional or international industry associations, such as pharma.be (General Association of the Pharmaceutical Industry in Belgium), PhRMA (Pharmaceutical Research and Manufacturers of America), EFPIA (European Federation of Pharmaceutical Industries and Associations) and the IFPMA (International Federation of Pharmaceutical Manufacturers & Associations), also employ various Regulatory Affairs professionals, where lobbying is an essential part of the job.

11.3   Regulatory Functions Within Regulatory Authorities

Apart from all the possibilities in the pharmaceutical and wider biomedical industry, there are also a lot of opportunities with the regulators or competent authorities, i.e. medicines and health product agencies (for drugs and related products), notified bodies (for medtech products) and health technology assessment (HTA) bodies (for negotiating reimbursement conditions).

In order to get the appropriate authorisations, e.g. a clinical trial authorisation, a marketing authorisation or a reimbursement status, the application dossiers have to be reviewed and evaluated. In each country or region, this is done by a team of assessors or reviewers, each expert in their own field of interest.

In the European Union, each member state has its own medicines agency and HTA body, each with a variable number of job opportunities as assessors or inspectors. On top of that, the European Medicines Agency (EMA) has regularly vacancies for EU citizens as assessors or inspectors, and in scientific jobs in regulatory science, either as traineeships or short- or long-term assignments.

The same goes for the European Commission's Directorate-General for Health and Food Safety (DG SANTE), employing experts in the fields of health and food safety, either as administrators for policy- and law-making or as inspectors for audits and inspections of national regulatory authorities.

11.4   Requirements for a Successful Career in Regulatory Affairs

11.4.1   Qualifications

For most of the described regulatory functions, a master or PhD in life sciences is the desired education. In the medtech sector, engineers, bioengineers and biomedical engineers might be preferred.

At entry level, a master degree is generally sufficient, or even a bachelor's degree will do for some more administrative jobs. For career advancement a PhD or an additional more specialised degree (e.g. in drug development, regulatory science, law, business administration or marketing) is an asset.

There are numerous opportunities out there for self-education in Regulatory Affairs. As an introduction, the following document of the EMA can be read 'From laboratory to patient: the journey of a medicine assessed by the EMA' (EMA 2019).

Probably the most extensive offer is found on the website of the Regulatory Affairs Professionals Society (RAPS 2022). Here you can find a series of books *Fundamentals of Regulatory Affairs* targeted by region (EU, USA or International) and products (medicines, biologicals or medical devices), online courses and (sponsored) webcast on various topics as well as their online magazine *Regulatory Focus*.

All these publications are freely accessible for members, and as a student you can join for a small yearly fee.

Some people prefer to boost their job and career opportunities in Regulatory Affairs by getting the Regulatory Affairs Certification (RAC), after passing the RAC Drugs and/or the RAC Devices exams, for which you can find all necessary information on the RAPS website.

And finally, to stay up-to-date with regulatory progress, frequent continuous training and attendance to congresses are very important.

11.4.2   Skills

A good scientific and technical background is certainly needed, but not enough to be successful in this field. On top of that, a number of personal skills are of paramount importance, such as:

- Strong negotiation and empathic skills.
- Ability to work in a complex matrix organisation.
- Ability to thrive in a cross-functional team environment with a global mindset.
- Be a trusted partner.
- Strong communication skills.
- Digital capabilities.
- Curious (in the asset, therapeutic area and in the environment), flexible and agile.
- Excellent command of English (written and spoken).
- Excellent verbal, written, organisational and time management skills and attention to detail.
- Ability to travel internationally occasionally.

11.4.3   Experience

To start as a regulatory professional in a more operational job, experience is not really a prerequisite, although a traineeship in the field (either in industry or in a regulatory agency) during or just after your academic education is certainly worth considering.

Expert knowledge is definitely gained on the job, so that career progression is possible starting from entry levels. 'Learning on the job' is supplemented with externally organised trainings and congresses and is a constant challenge but also an incredible opportunity for development. Most companies and organisations offer development opportunities within regulatory but also in other areas in R & D, leading to rewarding careers.

Some high-end jobs require special expertise that can only be acquired after several years of experience in the field, which is also the case for middle- and top-management functions.

11.5 Career Perspectives

Making the transition from academia to regulatory can be challenging. Some helpful reading can be found in *The PhD scientist's pathway into regulatory affairs* by DiMichele (2021).

As already mentioned before, you can start as a Regulatory Affairs/Science specialist in a particular area of interest, and become a real expert in the field over time. Others will quickly want to move to a leadership position, as leader, manager or director.

Some may want to advance their career in Regulatory Affairs/Science within one single company or a national agency, while others may want to switch regularly between organisations, e.g.

– From a (big) pharma company to a medtech company, a CRO or a biotech start-up, or vice versa.
– From a pharma company to a national medicines agency, the EMA or the EC's DG SANTE.
– From a medtech company to MedTech Europe (the European trade organisation for the medtech industry).
– From a pharma company to starting your own consultancy service company.

You can also decide to quit the Regulatory Affairs/Science scene, and progress your career in a different direction, still within the pharmaceutical or biomedical environment.

In this vast array of possibilities, everything seems possible, as long as you know for yourself where you want to go next, and where you finally want to end up. In this respect, preparing a personal career development plan, eventually with the support of a career coach, can be very useful.

11.6 Conclusion

As science and technology are evolving rapidly, the regulatory professional has to be curious, flexible and agile and to have continuously a learning mindset, be it in a large pharma company or a start-up, in a medical device company or at the side of the regulator. Interesting challenges and great opportunities are waiting for anyone who starts a career in Regulatory Affairs/Science.

References

DiMichele L (2021) Regulatory career development: the PhD scientist's pathway into regulatory affairs. Regulatory Focus. https://www.raps.org/RAPS/media/news-images/Feature%20PDF%20Files/21-4_DiMichele.pdf. Accessed 10 Mar 2022

European Medicines Agency (2019) From laboratory to patient: the journey of a medicine assessed by EMA. https://www.ema.europa.eu/documents/other/laboratory-patient-journey-centrally-authorised-medicine_en.pdf. Accessed 10 Mar 2022

European Medicines Agency (2020) Regulatory Science Strategy to 2025. https://www.ema.europa.eu/en/about-us/how-we-work/regulatory-science-strategy. Accessed 10 Mar 2022

European Medicines Agency (2021) Regulatory Science Research Needs. https://www.ema.europa.eu/en/documents/other/regulatory-science-research-needs_en.pdf. Accessed 10 Mar 2022

European Medicines Agency (2022) Regulatory science strategy. https://www.ema.europa.eu/en/about-us/how-we-work/regulatory-science-strategy. Accessed 10 Mar 2022

European Medicines Agency and Heads of Medicines Agencies (2020) European medicines, agencies network strategy to 2025. https://www.ema.europa.eu/en/documents/report/european-union-medicines-agencies-network-strategy-2025-protecting-public-health-time-rapid-change_en.pdf. Accessed 10 Mar 2022

Food and Drug Administration (2021) Advancing Regulatory Science at FDA: Focus Areas of Regulatory Science. https://www.fda.gov/science-research/science-and-research-special-topics/advancing-regulatory-science. Accessed 10 Mar 2022

Food and Drug Administration (2022) Advancing Regulatory Science. https://www.fda.gov/science-research/science-and-research-special-topics/advancing-regulatory-science. Accessed 10 Mar 2022

Johner C (2020) Regulatory Science: Europe is Flying Blind. https://www.johner-institute.com/articles/health-care/regulatory-science/. Accessed 10 Mr 2022

Molins R (2017) Regulatory science and regulatory affairs. J Regulat Sci. https://doi.org/10.21423/jrs-v05n02pi. (DOI assigned 3/11/2019)

Punia P (2013) Regulatory Affairs Vs Regulatory Sciences. https://pharmaceuticalmanufacturer.media/blogs/regulatory-affairs-column/regulatory-affairs-vs-regulatory-sciences/. Accessed 10 Mar 2022

Regulatory Affairs Professionals Society (2022). https://www.raps.org/. Accessed 10 Mar 2022

Chapter 12
Job Opportunities in Clinical Research Quality Assurance

Iris Gorter de Vries

Abstract The objective of quality assurance in clinical research is to promote and verify that clinical trials are executed according to all applicable rules and regulations, notably ICH GCP. These have been established in order to protect the safety and well-being of trial subjects and to ensure that trial results are reliable. Quality assurance is part of the much broader discipline of quality management, which is explained in this chapter. Several possible roles in the field of quality assurance and some suggestions how to get there are presented.

12.1 Introduction

We all assume that the drugs we are prescribed by our doctor will help us get better or at least cope with the problem for which we seek treatment. We would be very upset and indignant if it turned out that the treatment does not do what we were told it would or, even worse, is actively harmful.

How do we make sure this does not happen?

Prescription drugs need approval from the health authorities to be allowed on the market. In order to obtain this approval, the medicine should have been developed according to strict rules that have been created to protect patient safety and guarantee its stated efficacy. These rules are laid down by the International Council for Harmonisation (ICH; initially representing government and pharmaceutical industries in the EU, the USA, and Japan and being implemented by an increasing number of governments all over the world) in several guidelines of which E6 (good clinical practice, GCP) is directly relevant for the execution of clinical trials.

It is important to understand that the ICH guidelines and clinical trial regulations do not describe per se how to develop the most effective medicine or how to be most cost-efficient in the development process (although ICH GCP does point out the importance of efficient trial design). They describe the rules to be followed in order to protect the trial subject's safety and well-being and to guarantee the credibility of

I. Gorter de Vries (✉)
SGS-Life Sciences, Mechelen, Belgium

the trial data. In other words, it is possible to develop a medicine that is only marginally more effective than an already existing medicine, has cost a lot of money to develop, but whose development was transparent and yielded credible data while respecting subject rights and protecting their safety and well-being.

The focus of this chapter is on quality assurance (QA) in clinical research (CR): drug development from first-in-human till post-marketing trials, including all related manufacturing, laboratory, distribution, pharmacovigilance, and clinical activities.

Not discussed are many other activities that are also subject to ICH guidelines and to laws and regulations to ensure quality requirements are met, such as preclinical drug development, manufacturing, distribution and safety follow-up of commercial drugs, medical devices and technologies, and diagnostic processes, unless they are part of the clinical development process.

In order to understand quality assurance, the broader field of quality management is also touched upon.

12.2 What Is ICH GCP?

ICH is unique in bringing together regulatory authorities and pharmaceutical industry to discuss scientific and technical aspects of drug registration for human use. It aims to provide a unified standard for the ICH regions to facilitate the mutual acceptance of clinical data by the regulatory authorities in these jurisdictions. ICH GCP is a subset of ICH guidelines and addresses good clinical practice, an international ethical and scientific quality standard for designing, conducting, recording and reporting trials that involve the participation of human subjects while providing assurance that the data and reported results are credible and accurate and that the rights, integrity, and confidentiality of trial subjects are protected.

The ICH GCP guidelines describe the responsibilities of the independent ethics committees (IEC), the clinical investigator and the sponsor, as well as the requirements for protocol design, investigator brochure, and essential documents (for a more detailed description, see Appendix 1).

Other GXP guidelines include:

Good laboratory practice (GLP), good pharmacovigilance practice (GVP), good manufacturing practice (GMP), and good distribution practice (GDP)

12.3 Quality, Quality Management, and Quality Assurance

When we talk about "quality," we mean that the level of quality meets or exceeds pre-defined expectations. "Quality" needs to be built into the operational processes (quality by design). They have to be scientifically sound, well planned and executed, and compliant with regulations and contain quality control steps.

When we speak of quality management, we mean all process steps in clinical research that are aimed at achieving or exceeding the pre-defined level of quality, as well as the process of independently making sure that the trial is performed and the data are generated, documented, and reported in compliance with good clinical practice (GCP) and the applicable regulatory requirements. The latter is called quality assurance.

12.3.1   Quality Assurance

As already mentioned, quality assurance is part of quality management. While quality management should be everywhere in the organization, quality assurance is independent of the operational activities, advising the operations, as well as checking (auditing), at a given moment in time, a sample of the trial-related documents and activities against procedures, rules, and regulations, which are ultimately aimed at ensuring:

- Subject safety and well-being
- Credibility of trial data

12.3.2   Government and Ethics Committees

The independent ethics committees (IEC), associated with (university) hospitals, as well as the regulatory authorities play an important role in reviewing and approving (or rejecting) clinical trial designs, clinical trial conduct, and clinical trial reports. Regulatory authorities perform inspections to assure the public that the clinical trials were performed in accordance with all applicable laws and regulations.

12.3.3   Organization of Quality Management in Clinical Research

Each CR organization should have a quality management system or QMS in place. The QMS contains strictly controlled written procedures (standard operating procedures, SOPs) covering all activities. Roles and responsibilities are clearly defined, including training requirements. Deviations from SOPs or regulations are recorded and followed up with root cause analysis and corrective and preventive actions (CAPAs). Selection, qualification, and management of vendors is important since, like in most businesses, more and more tasks are contracted out to specialized organizations. Internal audits, performed by independent auditors of the QA department, assure management that the operational activities are performed in compliance with ICH GCP and all applicable rules and regulations. Internal audits are also an effective way to identify opportunities for improvement. To safeguard QA against operational bias, it is of crucial importance that the QA department is independent of the operational departments (i.e., reports directly to upper management and not to operational management and does not perform operational activities).

12.3.4 Keeping Up with Developments

Keeping up with developments and changes is of utmost importance to stay in business in any field, thus also in quality and compliance management in clinical research. This is a responsibility for both QA and operational teams. Professional organizations inform their members via websites, journals, conferences, and webinars, while ICH and regulatory authorities publish their requirements on their websites.

12.3.5 General Consideration on Quality Management

The high standards for quality in the development as well as the production processes of medicines in the European economic area and other high-cost countries (such as the USA) are at the basis of their continued production in these countries. They could be developed and produced at a lower cost if the quality standards were lowered. They could then no longer be used in humans without increased risk of complications and accidents.

12.3.6 Challenges in Quality Management

There are many challenges in quality management. Two prominent challenges are discussed here:

- Quality versus cost

    It is a challenge to balance the requirements from quality and regulatory point of view with those of the operational teams who have to deal with complex situations, short timelines, and tight budgets.

    In order to obtain the best balance between quality and cost and not to waste energy on things that are not very important, a risk-based approach needs to be followed. First, the most critical processes and data on which to focus have to be identified. Then, the risks (of an undesirable event happening) to these processes and data need to be identified and evaluated: how serious is the event if it happens, how likely is the event to happen, and how easily can it be detected when it happens. The next step is to decide what to do about the risk. It can be decided that the risk is acceptable and nothing is done. It can also be decided that the risk is so big that it needs to be avoided, i.e., the activity will not be performed. Another option is to transfer the risk to another party, e.g., an insurance company. Last, and most often applied, the risk can be decreased, or mitigated, by changing the process. Throughout the entire process of risk management, communication between all parties involved is important, and the approach and actual events must be reported in the final trial report.

- Data Integrity

Over the past 25 years, there has been an enormous increase in technological capabilities which has vastly impacted the field of clinical research. Trial data are now mostly collected in electronic records instead of on paper. Computerized systems have made their entrance in most processes, from temperature monitoring to data handling to statistics.

This computerization brings an increased risk to data integrity, such as loss of context, unnoticed and hidden changes to data, unauthorized access to systems, loss of data that are transitioned between systems, and loss of data because they are irretrievable due to changes of hardware or software.

12.4   Quality Assurance Roles and Career Options

12.4.1   Roles

- Quality and compliance manager (this role can have other names and can be divided over several positions):
  - Give independent advice to the business on quality and compliance topics.
  - Review operational procedures regarding quality and compliance topics.
  - Manage all aspects of audits and regulatory authority inspections of the business, including interaction with the auditor or inspector, setting the agenda according to the availabilities of the operational staff, making sure all required documentation is provided to the auditor or inspector, hosting the audit or inspection, following up on ad hoc requests, receiving the report, supporting the operational staff when dealing with the observations in the report, and finalizing and sending responses to the auditor or inspector.
  - Lead and support the business with the handling of deviations from procedures (as detected by auditors or inspectors or by own or sponsor staff): problem description, root cause analysis, and CAPA planning and execution.
- Author of procedures on quality and compliance.
- Computerized system validator: check and validate computerized systems.
- Data protection (related to General Data Protection Regulation – GDPR) manager.

- Auditor at sponsor or CRO.
- Inspector at government agency.

12.4.2 Educational Background and Personal Disposition

An education in medical sciences, medicine, pharmacy, pharmacology, nursing, laboratory techniques, or computer science can all give access to quality assurance or a related field in quality management. A "quality mind-set" is crucial and, as in many jobs, good mastering of the English language. A PhD is not required.

As to personal disposition, there is room for introverted as well as extraverted people. Some jobs are quite technical and do not require a lot of interactions with people; others are more team oriented or require very good people skills, in particular when interaction between QA and operations is taking place and in case of auditing or inspecting.

Good understanding and knowledge of the clinical research process, ICH, and applicable regulations is important, but a lot can be learned "on the job."

Some jobs require more or less extensive travel, such as auditor and inspector.

12.4.3 How to Start and Develop a Career in Quality Assurance

There are many possibilities to start a career in quality assurance. Some options are described here. A first job in the domain as a clinical research associate (CRA) in the sponsor organization, responsible for the oversight of the trial start-up and progress at the investigational site, will help you to really understand clinical research and ICH GCP and other guidelines and regulations. Another start could be as a clinical research project manager or as a trial coordinator at an investigational site. You can then decide to further develop yourself in "quality" topics, such as regulations on which you then can advise the business, writing of SOPs focussing on quality topics, or decide to train as an auditor. If you want to become an auditor, it is important to have a good knowledge of the field you want to be an auditor in, for example GCP, GLP, and GMP, but there are other important topics as well, such as data management and computerized systems. Training courses for auditor can be found at specialized institutes and organizations. On-the-job training with an experienced auditor at your side is a good way to complete your education. The same applies to inspectors at government agencies. Switching as an auditor between pharma and government is an option.

As you gain experience, you can grow in the organization and take on more responsibilities, including, eventually, senior management.

Appendices

Appendix 1: Topics in ICH GCP

- Clinical trial protocol, including but not limited to:
    - Subject in- and exclusion criteria
    - Study schedule
    - Data collection tools
    - Data management steps
    - Statistical methods
    - Study report

- Investigator's brochure of investigational product:
    - Nonclinical data
    - Clinical data

- Essential documents to allow evaluation of the:
    - Conduct of the trial
    - Quality of data produced
    - Compliance with GCP and applicable regulations

- Roles and responsibilities:
    - Investigator and staff
    - Sponsor and staff
    - Independent ethics committee/institutional review board

Appendix 2: Definitions

Audit

A systematic and independent examination of trial-related activities and documents to determine whether the evaluated trial-related activities were conducted, and the data were recorded, analyzed, and accurately reported according to the protocol, sponsor's standard operating procedures (SOPs), good clinical practice (GCP), and the applicable regulatory requirement(s). An audit is a snapshot in time of a sample of the data and documents.

CAPA

Corrective action and preventive action.

Compliance

Compliance in CR means compliance with ICH GCP, other GXP guidelines, legal requirements, and any other applicable rules and regulations.

Contract Research Organization

A person or an organization (commercial, academic, or other) contracted by the sponsor to perform one or more of a sponsor's trial-related duties and functions.

CRA

A clinical research associate is a representative of the sponsor or CRO responsible for the oversight of the trial start-up and progress at the investigational site.

EU Regulation 536/2014 (Effective Since January 31, 2022)

The goal of the clinical trials regulation is to create an environment that is favorable to conducting clinical trials in the EU, with the highest standards of safety for participants and increased transparency of trial information. The regulation requires:

- Consistent rules for conducting clinical trials throughout the EU
- Information on the authorization, conduct, and results of each clinical trial carried out in the EU to be publicly available

This will increase the efficiency of all trials in Europe with the greatest benefit for those conducted in multiple member states. It aims to foster innovation and research while helping avoid unnecessary duplication of clinical trials or repetition of unsuccessful trials.

GCP

Good clinical practice.

GDP

Good distribution practice.

GLP

Good laboratory practice.

GMP

Good manufacturing practice.

GVP

Good pharmacovigilance practice.

ICH

International Council for Harmonisation of technical requirements for registration of pharmaceuticals for human use. It aims to provide a unified standard for the ICH regions to facilitate the mutual acceptance of clinical data by the regulatory authorities in these jurisdictions.

ICH GCP

This document addresses the good clinical research practice, an international ethical and scientific quality standard for designing, conducting, recording, and reporting trials that involve the participation of human subjects while providing assurance that the data and reported results are credible and accurate and that the rights, integrity, and confidentiality of trial subjects are protected.

IEC

The independent ethics committee is an independent body (a review board or a committee, institutional, regional, national, or supranational), constituted of medical professionals and nonmedical members, whose responsibility it is to ensure the protection of the rights, safety, and well-being of human subjects involved in a trial and to provide public assurance of that protection, by, among other things, reviewing and approving/providing favorable opinion on the trial protocol, the suitability of the investigator(s), facilities, and the methods and material to be used in obtaining and documenting informed consent of the trial subjects.

Investigator

Person responsible for the conduct of the clinical trial at a trial site. If a trial is conducted by a team of individuals at a trial site, the investigator is the responsible leader of the team and may be called the principal investigator.

Quality Assurance

All those planned and systematic actions that are established to ensure that the trial is performed and the data are generated, documented (recorded), and reported in compliance with GCP and the applicable regulatory requirements.

Quality Control

The operational techniques and activities (i.e., built into the operational process) to verify that the requirements for quality of the trial-related activities have been fulfilled.

Sponsor

An individual, company, institution, or organization which takes responsibility for the initiation, management, and/or financing of a clinical trial.

Trial Subject

Subject in a clinical trial, either a healthy volunteer or a patient volunteer.

Some References and Further Reading

- International Council for Harmonisation www.ich.org
- Eur-Lex European legislation https://eur-lex.europa.eu/
- Food and Drug Administration (USA) https://www.fda.gov
- Research Quality organization www.therqa.com
- TransCelerate—Pharmaceutical Research and Development www. transceleratebiopharmainc.com

Chapter 13
Job Opportunities in Quality Assurance Related to Manufacturing of Medicinal Products

Maaike Gons

Abstract The world of manufacturing of medicinal products is fascinating and very dynamic and gives many opportunities for career development. Right after graduation one can start working at a plant. It is the role of the quality assurance (QA) department to have quality oversight over the manufacturing activities and the support activities that impact the quality of the product. Within quality assurance, different disciplines offer opportunities for starters or young professionals. Roles for starters will typically aim on support activities, while responsibilities can increase rapidly with growing knowledge of the regulations and processes, and the development of new skills. The career options are large, which includes development within the same quality team, but it is also possible to switch from quality into an operational role, or into a role at health institutes, at regulatory authorities or agencies like the EMA and the FDA.

13.1 Introduction

The pharmaceutical industry has a wide variety of job opportunities in several disciplines. In this chapter the focus is on the role of quality assurance related to the manufacture of medicinal products. A medicinal product is manufactured in multiple steps, from the manufacturing of active pharmaceutical ingredients (API) to the manufacturing of the final drug product. At the end of the chain, the product is labeled, in its final packaging, with its patient information leaflet, ready to be distributed and delivered to the patient. All these steps need to be performed in compliance with regulations and guidances, the so-called good manufacturing practice (GMP). Storage and distribution follow good distribution practice (GDP). The objective of these practices is to consistently produce, control, and distribute medicinal products to the quality standards appropriate to their intended use, so that patients timely receive a quality product.

M. Gons (✉)
Merus N.V., Utrecht, The Netherlands
e-mail: m.gons@merus.nl

© The Author(s), under exclusive license to Springer Nature Switzerland AG 2023
J. R. Thomas et al. (eds.), *Career Options in the Pharmaceutical and Biomedical Industry*, https://doi.org/10.1007/978-3-031-14911-5_13

The responsibility of quality assurance (QA) is to have oversight of all the activities needed to produce, store, and distribute a medicinal product, to ensure these are done in accordance with predefined processes and standards. The transversal character is key, as QA will work with all disciplines on the site to achieve this. The QA unit is a group independent from manufacturing, responsible to create, monitor, and implement a quality system.

Depending on the size and complexity of the organization, the size of the quality organization will differ, and certain functions may be combined. On a manufacturing site, in general the quality organization is around 20% of the total operational workforce, and consists of quality managers per activity, who each has a team with officers, coordinators, or experts. In terms of education, studies in life sciences are very suitable. Although certain roles require a specific background, like the role of qualified person to release the medicinal product, often profound knowledge of good manufacturing practice or good distribution practice are acquired on site. A scientific background and analytical and critical thinking skills are key to success in a role in quality assurance, as QA will have to decide at many occasions on the impact of an activity or event on product quality. To succeed it is important to acquire rapidly knowledge on the applicable regulations, like GMP, GDP, and the International Organization for Standardization (ISO) standards.

In this chapter insight is provided on the following:

- The activities on a manufacturing site.
- The regulatory framework that applies to these activities.
- The translation of requirements into a quality management system.
- A description of the responsibilities of the quality unit.
- Career options.

13.2 Manufacturing of a Medicinal Product

Manufacturing of a medicinal product takes place in multiple stages. Basically, two families exist, the classic products manufactured per chemical pathway and the biological products, manufactured from living organisms. The active pharmaceutical ingredient, the drug, is transferred into a product suitable for administration, for example, a tablet, a solution for injection, or a cream. After the compounding step, the product is packed in a primary packaging (vial, syringe, bottle, etc.), labeled, and placed in a carton with the patient information leaflet.

The manufacturing processes are very different when comparing the two families, or when comparing manufacturing of tablets and sterile products. Also, the size of the organization may vary from a small development site to a commercial, large-scale, multiproduct manufacturing plant. Nevertheless, from quality perspective, the same requirements apply, and the organizations are structured in a comparable manner with departments for production, supply, technical services, information

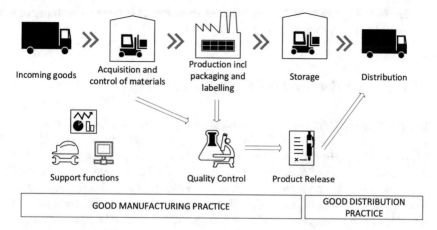

Fig. 13.1 Activities for commercial manufacturing

technology (IT), quality, and health, safety, and environment (HSE), supported by human resources and finances.

The environment is highly dynamic, focused on operational excellence at all steps to deliver a high-quality product in time. Science is important for the development of product and processes, and scientific approaches are used in many of the processes like the design of the manufacturing process, risk management, change management, or investigations in case of quality events. Both in operations and in the support functions, continuous improvements methods like Six Sigma and Lean are applied to increase efficiency and to make processes more robust.

The entire process as depicted in Fig. 13.1, from control of incoming materials up to distribution of the released product, is carefully designed with the aim to build quality into the process, also called "quality by design." As it is impossible to verify each single product on its quality, and as many tests are destructive, this quality by design is key to have confidence in the process, and to deliver products of constant quality. The design phase is followed by a validation process, where with documented evidence it has to be demonstrated that the manufacturing process will deliver the same product quality from one batch to another, in accordance with predefined specifications.

13.3 The Regulatory Environment

The manufacturing of medicinal products is highly regulated by health authorities, such as the European Medicines Agency (EMA) for Europe and the Food and Drug Administration (FDA) in the United States. The requirements keep evolving, to take into account new technologies and increased knowledge of processes, and also to create additional guidance for new types of therapies. It is the responsibility of the company to be in compliance with the regulations.

13.3.1 Directives and the EudraLex in Europe

In Europe, the legal framework for manufacturing of medicinal products is laid down in Commission Directives 91/356/EEC, amended by Directives 2003/94/EC and 91/412/EEC. The EudraLex Volume 4 (EudraLex 2010) contains guidance for the interpretation of these Directives. Part I describes the basic requirements for medicinal products, like personnel qualification, documentation, facility qualification, production, and supply chain. Part II contains the basic requirements for active pharmaceutical ingredients, used as starting materials. Part III contains documents related to GMP, and the annexes provide guidance for specific areas of interest, for example, Annex 1 focuses on requirements for sterile manufacturing.

13.3.2 Title 21 CFR in the United States

In the United States, it is title 21 of the Code of Federal Regulations, or "21 CFR," which governs food and drugs for the FDA. Different parts apply for the manufacturing of medicinal products, like part 210 that provides the requirements for good manufacturing practice for human medicinal products, and part 11 that establishes regulations on electronic records—key requirements related to computerized systems (FDA-CFR 2022).

13.3.3 The ICH

The ICH, or International Council for Harmonisation of Technical Requirements for Registration of Pharmaceuticals for Human Use, aims for harmonization of guidelines between pharmaceutical industry and regulatory authorities, and this on global scale. ICH's mission is to achieve greater harmonization worldwide to ensure that high-quality medicines are developed, registered, and maintained in the most resource effective way while meeting high standards. Starting small in 1990 with six member states, it is now a global, diverse organization, setting best practices to deliver safe and effective medicinal products to patients. Scientific discussions focus on advances in science and technology, and the challenges this may present. Many regulatory authorities have adopted these guidelines for their territory. The ICH establishes guidelines that cover safety, efficacy, quality, and multidisciplinary topics.

From manufacturing perspective, the quality series is important. These quality guidelines cover a variety of topics like stability, analytical validation, pharmaceutical development, and quality risk management (ICH 2020).

13.4   The Quality Management System

To translate these regulations and guidances, the activities of a manufacturing site throughout the product life cycle are described in a quality management system (QMS). The head of quality on site is responsible for this QMS. The objectives of a QMS are to manufacture a product of good quality, in a controlled manner, in compliance with the regulations. In addition, it aims to ensure performing stable processes by monitoring and use of control systems; and finally, continuous improvement is facilitated to improve processes, to improve the quality of the product, and to reduce variability. It needs to be a robust system that should be in place *and* in use, which means principles and processes are described, and evidence is provided to demonstrate the rules are complied with.

The quality management system is composed of documents with different level of detail, starting with the quality manual. It gives a description of the pharmaceutical quality system and describes the high-level responsibilities, the scope of the QMS, the quality policy, and all processes that ensure the controlled state. Increased detail is provided in standard operating procedures (SOPs) per quality system, and work instructions contain step-by-step instructions for a specific process.

Underlying procedures are constructed around the chapters in EudraLex Volume 4 (EudraLex 2010).

13.4.1   The Pharmaceutical Quality System

The pharmaceutical quality system or PQS defines the responsibilities and processes in place on a high level, needed to deliver a safe and compliant product. It covers the operational processes to manufacture the product, as well as the support processes needed. The PQS aims for consistency in the ways of working, with qualified personnel, and control over the activities to permit a careful decision on whether or not to release products to patients. Knowledge management and risk management are important enablers to ensure a robust system.

13.4.2 Personnel

People are a crucial factor in delivering a product of good quality. There should be sufficient personnel with clear responsibilities. Personnel needs to be qualified and trained on the processes they will perform.

13.4.3 Premises and Equipment

Premises and equipment need to be fit for use. For a sterile manufacturing plant, that means, for example, manufacturing areas with different degrees of cleanliness, and specifications for the number of particulates or microorganisms that can be found in the air. For storage areas specific requirements apply as well, like controlled temperature conditions, or the need to have specific areas for quarantined or rejected products. For equipment, it means that equipment needs to be qualified and a preventive maintenance program should be in place.

13.4.4 Documentation

Another key principle of the good manufacturing practice concerns control of documentation, aiming to establish, control, monitor, and record all activities. The requirements and instructions need to be described, which is done on high level to explain the principles, up to work instructions that are very specific. Records are generated to describe what has been done. This is needed to ensure compliant and reproducible ways of working, to deliver a product of quality.

13.4.5 Production

Production operations need to follow clearly defined procedures, laid down in the quality management system.

The following examples illustrate how this is done:

- Incoming materials and products need to be verified.
- Batches need to be distinguished one from another.
- Measures need to be taken to avoid cross-contamination.
- Yields and reconciliation may be required.
- Contamination should be controlled.
- Competent and qualified personnel is needed to perform these operations.
- Supervision needs to be in place.

- Any deviations from the procedures need to be investigated, to understand the root cause and the impact on product quality and patient safety.

13.4.6 Quality Control

Quality control is part of the quality unit. The control process ensures that materials, intermediates, and final product are in conformity with specifications. This is done by sampling at different process stages, and analyzing of these samples in laboratories. A formal release process will allow to state whether or not specifications are met, which is required prior to distribution of the product.

13.4.7 Outsourced Activities

Any activity that is outsourced to a third party, as well as the supply of materials for the manufacturing processes, need to be controlled and monitored. The manufacturing site is ultimately responsible for the quality of the outsourced activity or the supplied goods. Expectations and requirements are defined in a quality agreement between the parties. The third party or supplier needs to be qualified prior to engaging business, and an audit program should be in place to periodically assess their quality system and compliance of the activities. For raw materials and critical components, specifications are set up.

13.4.8 Complaints and Product Recalls

Processes need to be in place to address complaints in a timely manner—they need to be investigated to understand the nature of the complaint, and actions need to be taken in accordance. If a product is defective or not compliant, a recall process may need to be initiated, within very short timelines, and in collaboration with the health authority of the country where the product is distributed.

13.4.9 Self-Inspection

The self-inspection program is set up to assess the level of compliance of GxP activities. It also helps the organization to prepare for inspections by health authorities. If discrepancies are detected, against internal or external requirements, these need to be assessed, and a corrective action plan needs to be determined and implemented to resolve the issue.

13.5 The Quality Unit

13.5.1 The Quality Head

It is the role of the quality assurance (QA) department, or the quality unit, to have quality oversight over both manufacturing and support activities that impact the quality of the product, with the objective to ensure that the product is of the quality required for its intended use. The quality unit fulfills both quality assurance and quality control responsibilities. The head of quality has an independent role in the organization. He is overall responsible for the quality of the products manufactured on the site, and the maintenance of the quality management system. He pilots the management review, in which senior management evaluates the performance and effectiveness of the QMS and product quality.

The head of quality has a team that covers activities related to the product life cycle, quality systems, and compliance. A typical quality organization is depicted in Fig. 13.2.

Often, he is directly responsible for the release of the product as qualified person (see below), but this can be delegated; he needs to have exhaustive knowledge of the manufacturing operations, as well as of all supporting activities that together ensure the process is controlled and a product of consistent quality is delivered. The head of quality is part of the management team, and interacts a lot in particular with the operational colleagues as the manufacturing director or the supply chain manager.

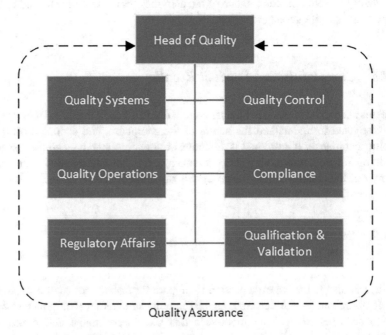

Fig. 13.2 A typical quality assurance organization

To translate regulations and guidances that are required for the manufacturing activities into a quality strategy, the head of quality is responsible to develop a quality manual and quality policies.

The head of quality will aim for "quality by design," a term signifying that quality should be built into the processes, as you cannot obtain consistent quality if the processes are poorly designed, and by testing only. A thorough design of a process, their validation and their transcription into documentation to allow for training of operators, will prevent errors, which is much more effective than finding rejects as it is impossible to find and eliminate all rejects.

The head of quality manages a team of experts to have quality oversight, to assess the impact of changes and deviations that may impact product quality or compliance, and to drive continuous improvement. He is supported by a process of quality risk management: a risk-based approach is used to understand where the risks on the site are, which exists of risk identification, risk analysis, and risk review. Based on the assessment, mitigation will be identified to lower the level of risk, and for the remaining risk the head of quality will decide whether it is acceptable or not, and how this outcome will affect the product and/or activities on site. An escalation mechanism should be in place, to ensure the head of quality will be informed of any serious issues, like critical deviations in manufacturing and situations that may lead to a recall.

13.5.2   Quality Systems

Quality system (QS) is responsible for the setup and maintenance of the overall quality management system, with a strong focus on continuous improvement of the quality systems. The quality system manager is responsible for specific elements of the QMS: training, the document management system, deviation management, corrective and preventive actions (CAPAs), change control, and management of third parties. With the help of quality performance indicators, the quality system manager will assess how the current processes perform, and where improvement is needed in terms of content and compliance, but also with regard to respect of timelines. The quality system manager also prepares the periodic quality system reviews.

The main quality systems managed by this team are as follows:

- *Training* of employees. All employees are trained on the GMP principles and company processes as part of the on-boarding process, and on yearly basis as GxP refresher training to stay up to date with changes and new developments. The team also trains on the quality systems described above, for example, on the deviation process: how and when to raise a deviation, tools to investigate, and how to identify successful corrective actions.
- *The documentation system.* One of the basic rules in good manufacturing practice is "when it is not documented, it did not happen." This implies that there is need

for a controlled documentation system, in which procedures and work instructions are maintained, but also records that allow to track actions along the way, for example, master batch records, or templates to register incoming goods and the controls performed, or logbooks to register use of equipment. The quality system team controls the document management system, which is generally an electronic system.

- *Data integrity (DI)*. The integrity of data is of high importance as important decisions will be made based on the data obtained that impact the patient: can the product be released or not? The attributes ALCOA+ are applied, which stands for attributable, legible, contemporaneous, original, accurate, complete, consistent, enduring, and available. Controls need to be defined to bring these in practice: this can be technical controls, for example, to ensure data cannot be deleted, or procedural controls to define what is and what is not allowed, if technical measures cannot be implemented. Sites need to have a data governance program in place to define what is needed to obtain reliable results, which allows to take the right decision on product release. It applies both to electronic and nonelectronic (paper) data. All GxP personnel need to be trained to have good understanding of the DI principles.

- *Change control*. Change control is the process to ensure that any change in the manufacturing process is carefully assessed, and will not impact the quality of the product. The quality system manager coordinates this process; he will establish a multifunctional team to assess the modification in terms of product impact, system impact, and regulatory impact. Once the change is approved, it can be implemented in accordance with the action plan.

- *Deviation management*. As the manufacturing, including quality control and other support processes, is fully controlled and is done against predefined processes and specifications, deviations to this process, or quality events, need to be assessed. Will the product still be of good quality; what is the extend of the event, does it concern one particular batch, only part of it, or maybe more batches, a defective equipment? The root cause needs to be investigated to understand why the event happened, and in order to define appropriate actions aiming to correct the event if possible, and to prevent the event from repeating itself in the future. The quality system team trains employees on this process, and monitors the process to understand the performance of the system.

- *CAPAs, or corrective and preventive actions*. Quality system is responsible for defining an effective process for corrective and preventive actions. Following several processes as deviations, audits, inspections, and annual reviews, the need for corrections may arise. The quality culture goes hand in hand with a strong culture for continuous improvement. Therefore, as soon as opportunities are identified to strengthen quality processes, a CAPA needs to be defined, describing a concrete action, an owner, and a timeline. If the CAPA is linked to a major or critical event, an efficiency review may be required. Quality system also defines how that process works.

- *Quality performance indicators*. To measure the performance of the different quality systems, a set of indicators is set up. This allows assessing whether the system functions correctly, or that actions are needed to improve it. Typical indicators measure numbers and respect of timelines and are a mix of leading and lagging indicators.

- *The quality management review (QMR).* The QMR aims for a periodic assessment of the different quality systems, which is presented to senior management, the direction of the site. It allows to identify any positive or negative trends, and to identify whether improvement is required to improve performance. For this, quality indicators are set up, and on monthly or quarterly basis, these are collected and assessed. The quality system team coordinates this, and the different sectors will contribute to assess their activity.

- *Management of suppliers and third parties.* To manufacture a medicinal product, a wide variety of materials and products are required, which need to be of consistent quality. The suppliers of these materials need to be qualified, and the materials have to be compliant with specifications. Some activities may be outsourced to other parties (contractors), for example, certain analytical tests, or the qualification of equipment. As the manufacturer is end responsible, there needs to be quality oversight on the outsourced activities, for which this team is responsible. They ensure suppliers or contractors are qualified prior to starting business, by assessing their level of quality during an audit. The extent of the qualification process will depend on the criticality of the activity outsourced or the material supplied. Expectations and responsibilities between the manufacturer and the contractor are defined in quality agreements. The third-party management team manages these; they will set them up with input from subject matter experts, and ensure periodic review and updates in case of changes in the agreement. Once qualified, the suppliers and third parties are monitored and audited, to ensure they continue to perform as expected and agreed. The team will set up this monitoring program as well as an annual audit program. They will also receive notifications in case the third party wants to modify something in his process that may affect the quality of the service or the product. The quality officer will do a pre-assessment, and then liaise with the relevant departments to perform a full assessment to define any potential impact on the product or the quality system. He will communicate and discuss the outcome to the third party. This is another transversal role, with interactions with all GxP departments on the site. There is also exposure to the suppliers or third parties to manage and monitor the activity, including the performance of audits.

This is a transversal role; the team interacts with all departments on site, and with all levels of employees from operators to the management team. It is office-based, however as there is a lot of interaction and it is key that QS understands the operational processes, and QS can regularly be found in the manufacturing and QC areas. The team typically consists of quality technicians, quality officers, and quality experts. One person can be responsible for one of more of the activities described above.

13.5.3 Quality Operations

Quality operations is responsible for oversight over the operational activities, from the supply chain to manufacturing and quality control. The team needs to make quality-driven decisions, based on objective facts. The team members interact on a daily basis with their colleagues in "Operations," and are often based in the same space to facilitate communication. The quality operations manager manages junior to experienced team members, who are responsible for a part of the process, where each team member is responsible for the same processes: document approval, batch record review, deviation management, and change assessment:

- *Batch record review.* Throughout the manufacturing process, a batch record is completed by the operators, to describe which action took place when, to describe any unexpected events, and to register results of in-process monitoring or in-process controls. This can be on paper or electronic. The Quality Operations team reviews these batch records after manufacturing is finished, including associated information like evidence that autoclaves are sterilized, or that line clearance took place.
- *Documentation and training.* Quality Operations reviews documentation related to the activities, like procedures or work instructions, whereby it is assessed whether the document describes correctly the activities and responsibilities, and also whether it is in compliance with regulations. The same goes for training materials. The team may provide training to the operational teams, and contribute to enhance the quality mindset.
- *Deviation management.* When deviations occur during manufacturing, these need to be documented and investigated. Quality Operations will approve the deviation, and assess the impact on product impact and compliance. If a deviation is estimated minor, little action is required. But if the deviation is major or critical, this involves heavy investigations by the operational team to understand what has happened, and to define the impact on the batch in question, as well as previously manufactured batches. In the worst case, the product cannot be released, or the product may even have to be recalled from the market if the deviation is detected after release of the product. Associated with the deviations, Quality Operations will assess the content of corrective actions defined following the investigation (will the action eliminate the cause or prevent it from re-occurring?), and they will measure the effectiveness of the implemented CAPA.
- *Environmental control.* Special requirements exist for the manufacture of sterile products, in order to minimize the risk of contamination, from microbiological nature or from particulates or pyrogens. The manufacturing happens in classified clean areas which have specific requirements for the level of cleanliness. This is obtained by the design of the areas, qualification of the facilities, a specific cleaning program, identification of the local flora, and a monitoring program to measure and trend the level of contamination.

    Environmental control includes temperature monitoring as part of cold-chain management, where for temperature-sensitive products such as vaccines or biologicals, it is key that the validated storage conditions are respected. This may be challenging, as temperature may be very low for such products. In particular maintaining the correct temperature range during transport can be a challenge, if you think about the loading/unloading process, and exposure of a truck to hot summer conditions.

13.5.4 The Qualified Person

The qualified person (QP) is responsible for the release of the finished medicinal product, which is defined as such in Directive 2001/83/EC and Directive 2001/82/EC (EUR-Lex 2001a, b). The certification of a batch is required prior to its release for sale or supply within the EU or for export. They are rigorously trained, and need to have in-depth understanding of pharmaceutical manufacture, the supply chain, and any factors that may affect the safety of medicines. This is well described in the Qualified Persons Study Guide published online by the Royal Pharmaceutical Society in the United Kingdom (RPS 2022).

The QP is legally responsible for batch certification before their use in clinical trials or before their availability on the market. This makes this an obligatory function for the manufacturing sites of the finished medicinal product. For intermediate steps, like the manufacturing of an API, this role is not required.

There is not a specific training to become a QP; a formal qualification in a scientific discipline like pharmacy, medicine, pharmaceutical technology, and biology, combined with gained experience on a manufacturing site, allows to submit an application.

13.5.5 Quality Control

Quality control (QC) is an operational department, part of the quality unit. It is responsible for the testing of raw materials and the product, and all lab management activities required to perform successful analysis with a reliable outcome. QC is a critical activity key to allow release of the product by the qualified person. Generally, there would be several labs like a microbiological lab, an analytical lab, and a lab for in-process controls, each of which is managed by a lab manager who reports into the QC manager. Each team is responsible for the following activities. There may be a support team to cover common activities, and that may provide scientific input for the validation of analytical methods, and in case of deviations or results that are out of specification or out of trend (OOS/OOT).

– *Sampling.* Sampling allows to collect the material to be tested, at different stages in the process: raw material, water, API, intermediate, in-process samples, and finished DP. For microbial analysis, samples of the environment are taken like samples of the air, of surfaces, of gowns, and of gloves. The samples are labeled with a specific identification, to ensure traceability. Sampling is done by trained personnel.

- *Testing and testing methods.* The samples are tested to confirm conformity with predefined specifications. This can be analytical testing or microbial testing. Methods are developed to perform testing in a consistent and reproducible way. For common analysis Pharmacopeias define the method, and for specific ones the company can develop and validate methods in house. Depending on the method required, equipment will vary, e.g., from simple pH meters to highly complex HPLCs.
- *Analytical records and results.* All data collected for and during the testing is documented in accordance with the good documentation practices. The record contains all information relevant to understand what activity has been performed, like the type of analysis, the sample tested, the analyst, the date, and the method that has been used. All along the analysis, the analyst will trace what is done, and what results are obtained. The results obtained of the analysis are joined to the analytical record. As results are mostly obtained in digital form, they can be reviewed either directly on the system or per printout. The entire record is reviewed as part of the release process. It is then archived for a legally defined period.
- *Handling of atypical results (OOS, OOT).* If a result is found to be out of specification (OOS), an investigation is needed. This consists of two steps. The first step is a laboratory investigation: is the OOS due to an error made in the lab? If this has not been confirmed, the second step orients on the manufacturing process to understand why this OOS occurred, and what the impact is. The same principle applies to out of trend (OOT), where in case of atypical results, an investigation will be started to understand what happened. Following the investigation, once a root cause is defined, the need for corrections is identified.
- *Release.* If the sample is in conformity with the specifications, the product can be released, or has to be rejected if not in conformity. After release, raw material can be used in the manufacturing process, drug substances can be further processed into a drug product, or the drug product can be released to the market. The QC Department prepares a certificate of analysis that contains an overview of all tests performed for a specific product, the specifications, and the results. It states whether or not the product is in conformity and is released or rejected.
- *Training.* All lab personnel need to be trained on general GMP principles. Analysts need to be qualified prior to performing a certain method themselves; this qualification permits to state the analyst understands the method, and is able to reproduce it in a reliable way. Periodically, requalification will take place. In addition, lab personnel is trained on all relevant SOPs on general quality concepts and on specific lab processes.
- *Management of reagents and reference standards.* For the analysis, reagents and reference standards are required. These are critical materials that need to be controlled. They can be bought or sometimes made in house. Aspects to control

include the storage conditions, the expiry date, what quality grade, and inventory management.
- *Equipment qualification, calibration, and maintenance.* Prior to any testing, the equipment on which the testing is performed has to be qualified and calibrated (where applicable). This is needed to ensure the equipment will give the correct outcome in a reliable way. For new equipment, a qualification process is defined, and on periodic intervals this will be repeated to ensure the equipment still functions as was intended. A maintenance program is in place for specific cleaning, replacement of parts, etcetera. These are also processes that are predefined, and described in SOPs.

The quality control team is composed of technicians/analysts, scientists, and lab managers. Work may be performed in shifts, to keep in pace with the manufacturing activities.

13.5.6   Compliance

The compliance team is responsible for the on-site audit program (internal audits), for the preparation and hosting of inspections by regulatory authorities or clients, for quality risk management, and for regulatory intelligence. The team also provides support to departments on how to interpret guidances and how to address complicated compliance topics, and may assist in assessing critical quality events or changes for the overall quality impact:

- *Internal and external auditing.* All critical activities are submitted to a self-inspection process, where internal, independent auditors assess whether the activity follows the procedures from the quality management system, and they also assess whether these procedures are compliant with the regulations. This allows for early identification of issues and allows for continuous improvement—any findings are investigated to understand the root cause, and then corrective or preventive actions (CAPAs) have to address the issue. Any external parties, for example, laboratories to which certain analysis are outsourced, but also suppliers of critical materials, need to be audited to ensure their quality system is compliant to internal regulations and the company's requirements. The compliance department sets up an external audit program following a risk-based approach, to audit the third parties on a periodic basis. Auditors are compliance experts, but are not necessarily part of QA. Candidates are selected, and then trained on the method of auditing by experienced auditors. After a few audits as contributor, they can become in the lead.
- *Inspection management.* Regulatory authorities will inspect on a regular basis for different reasons as described above. This can be to provide a manufacturing license, or to obtain a marketing authorization per product, or to allow commercialization. Then, routine inspections are performed on a periodic basis following a risk-based approach. The compliance team is responsible for the organization of

these inspections, which are often multiple day, with two or more inspectors. Almost the entire site is involved to provide their expertise on the topics audited. This makes that the organization needs careful preparation and good management during the inspections. The compliance team prepares the site for these inspections by means of "inspection readiness"—operators and experts are trained to understand what to expect, and the compliance team supports experts to prepare topics and rehearse them. For the organization of the inspection itself, a team is responsible to set up the infrastructure. They are are responsible for communications with the teams on site. Also they will set up the "front room" in which the inspectors are hosted, and a "back room" where requests are registered, the right expert is contacted, and the topic is prepared with the help of coaches.

- *Risk management.* Risk management is an enabler to ensure an effective pharmaceutical quality system. The compliance team is responsible for the process of risk management, such as development of the tools, training on the tools, and supporting departments to perform risk assessments. They also manage a risk profile for the site in which areas at risk are identified, with associated controls and plans to mitigate the risk. They will train departments on risk management, and assist them in identifying risks. These are then assessed with specific tools like failure mode(s) and effects analysis (FMEA). Following which mitigations are defined where needed to ensure the remaining risk is of acceptable level.

The team is typically composed of compliance specialists/experts.

13.5.7   Qualification and Validation

The qualification and validation department is responsible for the qualification of facilities, utilities, and equipment. Other processes need to be validated, like the manufacturing process, cleaning, and sterilization. Qualification and validation activities take place over the life cycle of products and processes, and aim to have documented evidence that the equipment or process is working as intended. The qualification team is responsible to identify which are the elements to be qualified, and to perform the qualification, initially for new equipment and then on a periodic basis. This applies to equipment used in quality control or production, but also to clean rooms, storage rooms with controlled temperature, or utilities. The Q&V team is responsible for the following topics:

- *Strategy.* The Q&V team is responsible for defining the validation strategy and the planning of the activities; this is described in validation master plans. A general site validation master plan gives the overall picture for the activities for the upcoming year. This is completed with smaller plans to describe the specific strategy for a project, for example, the validation of a new computerized system used in quality control.
- *Methodology.* The Q&V team is responsible for the methodology. The different phases of the qualification/validation process are design, installation, operational,

and performance qualification. Following the initial user requirements, a risk-based approach is applied to understand risks of the equipment or system, and tests are developed to confirm how the equipment is functioning. This provides a high degree of assurance that the equipment is functioning as expected.

- *Documentation*. The validation activities are captured in protocols and reports, written by the Q&V department.
- *Execution*. The team pilots the execution of the validation activities. If any events happen during the execution, the team will investigate in collaboration with the owner of the process or system. The team will assess the results of the execution, and if all acceptance criteria are met, the process or system is declared validated.
- *Change control*. To ensure the validated status of the process or system, the impact of changes on that process or system is assessed. When needed, revalidation may be required as part of change management.

Jobs in qualification and validation have a very transversal character, as the team will qualify or validate elements owned by other departments, like the equipment in quality control, or the manufacturing building. This requires good communication and planning. The team is typically composed of technicians, engineers, and life science graduates. The roles are office-based, but the team is also regularly present on the shop floor in the warehouse, manufacturing, or QC, to prepare Q&V activities and for execution of the protocols.

13.5.8   Regulatory Affairs

Manufacturing sites often have their own Regulatory Affairs Department, consisting of a manager with a team of RA Officers. The regulatory manager may report to the head of quality, or to the country—or global Regulatory Affairs Department. Regulatory Affairs on site level is responsible for the following topics:

- *Management of the site product portfolio*. The team is involved in preparations and submissions of applications to regulatory authorities of the countries where the product in question is or will be commercialized. Once a product is being commercialized, the regulatory dossier needs maintained so that it reflects the current operations.
- *Maintenance of the site master file*.
- *Contact with health authorities*. The RA team may be in direct contact with the health authorities regarding the registration dossiers, and will coordinate any questions that may arise following a submission of a regulatory dossier or a variation to an existing dossier.
- *Change control*. Once a product is marketed, changes may occur over time; the manufacturing process itself will evolve, specifications may change, the supplier of a critical material may change, etcetera. These changes are assessed by a multidisciplinary team, in which Regulatory Affairs assesses the regulatory impact. This has to be done prior to implementation of the change. If there is

an impact, the strategy needs to be defined. Depending on the nature and criticality of the change, this may be notification of a variation to the health authority, but in some cases official approval by the health authorities is required prior to release of the product to the market.

– *Labeling/leaflet requirements.* Information on labels and in patient leaflets is also regulated. RA needs to ensure that content on labels of products, and the content of the patient information leaflet, is complete and correct.

This role is typically office-based. The team can be composed of different levels of experience, from entry level to experts.

13.6 Qualifications and Skills

As the quality unit should have quality oversight over the activities, and be able to take decisions that will lead to the release of the medicinal product, most people within QA have a life science background. With a bachelor or master in life sciences like chemistry, chemical engineering, pharmacy, biology, and microbiology, there are multiple possibilities to find a role in manufacturing QA. Around 5% is pharmacist; however, this is not a required qualification apart from specific roles as the qualified person.

Typical skills for a QA role are:

– Critical thinking skills: this will allow understanding the impact on compliance or product quality of sometimes difficult and technical topics.
– The capacity to adapt to changes: as although controlled, changes occur permanently to correct, improve, and implement new ways of working.
– Rigor.
– A result-driven attitude will help in contributing to an efficient quality system.
– Strong reactivity is key to quickly address unexpected events, where decision-making may be fast when the product is at risk.

A good level of English is highly recommended, as the industry is so internationally oriented; in many companies this is the main language, written and spoken.

In particular for the external auditing team, the amount of travel may be important, up to 25% per year. For the other roles, this will be more marginal; there will be travel, for example, for training or benchmark activities.

In particular the production department often works in shifts, which may be two shifts (06 h00 to 14 h00 and 14 h00 to 20 h00, up to five shifts in which case production continues day and night, weekend included. Roles as QA operational officer may follow such a rhythm.

13.7 Career Perspectives

13.7.1 Evolving Within the Quality Organization on Site

Within the quality unit, many development options exist. With gaining experience, one can grow from a junior to a senior or expert role, or after 3–5 years into a manager role. A change from one quality team to another is also very feasible, as the principles remain the same, for example, from quality operations to a compliance role or to quality systems.

13.7.2 From Manufacturing to Quality and Vice Versa

The move to another discipline like production is also very interesting. This is possible from quality to production, or the other way around, and both have advantages. If you start in production, you get deep knowledge of the manufacturing process and the application of quality systems. You see the impact of training, the benefits of good written, and easy to follow work instructions. You would assess changes in the manufacturing process for impact on the product, and investigate deviations that may occur throughout the operations. At the same time, you have to ensure production schedules are respected and optimized, so that the time from start of production to the final step including review of documentation is as optimal as possible. It is very complementary to be able to bring in this experience in quality roles, where you would have an approver role. The other way around is not less interesting, being able to bring your knowledge on requirements and guidances in practice, and gain new experience on the shop floor. For the long-term perspective, it is a great benefit to have seen both operations and quality at the start of your career.

13.7.3 Transferring from One Environment to Another

In terms of work environment, there is a wide variety of options. Think about a manufacturing site to produce products for development, or the active pharmaceutical ingredient, a plant to produce biologicals, or a plant in which the drug product is manufactured, with tabletting lines or "fill and finish" for products in vials or ampoules. The next step in the supply chain also needs quality management, the warehouse, or transportation. An interesting development may be the role of responsible person for GDP.

Roles in quality management of medical devices or cosmetics are another good fit; there are specific regulations for these product categories; however, from quality perspective the same principles are applied.

13.7.4   Global Roles for Quality Assurance

On headquarter level quality organizations are headed by a global quality manager or chief quality officer. The global quality organization is often set up in a similar way as on a manufacturing site, with teams for compliance, third-party management, the quality management system, and operations. Within the global quality organization, the overall strategy and direction are defined. These are described in the global quality documentation system, shared with the sites or country organizations for local implementation.

13.7.5   Working for Regulatory Authorities/Agencies/Health Institutions

Another development option are roles in governmental organizations. Each country has its own agency for oversight on medicinal products. One of such agencies is the ANSM in France (National Agency for the Safety of Medicines and Health Products), responsible for evaluating the benefit/risk profile linked to the use of healthcare products (ANSM 2022). The ANSM assesses the safety, efficacy, and quality of these products. It assures surveillance and controls in laboratories, and performs inspections. The role of the inspectorate with its inspectors is to assess and control the entire chain, from development to manufacture and distribution. The inspections focus on organizations in the country itself, but also on organizations abroad for assessment of products for import into the European market.

Oversight on pharmacovigilance is another health agency responsibility, and an interesting area of development coming from QA.

13.8   Conclusion

Quality assurance is an interesting discipline with different options in starting positions and for further development. The transversal character is great as there is interaction with all operational departments, and at all levels within the organization. In all activities and decision-making, the ultimate goal is delivering a high quality of the product from which patients can benefit, which is a big driver for personnel in QA.

References

ANSM (2022) Agence Nationale de Sécurité du Médicament et des produits de santé. https://ansm. sante.fr. Accessed 13 Feb 2022

EudraLex (2010) Volume 4—Good Manufacturing Practice (GMP) guidelines. https://ec.europa. eu/health/medicinal-products/eudralex/eudralex-volume-4_en. Accessed 6 Feb 2022

EUR-Lex (2001a) Directive 2001/82/EC of the European Parliament and of the Council of 6 November 2001 on the Community code relating to veterinary medicinal products. OJ L 311:1–66

EUR-Lex (2001b) Directive 2001/83/EC of the European Parliament and of the Council of 6 November 2001 on the Community code relating to medicinal products for human use. OJ L 311:67–128

FDA-CFR (2022) Current Good Manufacturing Practice (CGMP) regulations. https://www.fda. gov/drugs/pharmaceutical-quality-resources/current-good-manufacturing-practice-cgmp-regula tions. Accessed 6 Feb 2022

ICH (2020) Quality guidelines. https://www.ich.org/page/quality-guidelines. Accessed 6 Feb 2022

Royal Pharmaceutical Society (2022) Qualified persons study guide 2022. https://www.rpharms. com/development/education-training/training/qualified-persons. Accessed 24 Mar 2022

Part IV
Other Opportunities in the Pharmaceutical and Biomedical Sector

Chapter 14
Careers' Perspective in a Science and Technological Park

Laura Aldrovandi and Simona Sbardelatti

Abstract Young researchers often believe that career paths can be constructed only in academia or companies, mainly multinationals; indeed, above all big life science companies are able to attract the interests of scientists. However, in this complex panorama, we would like to focus on a particular opportunity for experts in life sciences: the scientific and technology park. These entities, which can be considered a niche in respect of other career paths, offer some interesting opportunities for professional careers in the life sciences sector.

14.1 Brief Introduction on Science and Technology Parks

A science and technology park (STP) is an ecosystem in which business and research are in contact; this kind of structures can also favor the growth of new enterprises (in the form of start-up or spin-off). A STP may act as intermediary between technology developer and technology diffuser, helping the passage of research results from universities (research labs) to the market (Simsek et al. 2016). To better understand what a technology park is, we can report the characteristics described by Roldan (Roldan et al. 2018), who described a park as a structure able to provide support services, physical infrastructures, a relationship network with other companies or universities, and innovation (in product, process, marketing, organization) and improve performance of the industrial sector.

Several STPs exist at international level and they differ for their characteristics, i.e., they can differ for geographical localization, specialization (i.e., they can be multisectoral, focalized on life sciences or mechanicals or materials, they can host companies, and/or they can act as incubators, etc.), and management structure. Hence, it is difficult to have a common description, but to better describe STPs, we report some definition present in the scientific literature that can be adapted to the

L. Aldrovandi (✉) · S. Sbardelatti
Technology Park for Medicine (TPM), Mirandola, MO, Italy
e-mail: simona.sbardelatti@tpm.bio

majority of the STPs. The International Association of Science Parks and Areas of Innovation (IASP) reports that:

> A Science Park is an organization managed by specialized professionals, whose main aim is to increase the wealth of its community by promoting the culture of innovation and the competitiveness of its associated businesses and knowledge-based institutions. To enable these goals to be met, a Science Park: stimulates and manages the flow of knowledge and technology amongst universities, R&D institutions, companies and markets; facilitates the creation and growth of innovation-based companies through incubation and spin-off processes; and provides other value-added services together with high quality space and facilities. (JRC Technical Reports 2014)

Whereas the Organisation for Economic Co-operation and Development (OECD) reports that:

> (. . .) they concentrate high-tech industries and specialized service centers (. . .) they have at least one university department or institute of technology with which hosted companies can communicate with each other (. . .) they include an important component of research and development (. . .). (Guadix et al. 2016)

What we can report is that some elements could be identified as essential for establishing a successful STP:

- Presence of universities or research centers, promoting the spreading of new technologies, innovation, and knowledge.
- Establishment of collaboration between all the entities located in the STP (spanning from institution to companies) (McCormack et al. 2015).
- Integration of all the policies regarding education, development, and research. Policies may be tailored on the specific needs of the ecosystem.

For the purpose of this article, we would like to focus on the life sciences sector, which is quite different from the others. Indeed, the life sciences sector is characterized by a strong regulatory framework, products and services have direct consequences on the health status of the population, and the market is dominated by very big players (Ramlogan et al. 2007; Rosenberg 1994; Coffano 2016). These elements influence also the STPs specialized in the sector: expertise, competencies, infrastructures, equipment, etc. need to be properly selected to support companies and R&D activities.

14.1.1 Technology Park for Medicine (TPM) "Mario Veronesi": An Example of a Science and Technology Park

Technology park for medicine (TPM) "Mario Veronesi", despite its quite recent establishment, can be considered a STP, due to its characteristics: localization, specialization, management system, vision, and mission. We will describe TPM just to give an idea of how a STP is structured and because the professional profile described in the following section are strictly linked with our experience with TPM.

TPM "Mario Veronesi" is managed by Democenter-Sipe Foundation, a technology transfer center of the University of Modena and Reggio Emilia. Democenter-Sipe Foundation collects institutions, trade associations, banking foundations, and more than 60 local companies. It has separate branches at Modena (TPM located in Technopoles and it supervises Knowbel, a business incubator, located in Spilamberto).

TPM is located in the Mirandola Biomedical District (Modena, Italy) which comprises more than 90 enterprises specifically focused on the development and production of active and non-active medical devices for apheresis and plasmapheresis, hemodialysis, heart surgery, anesthesia, gynecology, infusion, transfusion, autotransfusion, continuous renal replacement therapies, and enteral and parenteral nutrition.

TPM, inaugurated in January 2015, is meant to be a place where both business and technological expertise can co-work and grow together. TPM helps leverage research and development for a strong biomedical presence in the region in collaboration with a network of acclaimed regional high-technology centers. TPM is a certified quality system according to ISO 9001 and ISO 13485.

TPM houses four laboratories, all organized and managed in partnership with the University of Modena and Reggio Emilia: toxicology and proteomics (TOP), polymer science lab chemical (POS), applied microscopy and cellular biology (MAB), and materials, sensors, and systems (MS2).

TOP provides support in evaluating response of hemo-components upon materials' interaction, and in analyzing release of potential toxic substances from packaging or biomedical devices. TOP has recognized and consolidated experience in the following macro-activities that are carried out according to the international regulations of the sector, and through advanced methodologies. Furthermore, the TOP laboratory supports the elaboration of study protocols for the identification of the best in vitro and in vivo analysis approach in order to evaluate the specific activity of the materials studied. Moreover, it has a wide experience in proteomic approaches. Main equipments are ultraperformance liquid chromatography (UPLC)/atmospheric pressure gas chromatography-mass spectrometry (APGC-MS) (Xevo G2 Qtof), Agilent 3100 OFFGEL Fractionator and climatic chamber.

POS chemical laboratory combines the need of scientific research on new materials with the study of new applications for "traditional" materials. The laboratory is equipped with ultraviolet/visible region (UV/VIS) and infrared (IR) spectrometer, both used in the field of polymer synthesis and instrumentation for chemical characterization, and the innovative electrospray, for the production of nanoparticles and nanofibers or coating.

MS2 aims at supporting companies in design, development, characterization, and validation of new materials, products, measuring systems, and equipment. Scientific expertise is supported by state-of-the-art instruments (such as 3D-Bioplotter used for realizing scaffolds and organ-on-a-chip).

Table 14.1 Activities carried out by TPM

TPM "Mario Veronesi": what we do			
Research services for innovation and industrial development	Design and co-design of medical and surgical devices	Support for product registration	Support in fund raising for enterprises and SMEs in the field of biomedical, cosmetology and food field
Technology transfer	Incubation and development of ideas and start up	Education	Business development

MAB offers know-how on cell biology on isolation and culture of adult mesenchymal stem cells (MSC) from fat and bone marrow, and on induced pluripotent stem cells (iPSC). Differentiated MSC are used for new biocompatibility and toxicity assays by label-free technology (EnSpire, Perkin Elmer). Cell interaction with materials can be studied through ex vivo and in vivo imaging (IVIS LUMINA, Perkin Elmer). Advanced microscopy instruments (Axiozoom V16, Axio Imager M2, Observer Z1, Zeiss) are available to investigate surfaces. Thanks to these advanced instruments, MAB offers the development of new protocols and new cell models for studies of biocompatibility, toxicity, and regenerative medicine.

Starting from 2015, TPM growth, an incubator (TPM Cube) was created, specialized on biomed, medtech, and biotech start-up; new labs were added, to respond to the market requirements (usability and chemical—POS). Also, services were adapted in function of the companies' requirements.

Moreover, education was reinforced in the area, through the creation of an *Istituto Tecnico Superiore-Nuove Tecnologie della Vita*—ITS (https://www.its-mirandola-biomedicale.it/, ITS Foundation) which is a course specifically dedicated to medtech.

Besides R&D activities, TPM carry out workshops, dissemination activities with the aim of spreading knowledge about new technologies, life science trends, etc. In Table 14.1, activities carried out by TPM are reported.

14.2 Medical Device Sector

Starting from the pharmaceutical sector model, the medical device sector in Italy generates a market worth 16.2 billion euros between exports and the internal market, and it has 4546 companies, which employ 112,534 employees. It is a very heterogeneous, highly innovative, and specialized industrial fabric, where small companies coexist with large groups.

There are several indicators with which we define the sector, such as:

– *Number of companies*: There are 2523 production companies that, together with 1643 distribution and 380 services companies, are directly involved in the production and/or distribution of medical devices in Italy. The biomedical device sector is characterized by a strong prevalence of small medium enterprises (SMEs) (about 94% of the total). Indeed, this sector is one of the most heterogeneous one present in Italy. In fact, there are at least 13 main compartments to which the companies belong: biomedical, technical equipment, electro-medical, dental, etc.

– *Import and export*: Currently, China is playing a leading role in the international trade. In particular, imports from this country have increased by 15.1% in 2021. The import of electro-medical devices from Asia also grew by 76.5% and +113.2% from South America. The import of technical equipment from Africa decreased by 100% and from North America by 38.7%. Considering the global biomedical market, Italy as importing country is at number 12 worldwide,

while exports saw a general decrease of 5.3%, toward the United Kingdom, followed by the −14.4% recorded toward Poland and −12.3% toward the USA. On the other hand, exports to Belgium (+50%) and to the Netherlands (+6.4%) and Spain (+6%) increased.

– *Employment*: The medical device sector is characterized by highly skilled employment. The number of employed women is 46% compared to the employed men 54%, and 7.4% of the employees are involved in research and innovation: these percentages are higher than the general average of the country. In particular, the qualification of the employees are 48.6% of university graduates, 37.6% with a high school degree, and 13.8% others. There is a strong concentration of this employment in Lombardy, Emilia-Romagna, and Veneto.

– *R&D investments*: Despite the Covid-19 pandemic, 682.8 million euros are the investments made in 2021, specifically, 72.6 million euros for basic and applied research and 610.2 million euros for the development of medical devices. This includes the prototyping, the development of the finished medical device, and its patenting.

– *Start-up and innovative SMEs*: In addition to the large enterprises, in Italy are present approximately 300 smaller companies, considering both innovative start-ups and SMEs. In particular, they have strong innovative competencies and huge investments in research and development.

The data described above are collected and processed by the Confindustria Medical Devices Study Center (https://www.confindustriadm.it/il-settore-in-numeri/).

Europe is an established leader in medical technology research and innovation (R&I), delivering major advances in areas including cardiac pacemakers, deep brain stimulation, intravascular ultrasound, next-generation sequencing, point of care diagnostic testing, and home dialysis care. The high number of patients filed by companies and the data on trade flows and employment statistics reflect the innovative nature of the sector. By turning scientific ideas into solutions for patients, health professionals, and health systems, industry has contributed to better outcomes and greater efficiency in healthcare. In the process, Europe's medical technology companies have helped the region to be a world leader in a highly competitive sector.

In Italy, specifically in Mirandola (MO), starting from 1962 is located the second biomedical district. Born thanks to the intuition of the pharmacist Mario Veronesi who invented one of the first infusion devices, the district is now recognized as the Silicon Valley of biomedical in Italy. An area that occupies a total of about 5000 employees, with a prevalence of medium or small size and only among the larger companies the form of joint-stock companies prevails (18% of the sample).

The numerous companies in the district now support a very wide range of healthcare areas, including hemodialysis, cardiac surgery, anesthesia and intensive care medicine, apheresis and plasmapheresis, blood transfusion, nutrition, and gynecology. The production specialization of the companies in the Mirandola Biomedical District concerns disposable plastic products for medical use and equipment for dialysis, cardiac surgery, transfusion, and other healthcare applications. The production of disposables accounts for more than 80% of the total, while biomedical equipment accounts for 13%. The district produces both finished products and the components needed to make disposables.

These data are an integral part of the Report on Production, Research and Innovation that the Confindustria Medical Devices Study Center published in January 2022.

14.3   Job Opportunities in Science and Technology Parks

In this section, we will analyze the specific professionals that can operate in STPs, specifically focused on the biomedical sector, due to our experience. Of course, some of these considerations can be extended to other sectors, such as the pharmaceutical or cosmetic sector, which have some common points, e.g., research activities, regulatory affairs, etc. In any case, the major part of the professionals described can also be employed (or are present) in companies, in particular big multinational ones, such as Medtronic and Fresenius; instead, SMEs (which are the majority of companies at EU level) employ directly only some of the professionals which will be described and have as consultants the others. Hence, we believe that this overview can be useful for all scientists looking for job opportunities.

To better describe the professional present in STP, starting from the experience of TPM, we will group their profile in five categories, which reflect the main activities carried out. In particular, we can identify the following professionals:

– High-tech profile: very focused on R&D activities
– Services profile: specialized on problem solving for companies
– Regulatory specialist and quality manager: specialized in the product/medical device and process compliance
– Communication and marketing: hybrid profiles with the aim to maintain and promote the dialogue with external stakeholders
– Project manager and technology transfer

14.3.1 High-Tech Profile

We identified these professionals as the ones involved mainly in the design and development of R&D projects, required by companies or carried out directly by the STP. For R&D definition, we consider the one reported by the OECD:

R&D development comprises creative and systematic work undertaken in order to increase the stock of knowledge—including knowledge of humankind, culture, and society—and to devise new applications of available knowledge.

R&D can have impact on process, service, and product of life science companies and on production. Professionals required for this kind of activities are highly specialized, mainly coming from academia, with a PhD or master on specific life science themes. They must have the knowledge and the capabilities of carrying out experimental processes, but may also know the market and its requirements, to develop new solutions that can be adopted by companies. Indeed, the R&D activities carried out by these professionals start from solutions which are almost at technology readiness level (TRL) 3 or 4 (TRL 3, experimental proof of concept, or TRL 4, technology validated in lab); hence, research carried out in STPs like TPM not only comprises basic research activities. The final TRL can reach the 7 or 8 (TRL 7, system prototype demonstration in operational environment, or TRL 8, system complete and qualified). TRL 8 requires the collaboration of professionals like the one described in the following chapter (regulatory). However, it is indispensable that also R&D staff is informed about medical device (or pharmaceutical) regulation, because also design and testing phases may be carried out in compliance with pharma or medical device regulation to reduce the time to market. Moreover, knowledge of the most important standards, like good manufacturing practice (GMP) or good laboratory practice (GLP), can be considered an important plus for researchers.

Hence, these professionals may be able to cover different stages of new product development. Another expertise needed is the ability to work and/or manage a team (with different specializations) and to respect time and resources at disposition to finalize the projects. Indeed, often economical resources are established before the project starting, and it is hard to obtain integration or other funds if the estimation is wrong. Moreover, the ability of interacting with companies' staff or other research centers is required.

Regarding the specific competencies and education, as anticipated when we described the sector, the competencies are several; teams must be multidisciplinary. High-tech professionals in STPs comprise:

- Biologists or biotechnologists, with experience in molecular biology and bio-chemistry, bioinformaticians, and biomedical scientists
- Pharmacologists, experts in pharmacokinetics or pharmaceutical technology
- (Clinical) toxicologists
- Chemists (with expertise in materials or analytical)
- Engineers (mainly but not exclusively, biomedical, mechanical, electrical, etc.)

14.3.2   Services Profile

Besides R&D projects, which requires huge investments and have a duration spanning from months to years, we consider services as activities required by companies to resolve problems or to develop only a small part of a product. In this case, service requires small investments and the duration are months (mainly 1 or 2 months of activities). The TRL of the activities are mainly from 5 to 8 (or sometimes 9). The competencies needed are not so different from the ones described in the previous section, considering that the professionals involved have a similar background (biologist, biotechnologist, figure graduated in pharmaceutical themes, chemists, or engineers). Different in respect of the previous profile can be the level of graduation; indeed for this kind of activities, PhD or masters are not so indispensable; on the other side, technical skills are very important. Different are also the dimensions of the teams, which are often smaller than the teams needed for R&D projects. Also, the multidisciplinary level required for services is less evident; indeed problem solving is often circumscribed to a specific issue requiring one or two specific competencies.

Industrial oriented mindset is required, because of the strong interaction with companies; also, a knowledge of medical device regulation is mandatory for these kinds of professionals, such as GMP and GLP knowledge.

In our case, clinical development, besides the activities strictly needed for obtaining the certification, is not so much treated; however, some STPs can offer also this kind of activities: other competencies may be added to the previous list, e.g., can be useful professionals as data managers and analysts, biostatisticians, or doctors to set up the clinical trial.

14.3.3   Regulatory Specialist and Quality Manager

Professions in the world of life sciences are evolving, and companies are increasingly careful to select their profiles. The regulatory affairs industry plays an important role in ensuring the safety of medical devices. The ubiquity of regulatory work makes it an ideal field for anyone interested in using scientific methods and analysis to make a difference in the world around them. Becoming a regulatory affairs specialist is one of the most common ways to break into the industry, especially after the entry in force of the new medical device regulation (MDR). Required from the new MDR, each medical device's manufacturers needs a specific professionals specialized in the regulatory field able to follow all the certification process from the very beginning with the definition of the conformity of the devices and with the check of the technical documentation up to the management of post-marketing surveillance obligations.

Becoming a regulatory specialist doesn't require a specific degree (law, medicine, pharmacy, engineering) or PhD, but lately due to the increasing importance of this role, several university masters were born. An example is the university master in "Regulatory sciences and quality management in the biomedical field," a postgraduate course with the aim of training professionals with adequate skills in the field of regulatory activities and the quality management system. In particular, knowledge of regulatory practices matches the management and marketing skills with the aim to understand the meaning and scope of the specific procedures.

A quality manager, or quality assurance manager, ensures that the product and all processes developed by the company or the STP in this case meet quality standards set by the organization before it is being launched into the market. The QM is in charge of supervising the production process to make sure that all products meet consistent standards, and the duties include developing and implementing quality control tests, inspecting products at various stages, writing reports, and documenting production issues.

14.3.4 Communication and Marketing

In our vision, communication and marketing in a STP comprise very different activities such as:

- Dissemination of results of research activities.
- Organization and promotion of thematic workshops or events; events and workshop can be directed to companies, the research sector, or to a nonspecialized audience (i.e., open day is organized to involve citizenship or young students).
- Participation to thematic trade fairs also with booths.
- Promotion of R&D and service activities carried out by the laboratories located in the STP. Promotion has several objectives: find new clients (companies, public and private entities, research centers, etc.) and establish new partnership with other research centers to carry out projects.
- Involvement of the public stakeholders (such as universities or chamber of commerce) to underline the activities and the results obtained by the STP.
- Management of website and social network of STP.

Communication & marketing profile, like in companies, is an important figure also for STPs, and it can be considered also a hybrid profile. Indeed, it is not essential that this role is covered by figure with a scientific background; however, in our experience, scientific background can be useful to communicate in a proper way with all the stakeholders, like companies, public entities, or other research centers. Probably, if this role is covered by a scientific profile, it will be necessary to have collaboration with experts in graphic design, website development and management, etc., to obtain dissemination and exploitation materials that can be used in different channels.

Due to the specific characteristic of the sector, we saw that this role can be covered by professionals with a degree in a biological or medical discipline or biomedical engineering. It is necessary to have a proper knowledge of the field of application of the R&D activities performed by the STP. Technical background can be supplemented with masters or courses on communication or marketing. It is probably not essential to have a deep knowledge of the technical aspects, because communication and marketing can involve, in case of necessity, for each activity, the expert of a specific theme or product or technology. On the other hand, this profile may be very proactive in the involvement of all the stakeholders, able to manage the relations and to tailor scientific contents in function of the targeted audience.

14.3.5 Technology Transfer and Project Manager

Technology transfer allows the deployment of science into society. It is an evolving field of knowledge combining science and business approaches. There are some essential parameters to consider in that process as the intellectual property aspects such as confidentiality, patenting, and individual and institutional commercial rights. The developmental stage of a technology is key to deciding what steps to take to increase the chances of success of the transfer, and to understand which partners are directly involved along the whole process. There are many mechanisms to add value to an invention disclosure to make it more amenable for a transfer in the forms of a license or a start-up. Some typical agreements are commonly used in technology transfer, such as confidentiality agreements, material transfer agreements, R&D licenses with or without commercial option, commercial license agreements, and creation of spinoff companies.

The person involved in the technology transfer needs to understand the drivers and the needs of a relevant market, which can prove to be difficult, and how to overcome this.

There is a cultural encounter between business and science; both fields of knowledge have to reach common goals.

This philosophy has been highlighted also for the role of the project manager. This role takes a different version if we describe it in the university or in the science and technology park. In particular, the project manager plays a primary role in standing between the R&D activities and their technology transfer.

In particular, the project manager collects all the innovative ideas and translates them in a R&D project, combining business and science, and bringing the research at a new stage. In fact, the project manager leads the team, helping the relationship between the members of the team and the partner of the project. Other duties of this role are to foster the development of the project aiming to achieve the objective and the results.

Table 14.2 summarizes for each of the different job categories which profile or degree is required, and which additional courses are recommended. It is important to underline that this is our personal view.

Table 14.2 Required degree and recommended additional training for the different job categories described in this chapter

Role	Profile/degree	Additional training opportunities
High-tech profile	Scientific degree	*Master and courses* on the regulatory field, in order to understand how to apply the quality and the regulatory affairs in the laboratory work. Updating training, participation to conference and meeting
Services profile	Scientific degree	*Master and courses* on the regulatory field, in order to understand how to apply the quality and the regulatory affairs in the laboratory work. Updating training, participation to conference and meeting
Regulatory specialist and quality manager	Scientific degree Law degree Economic degree	*Master and courses on the regulatory field* in order to be constantly updated to the new MDR and how to improve the quality management
Communication and marketing	Scientific degree Economic degree Communication degree	*Master or courses on communication or marketing*, to improve the knowledge and the skills in order to develop a specific communication tailored for the scientific public
Project manager and technology transfer	Scientific degree Economic degree	*MBA, master in business administration*. This will support the person to focus on accounting, applied statistics, human resources, business communication, business ethics, business law, strategic management, business strategy, finance, managerial economics, management, entrepreneurship, marketing, supply-chain management, and operations management

14.3.6   Career Perspectives

The entry point in STPs can differ in function of the different profiles.

Generally talking, starting from an easy entry point, researchers can ask for a graduate internship to enter in contact with a laboratory and starting a first approach with companies. In this case, often the university thesis is on applied research in collaboration with companies. In the same way, STPs can host students performing a PhD program. These programs are favored by the strict connection between STP and universities, which can facilitate the design of specific arguments for the PhD thesis.

For other profiles, in function of the management structures and of each country's labor regulation, the access to position in STPs can vary. Indeed, researchers can be appointed through public tenders or directly. What is important to know is the degree required for each position, as described in the previous sections: some positions require high level of education (such as PhD), other less skilled profiles. Moreover, in some cases, where the collaboration is well established, also university researchers can be dislocated in STPs to perform industrial R&D.

Concerning the careers' perspective, researchers can have three different choices:

- Growth inside the STPs. In this case, researchers or other profiles can stay in the STPs, specializing in each of the activities described; it is clear that the career growth depends on the dimension and characteristics of the STPs, big STPs can offer different paths of career, and other can offer a stable position.
- Return to university. Where the link with universities is strict, for researchers that maintain their role also at university can be possible to continue their careers in academia. In this case, the link with STPs can be maintained during years, favoring the cross-contamination between academia and STP.
- Passage to companies. It is very frequent that researchers, after some years of experience acquired in STPs, pass to work in companies of the sector. This is favored by two different phenomena: the first one is the experience acquired by the researchers in applied science, matching knowledge of the sector (such as regulation) with strong scientific background; the second one is the continuous contact between the researcher and the company, favoring the mutual knowledge.

These choices are available for all the profiles described, high tech, service, regulatory, communication and marketing, and PM/technology transfer. However, for researchers performing services, R&D and regulatory, passage into the industrial sector is much easier than for the others; R&D can easily passage also in a university environment. Other profiles, such as project manager, can be easier than the others who have a professional growth in STP.

At TPM we have evidence of all the described paths, professionals that stay at TPM or prefer to return to academia or other absorbed by companies. The choice depends mainly on the aspiration of the single researchers.

Another option for professionals working in STP who have a specific knowledge of market and sector requirements is the creation of a start-up/spin-off. This kind of phenomena is less frequent because it requires an innovative and profitable idea (it is required a "think out of the box" approach), and in the life sciences sector, entering into the market with a new solution (product or service) requires huge investment and time. However, STPs are often a proper ecosystem to development of new ideas, thanks to the strict contact with companies and because several STPs (like TPM) have specific areas for incubation of start-ups and are able to administer consultancy for business creation and growth. STPs can be also a great opportunity for external start-up and spin-off which would like to grow in a proper ecosystem.

14.4 Conclusion

Starting from our knowledge, this is our vision about the job employment in STPs. Indeed, we tried to transfer the lessons learned in our experience and analysis of life science STPs. However, as anticipated, each STP is a unique model, also in key aspects, such as management structure, revenue models, hosted laboratories, collaboration with stakeholders, etc. In a STP, the key roles are slightly different compared to the university or to the companies, but this is the strength of a structure like this.

The possibility to work directly with companies, universities, and research centers helps all the professionals described to understand the importance of the research in order to boost the innovation, especially in a sector as the biomedical and the medical technology. STPs are able to offer interesting opportunities for professional careers in the life sciences sector combining the knowledge acquired from an academic pathway with the traditional skills of a business.

In this scenario, the traditional professional figure is completely turned upside down. The contamination of the different environment creates a new professional profile adsorbed in a solid and advanced interconnection among researchers, clinics, biomedical experts, and quality and regulatory affairs.

References

Coffano M (2016) Innovation dynamics in the medical device sector. No. Thesis. EPFL

Guadix J et al (2016) Success variables in science and technology parks. J Bus Res 69(11): 4870–4875

JRC Technical Reports (2014) https://doi.org/10.2788/1795. ISBN: 978-92-79-43179-1 (PDF), ISSN: 1684-0917 (PDF), Other: EUR 26867 EN

McCormack B, Fallon EF, Cormican K (2015) An analysis of open innovation practices in the medical technology sector in Ireland. Proc Manufact 3:503–509

Ramlogan R, Mina A, Tampubolon G, Metcalfe JS (2007) Networks of knowledge: the distributed nature of medical innovation. Scientometrics 70(2):459–489

Roldan LB, Hansen PB, Garcia-Perez-de-Lema D (2018) The relationship between favorable conditions for innovation in technology parks, the innovation produced, and companies' performance: a framework for an analysis model. Innov Manag Rev 15(3):286–302

Rosenberg N (1994) Medical device innovation. In: Cepr/Aaas conference, Stanford University

Şimşek K, Yıldırım N (2016) Constraints to open innovation in science and technology parks. Procedia Soc Behav Sci 235:719–728

Chapter 15
To Be or Not to Be: Entrepreneurship and Enterprise Creation as a Way to Innovate in Life Sciences

Brian Cahill, Fabrizio Conicella, Eoin Galligan, and Miklós Györffi

Abstract New market opportunities in the life sciences will emerge in the next few years, thanks to scientific advancements and the need for entrepreneurs who can address these opportunities is following such a trend. The role of companies, in particular of innovative start-ups in contributing to the development and economic growth of society and in the development of healthcare-related solutions, has been extensively studied. Unfortunately it has been clear since at least a decade that there is a profound mismatch between the traditional role of doctoral education in preparing young researchers for an academic career. Particularly in life sciences the existence of pure scientific results, however excellent they may be, does not automatically entail their transformation into innovative activities. This is the reason why the role of the researcher within the entrepreneurial process of a high-tech start-up—particularly in the field of biotechnology—is fundamental, especially in the initial stages. Examples of focused training and supporting solutions are existing but still not standardised. On the other hand, the need to maximise the impact of scientific research on society requires curricula, particularly for STEM (Science, Technology, Engineering and Mathematics) students, which will explicitly include entrepreneurial and innovation management components as transformative tools to maximise their contribution to society.

B. Cahill
Leibniz Information Centre for Science and Technology, Hannover, Germany

F. Conicella (✉)
Life Science District Srl, Milano, Italy

E. Galligan
Technology Transfer Office, Aarhus University, Aarhus, Denmark

M. Györffi
Eötvös Loránd Research Network, Budapest, Hungary

© The Author(s), under exclusive license to Springer Nature Switzerland AG 2023   249
J. R. Thomas et al. (eds.), *Career Options in the Pharmaceutical and Biomedical Industry*, https://doi.org/10.1007/978-3-031-14911-5_15

15.1 Entrepreneurship as a Key Skill and Opportunity for Potential Innovators in Life Sciences

It has been clear since at least a decade that there is a profound mismatch between the traditional role of doctoral education in preparing young researchers for an academic career and the reality that a significant majority of researchers will pursue a career outside academia (Haynes et al. 2009; The Royal Society 2010). In 2010, *The Economist* magazine (The Economist 2010) described the rise in the number of PhD students as being an 'oversupply' and accused universities of regarding PhD students as 'cheap, highly motivated and disposable labour'. The traditional 'apprentice-master' model of doctoral training resulted in a focus on training for a job in academia: even now most early-career researchers continue to focus most strongly on carrying out research work that will lead to publications in scientific journals. The emphasis on purely academic outputs that are of most value for those who will pursue an academic career is evidenced by practices in academic hiring: research publication continues to be by far the most significant assessment criterion for academic careers (Saenen et al. 2019). This contrasts very sharply with the predominant long-term career trajectory of doctoral researchers into careers in the private sector, where publication record often plays no role in hiring decisions. A recent declaration by the Marie Curie Alumni Association and the European Council of Doctoral Candidates and Junior Researchers (Eurodoc) addressed the career prospects of early-career researchers by calling for (1) sustainable academic career prospects for researchers, (2) career management services at organisations employing researchers, (3) more emphasis on transferable skills training and (4) wider networking options (Kismihók et al. 2019).

Many measures have been undertaken to adapt the quality of doctoral education (Davies et al. 2019) to support doctoral researchers to find a career path out of universities into the private sector (Chong and Clohisey 2021) and address perceived skills gaps in their career development (De Grande et al. 2014). Doctoral programmes have begun to take responsibility for the career prospects of PhD candidates by providing courses in transferable skills. Early-career researchers are sometimes provided with skills training in entrepreneurship that helps them to assess the technological and commercial potential of research results and decide whether and how to transfer research into a potential invention. It is essential for researchers to acquire the communication skills necessary to convince potential investors and to negotiate contracts. Among these courses, entrepreneurship, communication, project management, leadership and negotiation are among the transferable skills training that are sometimes offered to some early-career researchers. Most often doctoral training is relatively generic rather than personalised to the career development wishes of early-career researchers and the needs of potential employers (Kobayashi et al. 2014). Eurodoc recently published a report that contained an infographic that illustrates the wide range of transferable skills that early-career researchers can choose to develop (Weber et al. 2018). Enterprise was represented by commercialisation, entrepreneurship, innovation/knowledge transfer, intellectual property rights (IPR), legal/business standardisation and patenting. Many of the skills under other headings, particularly interpersonal and communication skills, are also relevant for entrepreneurial careers.

Doctoral training programmes, particularly in STEM (Science, Technology, Engineering and Mathematics)-related disciplines, have the potential to promote entrepreneurship in such a way that relates directly to careers in innovation, product development, sales and marketing. Among EU-funded programmes, the European Institute of Innovation and Technology (EIT) (European Institute of Innovation and Technology 2020) has been leading in developing master's and doctoral programmes that are built around entrepreneurial education and focus on combining education, training, research and innovation with an entrepreneurial mindset. Nevertheless, although the EIT provides a model for master's and doctoral programmes, of the five EIT innovation communities, EIT Health is relatively poorly represented in this form of education with less than 1% of the currently enrolled EIT-labelled PhD students.

Many potential inventions in research institutions remain unexploited due to the lack of a coherent overall strategy for technology transfer within the organisation. This extends far beyond simple provision of skills training to early-career researchers. Some research institutions have developed support for a range of services for entrepreneurial training, protection of intellectual property and exploitation of innovations through licencing or founding a spin-off company. In the life sciences, the European Molecular Biology Lab (EMBL) plays an outstanding role in the support of career development of its early-career researchers (Woolston 2020). The EIPOD Postdoctoral Programme provides coherent career development support for a cohort of postdoctoral researchers with mandatory training in entrepreneurship in life sciences with optional entrepreneurship-targeted e-learning training modules (EMBL n.d.). In addition, EMBL founded EMBLEM GmbH that embeds technology transfer within EMBL by identifying, protecting and commercialising intellectual property-generated researchers.

15.2 Impact of Entrepreneurship and Entrepreneurs in Life Sciences on Our Society

In the course of the twentieth century, developments in the life sciences have had a vast impact on society and social well-being. Such developments have led to the extension of life expectancy, which has gone from an average of 47 years in 1950 to 73.2 years in 2020. Initially, the development of vaccines and the discovery of antibiotics contributed to a large degree to this increase in life expectancy (Worldometer 2020), thus boosting significantly social interest towards health management, and particularly healthcare delivery. Child vaccination resulted in the practical eradication of diseases that were a major factor in child mortality.

New discoveries within the life sciences significantly enlarged the spectrum of products in pharmaceuticals and medical devices. As a consequence, healthcare industries (pharmaceuticals and medical devices) diversified their product offerings with ever more reliable and efficient products that became important economic factors of developed societies. Healthcare delivery (Piña et al. 2015) is also increasingly gaining importance in the comprehensive provision of healthcare services.

The traditional approach towards healthcare delivery is centred on its health restoration function. However, scientific discoveries (particularly in physics, chemistry and biology) have also facilitated the development of more sophisticated diagnostic equipment and procedures with which health conditions can be monitored more reliably. In this line, we have also witnessed a more precise and diversified disease identification process, which opens the door for more refined products and services. The role of healthcare delivery has also been enlarged from the restoration of health to preservation and prevention. Within this, a number of factors—not immediately bound to healthcare delivery—gained significant importance, among which the most notable ones are those related to the environment. Currently, a large part of environmental policies are motivated by protecting health and preventing disease. Similarly, another area is that of production of healthy food and policies related to this.

In the developed societies with extended life expectancy, we also witness a new phenomenon, which is the ageing population and its needs. Such needs are not necessarily related to health, but they help in maintaining an honourable, full value life condition. However, the ageing society is a challenge since the market is defined by the continuously growing elderly population whose needs (expressed both in terms of the pharma, food and devices sector) are increasingly different from those of middle-aged and younger people.

The significant shift in technologies in all healthcare areas creates new market opportunities and is certainly a level playing field for entrepreneurs, i.e. for those who have the knowledge and capacity to develop and market products and services required within the new conditions. For instance, one of the major producers of electronic appliances in Europe, Philips, totally ceased producing lighting equipment and electronic devices (radio, television, etc.), and its main high-tech production line today is healthcare. The new technologies associated with artificial intelligence bear the promise of extensive use in healthcare, but raise intensive debate on the ethical and regulatory issues associated with assigning responsibility. For example, if a robot helps in a surgical intervention and the patient dies because of a malfunction, who is responsible: the manufacturer of the robot or the surgeon?

Cyber technologies also offer a much larger perspective on storage and later use of patient data, with associated market opportunities for data entrepreneurs. For instance, IBM has transitioned from being a major manufacturer of mainframe computers in the 1970s into a major healthcare data broker through its Watson Health data management system. However, handling patient data raises a number of concerns, from the use of personal data up to the reliability of healthcare decisions based on large sets of patient data, partly addressed by regulation. Regulation is becoming more sophisticated in all areas of life sciences which raises the question of the impact of regulation on entrepreneurship, as final products need to conform with an increasingly complex regulatory framework.

A particular regulatory aspect is standardisation, which in principle creates market opportunities for entrepreneurs to produce alternative products with higher technical performance, at a cheaper price. Nevertheless, standards are stricter in industries associated with the life sciences. Products and services addressing the general population may need to be tailored, in order to address the differing medical needs of individuals. The same disease can often have a completely different impact on different individuals. This leads to the use of technology to deliver personalised medicine, which is becoming more readily available as more refined technologies are entering the market.

A high level of healthcare delivery is not possible without an extensive and sophisticated healthcare system. The development of healthcare systems is an important indicator of social development. The organisation of healthcare systems goes hand in hand with the proliferation of health insurance, which is also highly regulated. This in itself represents an enormous market. Still, it differs from country to country, even within the EU, which results ultimately in extremely different conditions. The increasing cost of healthcare and increased budgets creates an opportunity for those who can lower the costs by developing new cheaper products or services.

Basically, these shifts have contributed to new market opportunities in the life sciences and the need for entrepreneurs who can address these opportunities. Conversely, the capabilities of health entrepreneurs to take advantage of scientific and technological developments, and produce and market products that meet the health regulatory and standardisation requirements, have boosted significantly the transformation of healthcare delivery in terms of health preservation, restoration and prevention.

15.3 From Science to Innovation: The Alternative Way Through Start-Up Creation

15.3.1 The Path from Science to Start-Up Growth

The role of companies, in particular of innovative start-ups in contributing to the development and economic growth of society, has been extensively studied (Skala 2019; Del Bosco et al. 2021). However, the role that STEM (Science, Technology, Engineering and Mathematics) researchers-turned-entrepreneurs play in contributing to this impact has not been equally emphasised (Samsom and Gurdon 1993; Audretsch and Kayalar-Erdem 2005; Wang et al. 2021). Entrepreneurship is not often included in the list of possible career paths for scientists (Oliver 2004; Miron-Shatz et al. 2014; Froshauer 2017; Goji et al. 2020); hence, relatively little attention has been placed in providing skills and knowledge related to entrepreneurship at a university level. On the other hand, the lack of awareness about the innovation process deriving from scientific results—which is particularly competitive, long and selective in sectors linked to human health and biotechnology—is perceived as an important obstacle that researchers themselves need to overcome to pursue entrepreneurial career paths.

The existence of pure scientific results in biotech, however excellent they may be, does not automatically entail their transformation into innovative activities (Patzelt and Brenner 2008; Patzelt et al. 2012; Shimasaki 2020). Usually an 'act of creativity' is needed (Amabile 1997, 2013; Rank et al. 2004; Edwards-Schachter et al. 2015) that serves as a conceptual and operational hub. The creative act, i.e. the identification of a technical solution to a problem in a unique and distinctive way, is a key step. It allows the identification of how to protect the invention and to foresee exploitation paths. It is the step that identifies the passage from the basic research activity (focused in creating new knowledge) to the innovation phase that will permit the development of a new product, process or service that will be made available to those that express the need.

Critical analysis is necessary before choosing to undertake technology transfer. There are different paths that could be followed: for example, the transfer of the invention, the filing of a patent that protects it and the finalisation of cooperative research projects (Wright et al. 2004; Weckowska 2015; Kergroach et al. 2018) with partners or the direct exploitation of the knowledge generated through the creation of an innovative start-up. The decisions to start a sustainable and clearly defined development path are not based exclusively on scientific excellence, but also on the active choice by the researcher, or of a team of researchers, to switch to a career path that supports the development of the invention. The personal characteristics and the aptitude for professional development, together with a clear awareness of the path itself, are the key factors to understand this decision of researchers to become entrepreneurs (Veeraraghavan 2009; Mas-Tur and Ribeiro Soriano 2014; Block et al. 2017; Kamid et al. 2020). However, the awareness of the path derives entirely from the knowledge and skills to which the potential entrepreneurs have been exposed to during their training experiences. Most often though, the potential entrepreneurs are left to find their way and learn the tricks of the trade the hard way, with little or no guidance.

The act of creativity can facilitate researchers to take that first step towards the exploitation of the created knowledge; nevertheless, creativity alone is not sufficient for undertaking an entrepreneurial path. How to make practical use of the acquired knowledge and how to protect it is also fundamental, as well as identifying the right support factors and sources of financing. Moreover, the development of technological products requires a continuous verification of the distinctive elements that make the product competitive in an existing marketplace, as compared to other products in the existing market or in advanced development.

Both of these activities must be based on the researcher's ability to use his own knowledge and skills and on his interactions with experts, technicians and users operating outside the academic environment. The existence of networks, ecosystems and other actors (technology transfer offices, incubators, science parks, etc.) working at the interface between the world of research and the world of industry greatly facilitates this activity. These entities play an important role in facilitating the initial development of the initiative and in defining the strategy that will allow the fundraising itself. The definition of the strategy and the distinctive and unique application of the research results to satisfy a need are often summarised in short documents ('pitch', 'executive summary'). These short documents will then form the basis of the business plan that illustrates the path that the innovative company intends to follow, and for the 'business model' which explains how the company itself will be sustainable by creating economic value. The "Value proposition description"[1] that will result from the development of business perspective analysis and the description of such perspectives and of the activities that will be realised to transform the idea in a real solution available for users and patients will constitute the "starting engine" of the entrepreneurial machine (Kaplan and Murray 2010; Gurău and Dana 2020).

It is evident that investors have a 'clear' goal: the transformation of the initial financial support into higher economic value at a certain stage of development of the funded initiative ('Exit'). They are providing financial resources in exchange for a percentage of ownership in the entrepreneurial initiative that they will 'sell' when the economic value created will be high enough to permit a good return on investment. As a consequence, the scientist-entrepreneur will be 'obliged' to offer part of the ownership to an external actor with the goal to have, in the near future, a greater economic value than the initial one.

Unfortunately, the risk of failure is quite high for such ventures, particularly in the health sectors, and investors are meticulously selective in their choices. To de-risk funded initiatives, they are not limiting activities in providing resources, but they act directly to ameliorate the competencies and existing networks to provide solutions to the issues linked to the industrial development of the possible products in an environment that is highly regulated and extremely competitive.

15.3.2   Key Roles Inside a Start-Up for Scientists

The role of the researcher particularly with STEM (Science, Technology, Engineering and Mathematics)-related background within the entrepreneurial process of a high-tech start-up—particularly in the field of biotechnology—is fundamental, especially in the initial stages. Not only is the entrepreneur the inventor of the technological solution at the basis of the possible new product, process or service, but the same initial validation and development-oriented experimentation activity requires

---

[1] The value proposition will include, at least, research of excellence description, its protection (the patent), the definition of a strategy and the formalization of these in documents to be shared (business plan, pitch and business model) will allow to introduce oneself to initially close and informal investors (the three '3F', family friends and fools 'and business angels') and then to more and more professional actors ('seeds and venture capitalists') in order to attract economic resources which, with additional public funding.

specific skills, knowledge and time dedicated for that activity/solution. The researcher, however, in this phase must necessarily reflect on the role he intends to play during the development process.

A first consequence of this reflection will be an increase in the focus and implementation of research activities, increasingly conceived to enrich the value of the future product and to accelerate its development. Legitimate scientific curiosity will have to make way for a justifiably more calculated approach. This takes on an increasingly important aspect to be assessed due to the ability to attract financial resources from risky investors clearly guided not simply by scientific interest but by the possibility of creating economic value.

The need to acquire more managerial skills and to interact extensively with internal and external stakeholders of the start-up operating in areas of knowledge adjacent but different from the scientific one obliges a choice. Dealing with administrative, regulatory, quality management, production, development of clinical programmes, human resource management, business development, etc. is a challenge. Hence, the researcher is often faced with two choices, to 'become a manager' or whether to continue operating in the start-up with a role more closely linked to science, often as CSO (chief scientific officer). Obviously, the choice to become a manager requires a training path (training on the job or institutionalised training such as participation in a master in business administration) and cultural adaptation that also requires the identification of new priorities for the activities. The initial choice is then repeated at the various stages of the start-up's development: the increase in complexity will require additional skills and knowledge, and will always lead to new choices and changes of role, responsibility and often organisational position within the company. Essentially the candidate has to receive changes, accept it and start living with it all for the greater good of a successful venture. Consequently, some typical aspects of the research world such as freedom of choice of research questions, ownership of the research results, the possibility of publishing freely, etc. will be increasingly questioned at the expense of other elements such as the ability to protect research results, possibility to publish only after an analysis of the intellectual protection possibilities, the need to focus on commercially relevant activities, etc. Obviously, the change can also have advantages, above all economic but also the ability to influence the development of a technological product/solution which, speaking of human health, will have a positive impact on the lives of all of us.

15.4   Training on Entrepreneurship and Life Sciences: From Hidden Gems to Standard Curricula

The growth of life science entrepreneurship programmes for early-stage researchers continues unabated, with two European examples being SPARK Norway and EIT Health. SPARK Norway (part of SPARK Global) is a 2-year innovation programme to further develop ideas within health-related topics in the life science domain. It is open to researchers at the University of Oslo, Oslo University Hospital and Akershus

University Hospital (SPARK Norway n.d.). EIT Health was established in 2015, as a 'knowledge and innovation community' (KIC) focusing on health, within the European Institute of Innovation and Technology (EIT). It is based in Munich, with regional hubs across the EU (EIT Health n.d.).

Such programmes have been triggered by the growth of 'research impact' demands from academic funding organisations such as Horizon 2020 (European Commission; Directorate-General for Research and Innovation 2015). These stakeholders promoted spin-outs and partnerships as a required research outcome and offered follow-on proof-of-concept funding to enable such activity. These programmes enable the final component—to train life science researchers to compete for proof-of-concept funding (or seed investment)—utilising appropriate business, development and regulatory concepts.

A range of models have been used, from the innovation programme based at a specific university to focused 'boot camps' that are open to many regional institutions. Most programmes demand a competitive application from the researchers and seek to mature a commercialisation case via training and mentors and may include proof-of-concept funding. There are typically two types of educational components: the standard curricula and more specialised life science 'hidden gems'. The former can be delivered by university or incubator staff, while the latter is often delivered by external guest instructors such as industry scientists, regulatory affairs consultants or experienced entrepreneurs. SPARK Oslo delivers their training at the university with specialised seminars every 2 weeks in the early evening. Alternatively, EIT Health offers a structured programme open to researchers from different universities.

What is included within the standard curricula of life science entrepreneurship? In crossing the boundary between research and innovation, many researchers need time to reflect. Important aspects of the curricula can focus on leaving the individualistic nature of academic culture towards the 'team culture' of innovation. Three important examples are language and communication, business models and the regulatory process.

As researchers enter this process of reflection, it is important to define terminology and explain how language is used within innovation. Take 'value proposition'. At a research conference, a postdoctoral researcher will present the experimental protocol that was used and the statistical quality and evaluate if the knowledge obtained validates (or invalidates) their hypotheses. Communication in innovation is different. The innovator has to interact with stakeholders to understand their perception of a problem. They propose to solve this problem and convince stakeholders that the value of their approach is superior—and could be the basis of a competitive business. The process is iterative: interact with stakeholders, refine approach and interact again. This finishes with a text defined as the 'value proposition'. This example is covered in more detail further below. It highlights how terminology, culture and the researchers' activity are deeply intertwined and emphasises the importance of communication in entrepreneurship programmes.

A second example is life science business models. Michael Porter developed the framework of the value chain defined as the process or activities by which a company adds value to an article, including production, marketing, and the provision of aftersales service (Porter 1985). By understanding the value chain and benchmark business models, entrepreneurship programmes seek to ensure that researchers are prepared to design the value chain of their own spin-out company. Take the following two examples of life science business models—the contract research organisation (CRO) and the fully integrated pharma company (FIPCo). The FIPCo is the largest organisation of all, with expertise at all stages of drug discovery. Alternatively, CROs enable larger companies to outsource drug discovery (or medical device activity) to specialist organisations. CROs typically specialise in a stage of clinical development (Phase I or II) or a disease area (Dixon 2019).

The third curricula example is the regulatory process for drug development and medical devices. Regulatory authorities ensure that clinical trial interventions with novel drugs or devices are subject to close scrutiny. Empowering researchers with this knowledge is important for three key reasons: the high capital investment created due to regulatory demands, the subsequent expectations from investors and the impact that such 'constraints' have on researchers that are familiar with the freedom of research.

Global health authorities such as the Food and Drug Administration (FDA) and European Medicines Agency (EMA) follow a set of principles called good clinical practices (GCPs) which are specified in a set of guidance documents, International Conference on Harmonisation (ICH) (Chiodin et al. 2019). Within a life science innovation programme, a researcher would need to build a team that includes staff responsible for the regulatory strategy and to understand the steps to their first applications to the authorities.

While curricula in life science entrepreneurship programmes is becoming standardised, a number of programmes propose specific activities that yield short-term, high-impact learning for researchers. An iterative, learning process with stakeholders was previously described. In NIH's I-Corps programme (Maloy et al. 2020), Steve Blank systematised this process into a series of interviews that sought to validate hypotheses. He termed this process as 'customer discovery'. Although PhD students and postdoctoral researchers were assigned industry mentors, the I-Corps programme ensured they took 'ownership' of validating their own hypotheses via interviews. These discussions would be with stakeholders linked to the value proposition or business model. A series of interviews would gain evidence, forcing the team to invalidate hypotheses across the business model (National Science Foundation 2013).

An additional tool to empower researchers' learning is the target product profile. This document is used throughout the industry. An example is displayed on the WHO websites, and they are used within the SPARK Oslo programme (Clarke et al. n.d.). In essence, the framework enables a team to improve their communication on the final goal of a life science company—the product. It states the steps and additional components that enable the original university invention to be commercialised as a product. It can include the indication, formulation, drug product characteristics and preclinical and clinical studies. By compiling all proposed characteristics, the team (including external consultants) shares a final product vision. The FDA offers guidance on how to develop the TPP and has recommended its use within advisory meetings. It enables FDA staff to understand the technical details of the product and allows them to formulate focused questions.

With the arrival of Horizon Europe and particularly the EIC Accelerator instrument, it is clear that research impact activity is here to stay and will only increase. The standard curricula have long been a part of undergraduate education and are growing within the deliverables of PhD graduate school programmes. The 'hidden gems' of obtaining stakeholder's perception on the value proposition and the target product profile will continue to enter the research practice, enabling researchers to communicate the impact of their research findings and to obtain research funding.

15.5   Conclusions, Suggestions and Future Perspectives: A Way Forward, Unlocking the Potential of Entrepreneurial Education

The creation of a supportive and dynamic innovation ecosystem linked to national, regional and local innovation systems has been proposed as a way to give an answer to the need to stimulate entrepreneurial attitudes. Different policies and initiatives have been launched and financed within the framework of the European Research Area (Ulnicane 2015) in order to facilitate the 'production of knowledge' and the diffusion and adoption of such knowledge through innovations in the society. However, we are still facing a fragmented system, where components on some of the key assets for development are working in different, and in some cases, not coherent ways. To overcome this situation, we need to align policies and regulations while supporting all initiatives that outline the positive social role of innovation and lift up the role of the entrepreneurial approach as the key element that drives the innovation process. We have to consider all such elements in a world where the real challenge is to define a global framework of continental systems. Among the different open issues (awareness of the role of innovation and entrepreneurship at societal level, better support to knowledge exploitation activities, increased resources to produce knowledge, lower fragmentation of infrastructural investments, better support schemes for knowledge exploitation, standard regulatory environments, etc.), we would like to outline the need for a new approach in educating the new generation of researchers in STEM (Science, Technology, Engineering and Mathematics)-related disciplines to provide them with a better set of competencies and knowledge to maximise the impact of their activities.

The society to maximise the impact of science and the transformation of scientific results in innovations among other things needs curricula for STEM (Science, Technology, Engineering and Mathematics) students that will explicitly include entrepreneurial and innovation management components as transformative tools to maximise their contribution to the society. We need to better evaluate the role of entrepreneurial education in creating a better environment for innovation and as a tool to create welfare and progress. Providing researchers with the right skillset will enable them to evaluate the knowledge produced in terms of impact and to identify the entrepreneurial path that is required to transform such into solutions fulfilling human needs. The inclusion of standard entrepreneurial education modules at different levels of education, the possibility for researchers to be evaluated also in terms of their capability to approach research activities in an entrepreneurial way and the creation of a common regulatory framework for researchers that are willing to exploit the knowledge produced are all transformative initiatives that have the potential to change the actual situation.

We do not have to change the culture but rather enrich the actual culture with a key component: the idea that we can solve the problems that surround us.

Acknowledgements This article has been conceptualised by EuroScience's Science Policy Workgroup on Innovation and Entrepreneurship. The authors wish to thank Teresa Fernandez, Nandakumar Krishnaswamy, Olayinka Osuolale and Violeta Greciuhin for their critical revision of the initial manuscript.

References

Amabile TM (1997) Entrepreneurial creativity through motivational synergy. J Creat Behav 31:18–26. https://doi.org/10.1002/j.2162-6057.1997.tb00778.x

Amabile TM (2013) Componential theory of creativity. In: Kessler EH (ed) Encyclopedia of management theory. Sage, London

Audretsch DB, Kayalar-Erdem D (2005) Determinants of scientist entrepreneurship: an integrative research agenda. In: Handbook of entrepreneurship research. Edward Elgar, Cheltenham

Block JH, Fisch CO, van Praag M (2017) The Schumpeterian entrepreneur: a review of the empirical evidence on the antecedents, behaviour and consequences of innovative entrepreneurship. Ind Innov 24:61–95. https://doi.org/10.1080/13662716.2016.1216397

Chiodin D, Cox EM, Edmund AV et al (2019) Regulatory affairs 101: introduction to investigational new drug applications and clinical trial applications. Clin Transl Sci 12:334–342. https://doi.org/10.1111/cts.12635

Chong ZS, Clohisey S (2021) How to build a well-rounded CV and get hired after your PhD. FEBS J 288:3072. https://doi.org/10.1111/febs.15635

Clarke DF, Pascual F, Ojoo A (n.d.) Module 7: target product profiles. World Health Organisation, Geneva, pp 126–143

Davies T, Macaulay L, Pretorius L (2019) Tensions between disciplinary knowledge and transferable skills: fostering personal epistemology during doctoral studies. In: Wellbeing in doctoral education. Springer, Singapore

De Grande H, De Boyser K, Vandevelde K, Van Rossem R (2014) From academia to industry: are doctorate holders ready? J Knowl Econ 5:538. https://doi.org/10.1007/s13132-014-0192-9

Del Bosco B, Mazzucchelli A, Chierici R, Di Gregorio A (2021) Innovative start-up creation: the effect of local factors and demographic characteristics of entrepreneurs. Int Entrep Manag J 17:145. https://doi.org/10.1007/s11365-019-00618-0

Dixon J (2019) RIPCO, FIPCO, NRDO, FIPNET, VIPCO. Trade secrets, bioengineering community. Nat Biotechnol. https://bioengineeringcommunity.nature.com/posts/45149-ripco-fipco-nrdo-fipnet-vipco

Edwards-Schachter M, García-Granero A, Sánchez-Barrioluengo M et al (2015) Disentangling competences: interrelationships on creativity, innovation and entrepreneurship. Think Skills Creat 16:27–39. https://doi.org/10.1016/j.tsc.2014.11.006

EIT Health EU (n.d.) Promoting innovation in health. (EU) EIT Health. https://eithealth.eu/. Accessed 15 Nov 2021

EMBL (n.d.) EIPOD4 Fellowship programme—postdoctoral programme. https://www.embl.org/about/info/postdoctoral-programme/eipod4-fellowship-programme/. Accessed 15 Nov 2021

European Commission, Directorate-General for Research and Innovation (2015) Horizon 2020. Assessing the results and impacts of Horizon

European Institute of Innovation & Technology (2020) European Institute of Innovation & Technology (EIT). https://eit.europa.eu/. Accessed 15 Nov 2021

Froshauer S (2017) Careers at biotech start-ups and in entrepreneurship. Cold Spring Harb Perspect Biol. https://doi.org/10.1101/cshperspect.a032938

Goji T, Hayashi Y, Sakata I (2020) Evaluating "start-up readiness" for researchers: case studies of research-based start-ups with biopharmaceutical research topics. Heliyon 6. https://doi.org/10.1016/j.heliyon.2020.e04160

Gurău C, Dana LP (2020) Financing paths, firms' governance and corporate entrepreneurship: accessing and applying operant and operand resources in biotechnology firms. Technol Forecast Soc Change 153. https://doi.org/10.1016/J.TECHFORE.2020.119935

Haynes K, Metcalfe J, Videler T (2009) What do researchers do? First destinations of doctoral graduates by subject

Kamid, Marzal J, Heriyanti et al (2020) Responding the integrated model of entrepreneur characteristic with STEM to enhance students creativity. In: AIP Conference Proceedings

Kaplan S, Murray F (2010) Entrepreneurship and the construction of value in biotechnology. In: Phillips N, Sewell G, Griffiths D (eds) Technology and organization: essays in honour of Joan Woodward. Emerald Group, pp 107–147

Kergroach S, Meissner D, Vonortas NS (2018) Technology transfer and commercialisation by universities and PRIs: benchmarking OECD country policy approaches. Econ Innov New Technol. https://doi.org/10.1080/10438599.2017.1376167

Kismihók G, Cardells F, Güner PB et al (2019) Declaration on sustainable researcher careers https://doi.org/10.5281/ZENODO.3082245

Kobayashi VB, Mol S, Kismihok G (2014) Labour market driven learning analytics. J Learn Anal 1: 207–210. https://doi.org/10.18608/jla.2014.13.24

Maloy S, Pucher C, Sedam M et al (2020) Opening doors for diverse talent in biotechnology with the BIO I-Corps experience. Nat Biotechnol 38:1099–1102. https://doi.org/10.1038/s41587-020-0663-4

Mas-Tur A, Ribeiro Soriano D (2014) The level of innovation among young innovative companies: the impacts of knowledge-intensive services use, firm characteristics and the entrepreneur attributes. Serv Bus 8:51. https://doi.org/10.1007/s11628-013-0186-x

Miron-Shatz T, Shatz I, Becker S et al (2014) Promoting business and entrepreneurial awareness in health care professionals: lessons from venture capital panels at medicine 2.0 conferences. J Med Internet Res 16:e184

National Science Foundation (2013) US NSF—I-Corps. https://www.nsf.gov/news/special_reports/i-corps/. Accessed 15 Nov 2021

Oliver AL (2004) Biotechnology entrepreneurial scientists and their collaborations. Res Policy. https://doi.org/10.1016/j.respol.2004.01.010

Patzelt H, Brenner T (eds) (2008) Handbook of bioentrepreneurship. Springer, New York, NY

Patzelt H, Schweizer L, Behrens J (2012) Biotechnology entrepreneurship. Found Trends Entrep 8(63–140). https://doi.org/10.1561/0300000041

Piña IL, Cohen PD, Larson DB et al (2015) A framework for describing health care delivery organizations and systems. Am J Public Health 105:670. https://doi.org/10.2105/AJPH.2014.301926

Porter ME (1985) Competitive advantage: creating and sustaining superior performance. Free Press, New York

Rank J, Pace VL, Frese M (2004) Three avenues for future research on creativity, innovation, and initiative. Appl Psychol 53:518–528

Saenen B, Morais R, Gaillard V, Borrell-Damián L (2019) Research assessment in the transition to open science: 2019 EUA open science and access survey results

Samsom KJ, Gurdon MA (1993) University scientists as entrepreneurs: a special case of technology transfer and high-tech venturing. Technovation. https://doi.org/10.1016/0166-4972(93)90054-Y

Shimasaki C (2020) What is biotechnology entrepreneurship? In: Biotechnology entrepreneurship. Elsevier, pp 3–16

Skala A (2019) The start-up as a result of innovative entrepreneurship. In: Digital start-ups in transition economies. Springer, Cham

SPARK Norway (n.d.) SPARK Norway—a two-year innovation programme. UiO:Life Science. https://www.uio.no/english/research/strategic-research-areas/life-science/innovation/spark/. Accessed 15 Nov 2021

The Economist (2010) Doctoral degrees: the disposable academic, Why doing a PhD is often a waste of time. The Economist

The Royal Society (2010) The scientific century: securing our future prosperity

Ulnicane I (2015) Broadening aims and building support in science, technology and innovation policy: the case of the European research area. J Contemp Eur Res 11(1):31–49

Veeraraghavan V (2009) Entrepreneurship and innovation. Asia Pacific Bus Rev. https://doi.org/10.1177/097324700900500102

Wang M, Soetanto D, Cai J, Munir H (2021) Scientist or entrepreneur? Identity centrality, university entrepreneurial mission, and academic entrepreneurial intention. J Technol Transf 47:119. https://doi.org/10.1007/s10961-021-09845-6

Weber CT, Borit M, Canolle F et al (2018) Identifying and documenting transferable skills and competences to enhance early career researchers employability and competitiveness

Weckowska DM (2015) Learning in university technology transfer offices: transactions-focused and relations-focused approaches to commercialization of academic research. Technovation. https://doi.org/10.1016/j.technovation.2014.11.003

Woolston C (2020) Uncertain prospects for postdoctoral researchers. Nature 588:181–184

Worldometer (2020) Life expectancy by country and in the world (2020). Worldometer

Wright M, Birley S, Mosey S (2004) Entrepreneurship and university technology transfer. J Technol Transf 29(3/4):235–246

Chapter 16
How to Become a Successful Hospital and Community Pharmacist

Lilian M. Azzopardi ⓘ

Abstract An imperative of a professional practice is to ensure transformations. Identifying opportunities in evolvements of healthcare systems and being cognisant of changes in expectations of society warrants validity and relevance of the professional practice. This is what we have witnessed in hospital and community pharmacy. The chapter briefly contemplates how clinical pharmacy and pharmaceutical care have shaped the provision of direct patient care services and expanded the scope of hospital and community pharmacy practice. Innovations in practice such as use of robotics and collaborative practice are put forward. Domains are outlined to describe relevant competences and provide an insight into professional characteristics that support practising as hospital and community pharmacists. Attributes that lead to professional fulfilment are considered, and experiences and prospects for specialisation and professional development to become advanced practitioners are described. Advancement in pharmacy education and participation in translational research and implementation science contribute to pharmacist capacity building and empowerment to approach the transformation of pharmacy practice for the next decades. Emphasis is given to describe attributes of successful hospital and community pharmacy practice by highlighting the patient-centric goal, collaborative model, safe culture, digitalisation and entrepreneurship.

16.1 Introduction

Traditionally, principal career options for pharmacy graduates were in community and hospital pharmacies (DiPiro 2011). Evolvements in the pharmaceutical industry and regulatory sciences, research and entrepreneurship opportunities led to an evolvement of career options. A characteristic of pharmacy education is that graduates are prepared for a range of career pathways through a combination of fundamental science-based background and a practical real-world approach.

L. M. Azzopardi (✉)
Faculty of Medicine and Surgery, Department of Pharmacy, University of Malta, Msida, Malta
e-mail: lilian.m.azzopardi@um.edu.mt

© The Author(s), under exclusive license to Springer Nature Switzerland AG 2023
J. R. Thomas et al. (eds.), *Career Options in the Pharmaceutical and Biomedical Industry*, https://doi.org/10.1007/978-3-031-14911-5_16

A global overview of workforce distribution carried out by the International Pharmaceutical Federation (FIP) 10 years ago indicated that community (55%) and hospital (18%) practice were the main areas of practice for pharmacists (International Pharmaceutical Federation 2012). It is estimated that a similar situation holds today. Transformation in the professional practice in hospital and later in community, towards a more patient-centric practice, impacted on educational needs and outcomes. To respond to the pharmaceutical workforce needs, a focus on the competences required of pharmacists that are equipped with skills and abilities required to deliver effective services ensued. Competency-based education re-gained attention as a means to provide needs-based education. Competency-based educational frameworks are developed by the International Pharmaceutical Federation and adopted in a number of countries including Australia, Canada, the United States and the United Kingdom (Katoue and Schwinghammer 2020).

One way to reflect on hospital and community practice is to characterise the transformation in the professional practice, to identify needs-based competencies and describe roadmaps to empower the pharmaceutical workforce to meet the expectations of society as prescribed by the evolving healthcare ecosystems.

Further exposition of the key points that may be elucidated in examining ways for becoming a successful hospital and community pharmacist includes the role of clinical pharmacy and pharmaceutical care in a patient-centric practice, the contribution of collaborative practice and specialisation and emphasis on translational research. Research investigated in the academic scenario is translated into practice and back again to be collaborated through evidence-based implementation science and practice. The role of multidisciplinary education and investigational practice, as well as advancements in medical devices contributing to diagnosis and therapy, assists in the expanding scope of practice involving the mitigation and prevention of diseases. All successful community and hospital pharmacy practices must contribute to the three pillars guiding pharmaceutical services, namely, safety, quality and efficacy.

16.2 Transformation of Hospital Pharmacy Practice

Hospital pharmacy traditionally was described as the practice undertaken in the pharmacy with a focus on ensuring safe, accountable distribution of medicines within hospital settings. Historically, there is documented evidence that hospital pharmacists were also involved in direct patient services with pharmacists participating with physicians in ward rounds as early as the 1600s in Malta and the 1800s in Paris (Azzopardi and Serracino-Inglott 2020; Erstad and Webb 2020).

The game-changing drug developments and subsequent industrialisation of the manufacture of drugs in the post-Second World War era provided hospitals with availability of medicines. At the same time, the larger availability posed challenges to handle these opportunities, for example, which drugs to include in the hospital formulary. In the United States, amidst this scenario, an audit of hospital pharmaceutical services was undertaken as a means to establish standards for good hospital pharmaceutical services (Higby 2014). The exercise was the beginning of a momentum towards a 'philosophy of service'. This is how the concept of clinical pharmacy, which presented a focus on direct patient pharmaceutical services, was introduced in the late 1960s in the United States (Francke et al. 1964). Clinical pharmacy practice in the hospital setting evolved in other developed countries at different rates (Azzopardi 2019). This transformation established a characterisation of hospital pharmacy that has a twofold perspective: (1) generalist hospital pharmacist providing indirect pharmaceutical services and (2) clinical pharmacist services engaged in direct patient care pharmaceutical services.

According to the European Association of Hospital Pharmacists, hospital pharmacy practice covers the broad perspective and includes procurement and distribution of medicines and medical devices, compounding, clinical pharmacy services, patient safety and quality assurance (EAHP 2014). This statement resonates the concept of hospital practice which embraces seamlessly direct patient care services and indirect pharmaceutical services. As opposed to the United States, in Europe it is less common practice to have hospital pharmacists engaged in providing exclusively clinical pharmacy services (Frontini et al. 2013). Globally, in low-income countries, the lack of human resources may be a constraint towards having pharmacists dedicated to deliverly of clinical services on a daily basis (Bronkhorst et al. 2020).

In the United States, direct patient care services provided by hospital pharmacists became centre-front in consolidating quality patient care. Early studies demonstrated pharmacoeconomic benefits of clinical pharmacy services (Schumock et al. 1996). The patient care and pharmacoeconomic benefits contributed to the evolution of clinical pharmacy services to a distinct speciality and later to further ramifications of specialities such as pharmacotherapy, psychiatry and oncology (Carter 2016; Erstad and Webb 2020). Standards of practice were developed by the American College of Clinical Pharmacy highlighting the process of care, required documentation and emphasis on collaborative practice (ACCP 2014). The publication of these Standards was a milestone as an attempt to standardise and support reproducibility of clinical pharmacy practice. The standards put an emphasis on a comprehensive patient-focused approach in medication management within the context of multidisciplinary practice (Yee and Haas 2014). Standardisation practices of direct patient care pharmaceutical services serve to identify educational and training requirements to support competency development (Mamo et al. 2013). In Australia, performance measures were developed for clinical pharmacy practice, and a competency assessment framework was developed by the Society of Hospital Pharmacists of Australia (Lloyd et al. 2015).

16.2.1 Quality Standards

An argument brought forward by hospital administrators is that to be able to provide effective clinical pharmacy that contributes to patient outcomes, the provision of quality pharmaceutical services which support the medication use processes is fundamental. Examples of minimum standards for hospital pharmacy practice are established that address pharmacy management, procurement and formulary management, compounding for sterile and nonsterile products (American Society of Health-System Pharmacists 2013). Competences of quality assurance, accountability and documentation are key for hospital pharmacists. The development of competences related to handling and management of quality systems is a generic competence relevant to pharmacy graduates for different areas of practice including hospital practice (Muscat Terribile et al. 2013).

16.2.2 Dispensing and Administration

In hospital practice, the management of dispensing and administration are instrumental services to ensure access to medicinal products. With regard to administration of medicines, prescription validation or what is also referred to as medication order review contributes to patient safety by reducing medication errors due to inappropriate drug therapy. Through medication use review, hospital pharmacists appraise prescriptions prior to dispensing. The logistic challenges in the provision of prescription review service are mostly related to the availability of a 24-h pharmacy service for continuous and timely cover. Round-the-clock pharmacy service provision may be constrained in small hospitals. Pharmacists require the ability to mobilise scientific knowledge, adopt a systematic approach during prescription review, seek and interpret drug information as necessary and communicate with other colleagues from the healthcare team (Atayee et al. 2016). Prescription validation, which is mandatory in France, was shown to contribute in the short term to reducing prescribing errors (Estellat et al. 2007).

The use of medication distribution technology is gaining ground in hospitals with around 75% of hospitals in the United States making use of automated dispensing cabinets to support dose distribution (Pedersen et al. 2021). Technology is also becoming instrumental in intravenous preparations through the use of bar coding, intravenous robotics and management systems to reduce errors (Bhakta et al. 2018). Pharmacists are involved with validation and qualification of technology-driven processes to ensure patient safety. Independent of the extent of technology-driven processes of storing and distributing medicinal products within the hospital setting, the process needs to be aligned with established guidelines of Good Distribution Practice (GDP) (Jeong and Ji 2018). Pharmacists function as team leaders of the pharmaceutical workforce and are instrumental in facilitating standard operating procedures and pharmaceutical workforce resources that satisfy the requirements of GDP to ensure that safe, quality and effective medicines are dispensed and distributed through the hospital network.

The dispensing process includes medication preparation comprising extemporaneous formulations. Extemporaneous preparations are particularly required to adjust present pharmaceutical dosage form so as to address patient requirements especially in the paediatric and older population and patients with nasogastric tubing. There are limitations in terms of availability of liquid formulation products especially in particular therapeutic classifications such as in cardiovascular therapeutics. The preparation of oral liquid from capsules or tablets is required to ensure patient access to the medication. This process has to be directed to limit contamination and ensure the right medication is being used, at the right dose. Ensuring appropriate process application, documentation, traceability, human resource training and competence and the elaboration of specific formulae are functions that pharmacists are involved in and is an example where the knowledge and leadership in Good Manufacturing Practice is relevant to hospital pharmacy practice.

Within the hospital pharmacy setting, it is appropriate to reflect on the dispensing and administration of particular medicinal products that require specific procedures. These include antineoplastic drugs that require reconstitution, radiopharmaceuticals, specials and investigational medicinal products. The dispensing of these medicinal products requires specific protocol-regulated procedures that cover drug preparation and reconstitution, documentation and personnel training (Bayraktar-Ekincioglu et al. 2018; Hendrikse et al. 2022). Specials are medications that are unlicenced within the setting that they are being used, for example, a medicinal product that carries a marketing authorisation in the United States and not in the EU and is being used in an EU hospital. Since the medicinal product does not comply with the requirements of a marketing authorisation in the setting being used, pharmacists together with the clinical team have to consider manufacturer and sourcing suitability, clinical suitability and control risks. With regard to investigational medicinal products (IMPs), these products are used within a clinical trial framework. Pharmacists are required to fulfil obligations required when handling IMPs including rigorous documentation trail in terms of storage, dispensing and handling of unused products. Moreover, in many instances where clinical trials are undertaken within a hospital setting, pharmacists are involved in overseeing the quality assurance arm of the clinical trial process. Very often in hospitals where clinical trials are regularly being carried out, a pharmacy clinical trial unit is established where the pharmacists are supporting the implementation of Good Clinical Practice. Future technology that is currently being explored includes 3D printing of medications to allow for personalised medicine.

Standardisation and improving efficiency of the dispensing and administration services reduce pharmacists' time and allow for the process to be carried out by trained pharmaceutical workforce such as pharmacy technicians. Such evolvements have led to the number of hospital pharmacists directly involved on a daily basis to carry out processes of distribution and administration to be on the decline. It is imperative for pharmacists to understand the scientific basis for formulation development as much as the need to have the competences to manage a team of trained professionals to undertake the day-to-day work and to maintain systems that ensure quality and safety of the processes.

16.2.3 Medication Monitoring Activities

Medication monitoring services include compiling pharmacovigilance data and participation in therapeutic drug monitoring. With regard to pharmacovigilance, pharmacists are in a position to facilitate spontaneous reporting of adverse drug reactions in collaboration with the healthcare team. Awareness and attitude towards responsibility to contribute to safety signals within the pharmacovigilance framework are competences pertinent in pharmacy education (Yu et al. 2019). A number of hospital pharmacies provide measuring drug concentrations services. The transformations witnessed in hospital pharmacy support the involvement of the pharmacist not only in the measurement of drug concentrations but rather in the entire patient process (Almohammde et al. 2021). Liaison with the ward team is required to ensure appropriate timing of biological sampling, follow-up of laboratory processes including quality control principles that are built into the service, communication of the result in a timely manner and contributions to therapeutic decisions within the healthcare team. Interpretation of therapeutic drug monitoring requires application of pharmacokinetic knowledge within the context of appreciating the comprehensive individual patient clinical picture (Firman et al. 2021). In the United States, in around 70% of hospitals pharmacists monitor three quarters of patients in the hospital (Pedersen et al. 2019). Pharmacists liaise and in some settings practise in clinical toxicology units within hospitals. The overlapping areas of expertise of pharmacists and toxicologists allow for pharmacists to be in a position to pursue careers in toxicology centres. Within this context, pharmacists are participating in poisoning handling, medicolegal advice including forensic aspects as well as analytical services within the toxicology laboratory.

16.2.4 Medication Use

In medication use activities, the spectrum varies from participation in formulary system management and drug policies to the participation of pharmacists in therapeutic decisions. Interprofessional communication is focal to ensure sound and successful implementation of formulary and drug policy decisions. Pharmacoeconomic appreciation and scoping of clinical evidence to support decisions are elements that support pharmacists to validly contribute to rationale medication use discussions. Implementation of clinical decision support systems has been evolving over the past years where computerised modelling and knowledge integration are applied to enhance the healthcare provider with recommendations that are specific to the patient case being considered. Alarm settings are built-in to allow for identification of patient risks as a result of medication use, for example, due to comorbidities, dosing and interactions. This digitalisation in the provision of clinical decision-making enhances the participation of the pharmacist in the therapeutic decisions (Sutton et al. 2020). It is imperative to recognise that the digitalisation presents knowledge and supports optimisation and requires interpretation of the proposals in the context of the care setting, service provision and clinical care plan. Tools that focus specifically on medication appropriateness are available to support the pharmacist when navigating treatment guidelines, hospital protocols and reconciling this data against individual patient needs. Such medication assessment tools are particularly relevant when protocols and guidelines are applied in special populations such as older persons (Gauci et al. 2019) and in disease states requiring multiple drug therapies or relying on biological agents (Grech et al. 2016).

The intervention of pharmacists in medication use processes may include authority to order laboratory tests, prescribing and adjustment of medication therapy. The extent of authority varies across countries, may be drug class specific and may rely on protocol or collaborative prescribing practices (Pedersen et al. 2020). Prescribing authority includes antibacterial drugs such as vancomycin and aminoglycosides in the context of antimicrobial stewardship led by pharmacists. Monitoring compliance was shown to be higher with pharmacist involvement (Joseph et al. 2021a). As much as it is essential to recognise drug therapy required to achieve patient care goals, deprescribing of drugs that are irrelevant or adding burden to patient medication is an essential practice in therapeutic planning. Deprescribing is often a task led by pharmacists in collaboration with other healthcare professionals since the pharmacist has the opportunity to assess each medication within a patient's profile. Deprescribing recommendations require pharmacotherapeutic knowledge and liaison within the healthcare team (Scott et al. 2021).

16.2.5 Domains of Hospital Pharmacy Practice

Hospital pharmacy practice constitutes two domains, namely, the direct patient care services which rely on the provision of clinical pharmacy and the pharmacy-based activities that constitute processes of distribution and administration. For both domains the common denominator is patient safety (Fig. 16.1).

Activities of prescription review, therapeutic drug monitoring, pharmacovigilance and formulary development within a hospital environment can be shaped to evolve from a strict process-focus to a patient-centred service. An appreciation of the different domains in hospital pharmacy practice strengthens the individual's ability to perform in a respective domain. Successful development of a career pathway should include opportunities to interact, network, observe and reflect on experiences from the other domains of practice within a hospital setting.

Fundamental to the competencies for hospital pharmacists is recognition of the generalist knowledge and skills that are essential (Table 16.1). It has to be emphasised that valid hospital pharmacist contributions need to be based on scientific knowledge which relies on a broad perspective of pharmaceutical and clinical sciences including pharmacotherapy, quality systems and regulatory aspects that encompass Good Distribution Practice, Good Manufacturing Practice, Good Clinical Practice and Pharmacovigilance. To be able to mobilise the knowledge into an

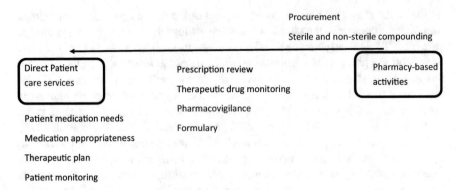

Fig. 16.1 The domains of hospital pharmacy practice

Table 16.1 Knowledge and skills for hospital pharmacy practice

Knowledge	Skills
Pharmacotherapy	Communication
Pharmacokinetics	Lifelong learning
Pharmaceutical regulatory sciences	Critical analysis and evidence-based practice
Quality improvement	Research

impactful contribution, transferable skills are required to ensure teamwork and to maintain relevance of knowledge to contemporary needs through lifelong learning, critical analysis and participation in research.

16.3 Transition of Care

As patients move across healthcare settings, the risk for medication errors increases as a result of disjointed patient care (Slazak et al. 2020). One of the accomplishments of pharmacists is that they can act as facilitators of patient care as the patient moves across the continuum of care particularly from secondary care to primary care. A pertinent example is when patients are discharged from hospital and return home, with updated medications. Patients and their carers have to face the challenges brought about by new medication intake schedules, overcome barriers to access of new medications, understand new treatment regimens and identify no longer required medications.

Healthcare professionals in the primary care setting are the resource to whom patients resort to. Despite the opportunities provided through digitalisation of healthcare, transition of information to the primary care healthcare professionals may be ineffective. Planned pharmacist-led transition of care services especially within a collaborative healthcare professional model has been shown to improve patient outcomes such as blood pressure control, diabetes management and anticoagulation therapy control (Njonkou et al. 2021).

Besides the domains identified for the provision of direct patient services, championing smooth transitions of care to patients requires establishment of partnerships with pharmacists in other specialities and practice settings, care managers and social support organisations (Stranges et al. 2020). Transmitting a message to colleagues and patients of availability and open communication together with an ability to detect high-risk patients or situations that require prioritisation are competences that support a successful transition of care pharmacist intervention. With the evidence in favour of improving patient outcomes through investing in pharmacists dedicated to provide transition of care services during hospital discharge, pharmacist-led transition of care services are expanding (Joseph et al. 2021b).

16.3.1 Domains of Transition of Care

Hospital and community pharmacists require clinical pharmacy skills as well as particular competences that contribute to an effective transition of care service (Fig. 16.2). Competences include:

(a) Adaption of communication skills according to patients' needs, for example, vulnerable patients, patients with disability and patients with social constraints

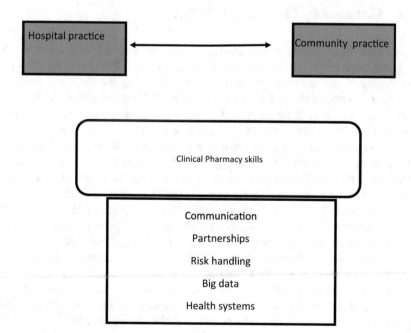

Fig. 16.2 Skills and competences to facilitate transition of care

(b) Fostering of partnerships with colleagues in different practice settings
(c) Undertaking risk analysis and stratification to identify priority patients and significant issues that require highlighting
(d) Handling of big data so as to navigate through the patient information including laboratory results, patient profile and medication history updates
(e) Navigating health systems including administrative tasks to ensure patient access to medication and identification of opportunities presented through digital platforms.

Quantitative outcomes research of transition of care services contribute to demonstrate effective hospital and community pharmacists' intervention in providing this service. The metrics measured include reduction of medication errors, hospital readmission rates, adherence to treatment and implementation of secondary prevention measures (Clay 2016). Beyond the metrics, it is appropriate to reflect on the value of the service according to pertinence, namely, introducing the service for patients who are at higher risk of effects of incomplete transition. Cardiovascular disease is an area where impact of transition of care has been particularly studied mostly due to the high chronic medication use burden and risk of readmission (Weeda et al. 2021). Older persons also present with a higher need due to multiple drug therapy and complex pharmaceutical needs (Villeneuve et al. 2021).

16.4 Community Pharmacy Practice

A paradigm shift in community pharmacy practice occurred as a result of the industrialisation of the production of medicines. This shift brought to light the real contribution of the community pharmacist by removing the limelight from the product and exposing the patient service (Azzopardi 2000). The clinical pharmacy philosophy introduced in the hospital pharmacy setting was a trigger for community pharmacy practice patient services to become established. In some countries, for example, in Malta, pharmacy education and practice research supported the development of clinical community pharmacy services (Azzopardi and Serracino-Inglott 2020). Clinical interventions by community pharmacists have been shown to contribute to patient self-care and to the management of chronic diseases (Wirth et al. 2011; Galea et al. 2014; Ungaro et al. 2015; Vella et al. 2015; Mifsud et al. 2019). The pace of evolvement of clinical community pharmacy practice is much slower than what we have witnessed in the hospital setting. There are barriers to implementing clinical pharmacy services in the community setting including physical constraints such as private areas for consultation, financial models and data accessibility (Bauman and Manasse 2019). Digitalisation provides an opportunity to overcome data accessibility barriers by linking primary and secondary care settings and also connecting physicians with community pharmacies (Eickhoff et al. 2021). Practice models vary across Europe, and in some countries, such as Germany,

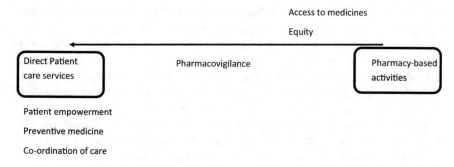

Fig. 16.3 The domains of community pharmacy practice

provisions are in place for remuneration of specific clinical services provided by community pharmacists (Eickhoff and Schulz 2006).

Reflecting on characteristic domains of community pharmacy practice, two domains are identified: the pharmacy-based activity and the direct patient care services (Fig. 16.3). For the pharmacy-based activities, access to medicines is a crucial aspect. Access considerations include availability of the product as well as financial support, whether the product is covered by a health insurance and to what extent. The community pharmacist may need to provide information to the patient about availability of generic medications, suggest substitution when medication is not available and discuss options with the patient. Patients require information about generic medicines to gain confidence and to switch to generic products so as to improve accessibility and increase equity (Sammut Bartolo et al. 2020). The direct patient care services can be described as patient empowerment, preventive medicine and coordination of care. In the context of direct patient care service, the positioning of the pharmacist as a healthcare provider is explicitly being put in focus. Especially in the community setting, such a provider role may be seen as somewhat being independent from other professionals. At the same time, independence does not mean non-communication, and emphasis has to be placed that whilst providing the patient service, it is crucial for pharmacists to collaborate with other healthcare professionals in the interest of patient safety. Such communication may rely on documentation through digital and remote platforms.

16.4.1   Patient Empowerment

With respect to the direct patient care services, community pharmacists are in a prime position to facilitate patient empowerment. The relationship between community pharmacists and their patients and the environment within a primary care setting is conducive for patient education on the management of disease states, how to recognise signs and symptoms which require seeking help and information about medications. Empowering patients with information strengthens patient compliance with pharmacotherapy and behavioural changes and contributes towards patient safety. An example of a patient empowerment service developed in Switzerland for fingolimod patients was combined with pharmacovigilance to monitor occurrence of serious adverse reactions and contributed to adverse drug reaction reporting (Bourdin et al. 2019). This model demonstrates how in the community setting, when clinical pharmacy interventions are connected with the provision of pharmaceutical services, the impact of the outcome of the intervention is magnified.

Patient empowerment is an important dimension within the self-care domain. Whilst self-care is encouraged as a means to relieve undue pressure on healthcare systems, community pharmacists are in a crucial position to provide the patient with support to ensure rational and safe use of quality medicines (Bell et al. 2016). Pharmacists support patient autonomy and at the same time influence patient decisions in self-care (Rajiah et al. 2021). The dimension of patient empowerment actually provides a strong metric to demonstrate accomplishments of community pharmacists. In education, quality of teacher workforce is associated with the potential of promoting students' attitudes and behaviour as a long-term impact (Blazar and Kraft 2017). By the same corollary, successful impact of community pharmacists can be evaluated through patient behavioural attitudes to health. The reflection can be approached from a macro dimension effect as a measure of successful contribution by community pharmacists towards the health status of society as well as at the micro level, on an individual community pharmacist level, for personal career satisfaction and fulfilment.

16.4.2 Preventive Medicine

In the European Union, the health strategy for Europe 2020 puts a focus on prevention of disease and protecting society from health threats as a pillar for economic strategy and growth (Seychell and Hackbart 2013). The term 'preventive medicine' is here coined to describe the contribution towards preventing disease. The outcomes have both an individual impact and a societal impact through the reduction of disease burden on the healthcare system. The outreach is through a broad spectrum. On one end, preventive medicine provides for the prevention of infectious diseases. Through this intervention, pharmacists promote vaccination information (Jusufoska et al. 2021). The intervention of community pharmacists in vaccination, including vaccine administration, was extended in many countries particularly due to the COVID-19 pandemic and the need for vaccination strategies (Paudyal et al. 2021; Yemeke et al. 2021). HIV pre-exposure prophylaxis is an approach used to control HIV spread and is an example of potential extension of community pharmacists' contribution to preventing infectious diseases (Tung et al. 2018). At the other end of the spectrum is non-communicable disease prevention. Community pharmacists are accessible health professionals who engage in macro and micro health promotion and disease prevention strategies. When interacting at the micro level, with individual patients, community pharmacists have the potential to direct advice specific to patient risks and needs, for example, patients with prediabetes, recommending smoking cessation and body weight management (Katangwe et al. 2020). Policymakers recognise the contribution of community pharmacists towards public health priorities (Almansour et al. 2021). In terms of metrics, positive interventions contributing towards public health interventions have been reported through community pharmacist services (Thomson et al. 2019).

16.4.3 Coordination of Care

Lessons learnt from the COVID-19 pandemic include impact on the healthcare ecosystem. During the pandemic, health services were strained, and some providers, including physicians, were not accessible to patients. At the same time, community pharmacists provided the support to patients to manage the constraints of the pandemic as well as to facilitate management of chronic diseases (Strand et al. 2020). This scenario highlights the contribution of community pharmacists as providers of care and particularly their function as coordinators of patient care. Pharmaceutical service provision may occur during informal patient counselling or through formal medication use reviews exercises. Monitoring patients with chronic disease, such as diabetes, and liaising with physicians through collaborative management, so as to perform repeat prescribing and follow-up dose adjustments, contribute to patient satisfaction and seamless care (Siaw et al. 2018). In the United States, the establishment of formal collaborative practice agreements between physicians and pharmacists allows for the expansion of services beyond the conventional scope of practice (Kiles et al. 2021). Such agreements are evolving particularly between physicians and community pharmacists for joint decision-making on point-of-care testing, whereby the pharmacists action results of point-of-care tests (Bacci et al. 2018).

Successful coordination of care requires professional communication as well as trust and maintenance of professional relationships. A common vision of philosophy of patient care between pharmacists and other healthcare professionals is essential towards a fruitful coordination of care.

16.5 Patient-Centric Hospital and Community Pharmacy Practice

The introduction of the concept of clinical pharmacy was established at a time when hospital pharmacists developed an intent towards a service provision of care rather than a product-based delivery. In 1985, Charles Hepler argued that pharmacists are performing clinically oriented services and providing informative advisory functions through 'highly personalised non-transferable services' (Hepler 1985). The need to highlight the responsibility of pharmacists towards patients through the delivery of clinical pharmacy services, to ensure responsible use of medicines and achievement of patient outcomes, culminated in the philosophy of pharmaceutical care (Hepler and Strand 1990). The philosophy of pharmaceutical care was an opportunity to support clinical pharmacy services. The development of pharmaceutical care models in hospital settings emphasises the clinical contribution to patient care within a collaborative context (Falzon et al. 2021). Pharmaceutical care models spotlight the professional clinical service provision in community pharmacy, overriding the importance that tends to be attributed to the business model in this practice setting, which is associated with the repetitive distribution of medicines (Ulrick and Meggs 2019). The pressures from payer organisations such as governments, health-insurance providers as well as consumers led to requirements to demonstrate the effective and valid contribution of pharmacists. Processes that highlighted the professional contribution of the pharmacists were seen as a means to position the pharmacist as a service provider. These were particularly relevant for community pharmacy practice, due to the convergence with the business model, which many times obliterates the professional model (Azzopardi 2000). Against this backdrop we are now witnessing a move from provision of services to a *patient-centric* vision for pharmacy services. The bicycle model of pharmacist professionalism described by Dubbai et al. (2019) emphasises the patient-focused approach within the delivery of professional pharmacy services.

So how can one inject the patient-centric focus in one's practice as a hospital or community pharmacist? The mantra is providing clinical pharmacy services and implementing pharmaceutical care models. Shaping the services according to society's needs is what contributes to effectiveness of the professional intervention and achievement of personal professional fulfilment and reward. When bringing in society's needs and expectations within the formula, to establish dimensions of professional service provision, current and future perspectives of the healthcare ecosystem should be taken into account (Felkery and Fox 2012). A pertinent dimension to be considered is digitalisation: how are you as a pharmacist providing professional services that meet the expectations of the digitally savvy and the digitally orphaned patients at the same time? The pharmacist is no longer the sole gatekeeper to information about medicine but rather the service provider for the individualised interpretation of evidence. Patients access medicine information through digital platforms, and the pertinent intervention of the pharmacist is to support the patient to navigate through the myths, the evidence, and interpret the information in the light of the patient's own clinical scenario.

The elaboration of telepharmacy and patient monitoring through smart medical devices are creating expectations for the pharmacist to provide real-time decisions. At the same time, relying exclusively on the opportunities provided by digitalisation goes against the patient-centred vision mostly because a professional service is required to interface with the patient and provide a patient-tailored approach. Digital literacy in the context of digital health is a competence that makes the patient-centric vision relevant in the context of today's scenario (Mantel-Teeuwisse et al. 2021). Communication strategies that foster trust, understanding of health concerns, tailoring of information and effective patient-pharmacist relationship are markers of what patients expect during pharmacist interactions (Scala et al. 2022).

The concept of patient-centricity in healthcare provision is also being embraced in the medicinal product development. Attempts in the pharmaceutical industry and regulatory landscape include understanding patient needs and actioning product development to meet disease area strategies that address access to medications (Yeoman et al. 2017). The advent of biological drugs provided an opportunity for personalised medicine (Kiely 2016). Biological drugs paved the way for biosimilars, which created the convergence of hospital and community pharmacists to discuss personalised patient needs when addressing equity, access to treatment, interchange-ability, switching and policy development (O'Callaghan et al. 2019). At the indi-vidual patient level, hospital and community pharmacists are expected to contribute to collaborative decision-making when starting treatment and when advising and monitoring patients during therapy switching.

Clinical practice of personalised medicine can be supported through precision pharmacotherapeutics based on clinical pharmacogenomics (Hicks et al. 2019). The example of clopidogrel is an example where the application of pharmacogenetic testing could support the patient-centric therapeutic decision to identify the patient population who will be vulnerable to major adverse cardiovascular events such as occurrence of in-stent restenosis as a result of genetic profile (Osama et al. 2021). Practitioners are gaining awareness and confidence in pharmacogenetic testing (Bruno Xuereb et al. 2022). A scientific approach to appreciating opportunities where pharmacogenetic testing has practical significance, identifying ethical barriers and leading innovations to incorporate service development are modalities through which hospital and community pharmacists operate in the contemporary and future healthcare landscape.

In the field of precision medicine, the use of particular medicinal products relies on the application of specific diagnostic testing to identify patients' suitability for the medicinal product. One of the earliest examples is the use of trastuzumab in breast cancer where the expression of HER2 (human epidermal growth factor receptor 2) is an important biomarker that identifies patients eligible for trastuzumab therapy. Pharmacists are key players to contribute to the appraisal of the companion diag-nostics that are required to support specific drug therapy use. Through their phar-maceutical regulatory science knowledge, they are in a position to appreciate requirements for quality, safety and effectiveness of companion diagnostics in the context of regulation according to the In Vitro Diagnostic Devices Regulation in the EU. From a practice position, pharmacists are normally frontline negotiators leading the clinical team to support procurement practices of companion diagnostics when the medicinal product is included in the formulary. Pharmacists are becoming more involved in the provision of pharmacogenetic and precision medicine speciality including implementation and interpretation of diagnostic testing to guide pharmacotherapeutic plans.

The patient-centric approach of hospital and community pharmacy practice puts forward a paradigm shift from a compartmentalised professional setting description to a comprehensive care delivery. It is, maybe, no longer apt to compartmentalise

Fig. 16.4 Patient-centric hospital and community pharmacy practice

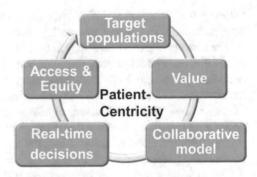

practice according to hospital and community setting but rather to put at the centre-front the *clinical service provision*. The clinical service provision relates to putting the patient needs in focus whilst ensuring access and equity to medications and the service and elaborate personalised interventions that create value through patient outcomes within the context of real-time decisions in relation to collaborative care (Fig. 16.4).

16.6 Measurement of Success

This chapter attempts to describe evolvements in hospital and community practice and highlights expectations of practice. In addition to describing skills and competences required to fulfil the dimensions of practice, an endeavour is made to put forward strategies that lead to successful practice. The question is how to describe success as a hospital and community pharmacist. Career success is difficult to describe in a definite manner since it is measured by young professionals, both at an individualistic level, with the opportunity to define one's own satisfaction markers, and through multidimensional constructs (McDonald and Hite 2008).

An example of a study that reflected on career success for hospital pharmacists identified acknowledgement, self-confidence and professional autonomy as metrics described by pharmacists (Jepsen and Spooner 2013). These metrics are strongly interrelated and are used in the development of postulated dimensions of successful hospital and community practice which are being proposed (Fig. 16.5). Employing the skills and competences to provide a patient-centric service leads to individualistic satisfaction and successful contribution to patient care. At a professional level, autonomy is commensurate to the ability to provide quality services that are directed towards ensuring safety and mitigating risks. Autonomy does not mean independent practice. To develop professional autonomy, one needs to ensure collaboration with other professionals. In the construct of future practice, responding to digital challenges and opportunities and nurturing entrepreneurship in developing innovative clinical pharmacy services are additional markers of success.

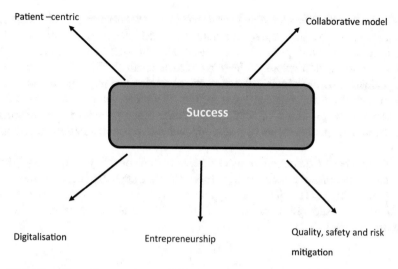

Fig. 16.5 Dimensions of successful hospital and community pharmacy practice

16.7 Pathways to Success

The European Association of Faculties of Pharmacy identified the domains of pharmacy education to prepare graduates with the appropriate skills mix that enables them to join and contribute to diverse areas of practice including hospital and community settings. The domains are science-practice balance, effective teaching methods, preparedness for lifelong education and becoming team players (European Association of Faculties of Pharmacy 2018). To progress to professional success, postgraduate learning and education are recommended. Career progression may rely on postgraduate formal education and specialisation. Postgraduate learning and professional development contribute to enhance competences as the graduate progresses to a decision-maker and seeks renewal of knowledge, which is extremely essential in the dynamically evolving healthcare landscape. In the United States, 2-year postgraduate pharmacy residency programmes lead to an advanced speciality focus. Scholarly activities and participation in professional organisations have been identified as a preferred modality to extending the residency programmes by another year (Dang and to-Lui 2020). In Europe, examples of specialisation programmes for community (Westein et al. 2019) and hospital practice (Sule et al. 2021) are available. Programmes that are based on inspiring graduates to develop the domains of successful hospital and community practice without delineating practice setting limits provide the opportunity to the individual of a wider competency advancement (Vella et al. 2021).

Research skills development in undergraduate years is a transferable skill that is also relevant to community and hospital pharmacy practice because it enables critical thinking and rigorous evidence-based assessments. In the United States, where the undergraduate degree provides a strong clinical knowledge and skills focus, standardisation of research training across curricula is weak (Karnes et al. 2022). The research perspective in postgraduate clinical-focused education may be viewed by candidates as challenging due to the unstructured nature of the learning methodology and the associated freedom of learning (Pham et al. 2019). In the long term, postgraduate training, which includes practice research and implementation science experiences, provides an added-value feature. The added value contributes to competences for the provision of advanced evidence-based patient-focused pharmacy services and supports a vision of leadership and entrepreneurship (Serracino-Inglott 2021).

Effective postgraduate programmes that support the development of hospital and community pharmacy practice competences should merge experience-based learning by engaging role models with the intent of not only providing knowledge and skills but also supporting engagement of the students in the learning process (Sternschein et al. 2021).

16.8   Career Opportunities in Hospital and Community Pharmacy Practice

In many countries vacancies in community pharmacy are widely available. Legal frameworks vary from one country to another in the context of possibility for a new graduate to fill management positions. Within community pharmacy, models of practice include scenarios where one pharmacist is considered to be the responsible professional to oversee safe and effective service provision from the pharmacy including pharmaceutical workforce, provision of services and ethical and legal obligations. Different nomenclatures are in use to describe the position, including managing pharmacist or responsible pharmacist. In some countries, a number of years of experience as a community pharmacist are required prior to taking up a professional management position. The other aspect in consideration within community pharmacy is the prospect of taking up ownership of a pharmacy. Owning a pharmacy may be restricted in some countries to being a pharmacist, and opening of community pharmacies may be population-based or dependent on geographical positioning. Career opportunities in community pharmacy are nowadays also evolving to positions which emphasise more the clinical pharmacy service provision. Pharmacists may wish to plan to consider clinical pharmacy positions in community pharmacies or in primary care healthcare settings. Most often these positions require that the applicant has undergone or is willing to undertake specialisation academic or professional training.

For the hospital pharmacy perspective, it is highly likely that graduands first join general positions that provide an exposure to varying extents of the professional services described in this chapter. During career progression pathways, opportunities are presented for the hospital pharmacist to take up particular focus such as in medicine information, clinical pharmacy, patient discharge planning and pharmacovigilance. Pathways of career development may be guided by the professional training that one pursues or by opportunities in career progression that are available.

Within hospital pharmacy structures, there are models which employ a distinctive career progression into a clinically based or pharmacy-based service. In the context of clinically based positions, opportunities to specialise in particular areas may be available through residency programmes. For pharmacy-based positions, there is also a wide spectrum of practice settings and specialities including clinical trials and research units, quality assurance unit, partial manufacturing and extemporaneous preparation units. Other models maintain a fusion of clinical and pharmacy-based practice and differentiate more through leadership and managerial levels. Managerial responsibilities include participation in administrative tasks that go beyond strategic and financial planning such as contribution to hospital committees, e.g. emergency preparedness, antibiotic stewardship, drug and therapeutics committee, formulary management and health technology assessments, patient safety taskforce, ethics committee and hospital accreditation. Career progression towards leadership positions relies on participation in scholarly and academic experiences, and in turn pharmacists in leadership positions are expected to dedicate time and resources to training, education and research of students and staff.

In contemporary practice, career progression and pathways maybe more clearly elaborated in the hospital setting when compared to the community setting. In the community setting, career structure is highly dependent on the particular setting. Relevant considerations include enterprise description such as whether the pharmacy is independent or part of a multiple chain, the location and area served. Turnout of career prospects may also be dependent on the readiness for entrepreneurship within the context of participating in new healthcare provision. For example, during the COVID-19 pandemic, a number of examples in different countries can be drawn on how pharmacists participated in the provision of care for COVID-19 detection through rapid antigen testing, in vaccination strategies and in patient management including access to hospital-only medicines via community pharmacies and with extended rights to ensure patient access to medications (PGEU Position Paper).[1]

16.9   Conclusion and Future Perspectives

Community and hospital pharmacists have remained remarkably resilient and strong through the transformations, including through the evolving technical digitalised world. Along the developments, the constantly changing regulatory environment alongside developing ethical and data protection requirements challenges the making of a successful hospital and community pharmacist. Further influences on

---

[1] Pharmaceutical Group of European Union. Position paper on the role of community pharmacists in COVID-19—Lessons learnt from the pandemic. www.pgeu.eu

pharmacy practice are marketing and financial revolutions presenting new opportunities which yet could cause a sustainable solid ground become softer. Digitalisation and complementary innovations must be utilised as a tool for good pharmacy practice. Pharmacists need to develop wisdom and hence a word to the wise: use your invaluable experiences to transform information into knowledge and change that into wisdom.

How will a successful hospital and community pharmacist be in 2030? By 2025, the evolvements will be governed by digitalisation. The successful pharmacist perhaps, through an ability of networking, will need to utilise wisdom pitched into practice to be able to identify problems, and more importantly validate solutions. Let us take the example of transition from dispensing to prescribing concepts. This development requires bridging traditional pharmacy practice with contemporary patient needs. This action may require the establishment of a new economic structure as well as new regulations. Pharmacy economic structures are often linked to dispensing services, and a prescribing model may require disruption to be successful. Pharmacists must prepare themselves to be a major player in such a transformation. Healthcare is moving at an impressive speed. Already we are witnessing a great evolution in the way digitalisation and self-care are advancing. Healthcare could witness infinite growth, but all this will be responsive to real-world needs.

The biggest advantage that the pharmacy profession has is that we are a profession that has succeeded to connect scientific evolutions with practice.

Pharmacy now needs to accelerate research and facilitate projects contributing to pharmacy practice to achieve the new goal in becoming a patient-centric profession. The concepts of clinical pharmacy and later of pharmaceutical care have presented the tools required for reaching this goal. The ideas are there and have been progressing in the last decades. What is needed now is to advance trust, education and ease of implementation. Trust is gained by being transparent including adopting a safety culture that spans through risk mitigation, near misses and errors reporting, and corrective actions. The relevance of teamwork, networking and collaboration between pharmacists and with other healthcare professionals should be emphasised rather than keep focusing on 'independent' practitioners, for example, is independent prescriber the right term that we should aspire to the describe pharmacist contribution in medicine use?

As far as education is concerned, the need for research in educational techniques and curricula cannot be overemphasised. Such an exposure strengthens confidence in pharmacists to participate in disruptive pharmacy practices to lead evolvements in the profession to match expectations for the next decades. In health, it is the outcomes that count most. It is relevant that the decision to trust the pharmacist needs to come from the people – society. The more that the people feel they are benefitting, the better the trust rating. The patient must remain at the centre of all the activities, and this includes accessibility of the pharmacist to the patient and to other healthcare professionals. We need to transform our traditional drug information centres.

References

Almansour HA, Aloudah NM, Alhawassi TM, Chaar B, Krass I, Saini B (2021) Cardiovascular disease risk prevention services by pharmacists in Saudi Arabia: what do policymakers and opinion leaders think? J Pharm Policy Pract 14:42

Almohammde S, Alhodian H, Almofareh S, Alshehri S, Almasri DM, Ghoneim RH (2021) A survey of therapeutic drug monitoring in a teaching hospital. Saudi J Biol Sci 28:744–747

American College of Clinical Pharmacy (ACCP) (2014) Standards of practice for clinical pharmacists. Pharmacotherapy 34(8):794–797

American Society of Health-System Pharmacists (2013) ASHP guidelines: minimum standard for pharmacies in hospitals. Am J Health Syst Pharm 70:1619–1630

Atayee RS, Awdishu L, Namba J (2016) Using simulation to improve first-year pharmacy students' ability to identify medication errors involving the top 100 prescription medications. Am J Pharm Educ 80(5):article 86

Azzopardi LM (2000) Validation instruments for community pharmacy: pharmaceutical care for the third millennium. Pharmaceutical Products Press, New York

Azzopardi LM (2019) Pharmacy practice in Western Europe. In: Babar Z (ed) Encylopedia of pharmacy practice and clinical pharmacy. Elsevier, Oxford, pp 478–487

Azzopardi LM, Serracino-Inglott A (2020) Clinical pharmacy education and practice evolvement in Malta. J Am Coll Clin Pharm 3:973–979

Bacci JL, Klepser D, Tilley H, Smith JK, Klepser ME (2018) Community pharmacy-based point-of-care testing: a case study of pharmacist-physician collaborative working relationships. Res Soc Adm Pharm 14:112–115

Bauman JL, Manasse HR (2019) Clinical pharmacy practice in community pharmacies: a frontier with promise? J Am Coll Clin Pharm 2:326–329

Bayraktar-Ekincioglu A, Korobuk G, Demirkan K (2018) An evaluation of chemotherapy drug preparation process in hospitals in Turkey—a pilot study. J Oncol Pharm Pract 24(8):563–573

Bell J, Dziekan G, Pollack C, Mahachai V (2016) Self-care in the twenty first century: a vital role for the pharmacist. Adv Ther 33:1691–1703

Bhakta SB, Colavecchia AC, Coffey W, Curlee DR, Garey KW (2018) Implementation and evaluation of a sterile compounding robot in a satellite oncology pharmacy. Am J Health Syst Pharm 75:S51–S57

Blazar D, Kraft MA (2017) Teacher and teaching effects on students' attitudes and behaviors. Educ Eval Policy Anal 39:146–170

Bourdin A, Schluep M, Bugnon O, Berger J (2019) Promoting transitions of care, safety, and medication adherence for patients taking fingolimod in community pharmacies. Am J Health Syst Pharm 76:1150–1157

Bronkhorst E, Gous AGS, Schellack N (2020) Practice guidelines for clinical pharmacists in middle to low income countries. Front Pharmacol 11:article 978

Bruno Xuereb A, Wirth F, Mifsud Buhagiar L, Camilleri L, Azzopardi LM, Serracino-Inglott A (2022) Pharmacist and physician perception of pharmacogenetic testing. Int J Pharm Pract 30(2):188–191

Carter BL (2016) Evolution of clinical pharmacy in the US and future directions for patient care. Drugs Aging 33(3):169–177

Clay PG (2016) "Pitching" pharmacists as improvers of transition-of-care outcomes. J Am Pharm Assoc 56:348

Dang YH, To-Lui KP (2020) Pharmacist perceptions of and views on postgraduate year 3 training. Am J Health-Syst Pharm 77(18):1488–1496

DiPiro J (2011) Preparing our students for the many opportunities in pharmacy. Am J Pharm Educ 75(9):article 170

Dubbai H, Adelstein BA, Taylor S, Shulruf B (2019) Definition of professionalism and tools for assessing professionalism in pharmacy practice: a systematic review. J Educ Eval Health Prof 16:22

Eickhoff C, Schulz M (2006) Pharmaceutical care in community pharmacies: practice and research in Germany. Ann Pharmacother 40:729–735

Eickhoff C, Griese-Mammen N, Mueller U, Said A, Schulz M (2021) Primary healthcare policy and vision for community pharmacy and pharmacists in Germany. Pharm Pract 19(1):2248

Erstad BL, Webb CE (2020) A brief history of pharmacy specialization in the United States. J Am Coll Clin Pharm 3:1464–1470

Estellat C, Colombet I, Vautier S, Huault-Quentel J, Durieux P, Sabatier B (2007) Impact of pharmacy validation in a computerised physician order entry context. Int J Qual Health Care 19:317–325

European Association of Faculties of Pharmacy (2018) EAFP position paper. EAFP, Parma

European Association of Hospital Pharmacists (EAHP) (2014) The European statements of hospital pharmacy. Eur J Hosp Pharm 21:256–258

Falzon S, Galea N, Calvagna V, Pham JT, Grech L, Azzopardi LM (2021) Development and use of an innovative gap finding tool to create pharmaceutical care model within a paediatric oncology setting. J Oncol Pharm Pract. https://doi.org/10.1177/10781552211053249

Felkery BG, Fox BI (2012) Pharmacy automation and technology: how patient-centric is your practice? Hosp Pharm 47:310–311

Firman P, Whitfield K, Tan KS, Clavarino A, Hay K (2021) The impact of an electronic hospital system on therapeutic drug monitoring. J Clin Pharm Ther 46:1613–1621

Francke DE, Latiolais CJ, Francke GN, Ho NF (1964) Mirror to hospital pharmacy. American Society of Hospital Pharmacists, Washington, DC

Frontini R, Miharija-Gala T, Sykora J (2013) EAHP survey 2010 on hospital pharmacy in Europe: parts 4 ad 5. Clinical services and patient safety. Eur J Hosp Pharm 20:69–73

Galea S, Zarb-Adami M, Serracino-Inglott A, Azzopardi LM (2014) Pharmacist intervention in non-prescription medicine use. JPHRS 5:55–59

Gauci M, Wirth F, Azzopardi LM, Serracino-Inglott A (2019) Clinical pharmacist implementation of a medication assessment tool for long-term management of atrial fibrillation in older persons. Pharm Pract 17(1):1349

Grech L, Ferrito V, Serracino-Inglott A, Azzopardi LM (2016) Development and validation of RhMAT, as medication assessment tool specifically designed for rheumatoid arthritis management. JPHRS 7:89–92

Hendrikse H, Kiss O, Kunikowska J, Wadsak W, Decristofor C, Patt M (2022) EANM position on the in-house preparation of radiopharmaceuticals. Eur J Nucl Med Mol Imaging 49:1095–1098

Hepler CD (1985) Pharmacy as a clinical profession. Am J Hosp Pharm 42:1298–1306

Hepler CD, Strand LM (1990) Opportunities and responsibilities in pharmaceutical care. Am J Hosp Pharm 47:533–543

Hicks JK, Aquilante CL, Dunnenberger HM, Gammal RS, Funk RS, Aitken SL, Bright DR, Coons JC, Dotson KM, Elder CT, Groff LT, Lee JC (2019) Precision pharmacotherapy: integrating pharmacogenomics into clinical pharmacy practice. J Am Coll Clin Pharm 2:303–313

Higby GJ (2014) A cornerstone of modern institutional pharmacy practice: mirror to hospital pharmacy. Am J Health Syst Pharm 71:1940–1946

International Pharmaceutical Federation (FIP) (2012) FIP global pharmacy workforce report, vol 2012. FIP, The Netherlands, p 18

Jeong S, Ji E (2018) Global perspectives on ensuring the safety of pharmaceutical products in the distribution process. Int J Clin Pharm Ther 56:12–23

Jepsen DM, Spooner O'Neill M (2013) Australian hospital pharmacists reflect on career success. J Pharm Pract Res 43:29–31

Joseph K, Ramireddy K, Madison G, Turco T, Lui M (2021a) Outcomes of a pharmacist-driven vancomycin monitoring initiative in a community hospital. J Clin Pharm Ther 46:1103–1108

Joseph T, Hale GM, Moreau C (2021b) Training pharmacy residents as transitions of care specialists: a United States perspective. Int J Clin Pharm 43:756–758

Jusufoska M, Abreu de Azevedo M, Tolic J, Deml MJ, Tarr PE (2021) 'Vaccination needs to be easy for the people, right?' A qualitative study of the roles of physicians and pharmacists regarding vaccination in Switzerland. BMJ Open 11:e053163

Karnes JH, Asempa T, Barreto JN, Belcher RM, Bissell BD, Gammal RS, Kier KL, Lee CR, Liu L, McCune JS, Minhaj FS, Sikora Newsome A, Ning J, Bookstaver PB (2022) The essential research curriculum for doctor of pharmacy degree programs 2021. J Am Coll Clin Pharm 5:358–365. https://doi.org/10.1002/jac5.1603

Katangwe T, Family H, Sokhi J, Kirkdale CL, Twigg MJ (2020) The community pharmacy setting for diabetes prevention: a mixed methods study in people with 'pre-diabetes'. Res Soc Adm Pharm 16:1067–1080

Katoue MG, Schwinghammer TL (2020) Competency-based education in pharmacy: a review of its development, applications, and challenges. J Eval Clin Pract 26:1114–1123

Kiely PDW (2016) Biologic efficacy optimization- a step towards personalized medicine. Rheumatology 55:780–788

Kiles TM, Patel K, Aghagoli A, Spivey CA, Chisholm-Burns M, Hohmeier KC (2021) A community-based partnership collaborative practice agreement project to disseminate and implement evidence-based practices in community pharmacy. Curr Pharm Teach Learn 13: 1522–1528

Lloyd GF, Bajorek B, Barclay P, Goh S (2015) Narrative review: status of key performance indicators in contemporary hospital pharmacy practice. J Pharm Pract Res 45:396–403

Mamo M, Wirth F, Azzopardi LM, Serracino-Inglott A (2013) Standardising pharmacist patient-profiling activities in a rehabilitation hospital in Malta. Eur J Hosp Pharm 21:49–53

Mantel-Teeuwisse AK, Meilianti S, Khatri B, Yi W, Azzopadi LM, Acosta Gomez J, Gulpinar G, Bennara K, Uzman N (2021) Digital health in pharmacy education: preparedness and responsiveness of pharmacy programmes. Educ Sci 296(11):296

McDonald KS, Hite LM (2008) The next generation of career success: implications of HRD. Adv Dev Hum Resour 10:86–103

Mifsud EM, Wirth F, Camilleri L, Azzopardi LM, Serracino-Inglott A (2019) Pharmacist-led medicine use review in community pharmacy for patients on warfarin. Int J Clin Pharm 41: 741–750

Muscat Terribile C, Wirth F, Zammit MC, Vella J, Azzopardi LM, Serracino-Inglott A (2013) Evaluation of a quality system developed for pharmacy teaching laboratories. Pharm Educ 13(1):134–139

Njonkou G, Gbadamosi K, Muhammad S, Chughtai I, Le G, Fabayo A, Tran H, Lam B, Senay M, DeLaine L, McSwain C, Price DA (2021) Assessment of the impact of pharmacist-led transitions of care services in a primary health center. Hosp Pharm 56(3):187–190

O'Callaghan J, Barry SP, Bermingham M, Morris JM, Griffin BT (2019) Regulation of biosimilar medicines and current perspectives on interchangeability and policy. Eur J Clin Pharm 75:1–11

Osama S, Wirth F, Zahra G, Barbara C, Xuereb RG, Camilleri L, Azzopardi LM (2021) CYP2C19*2 genetic polymorphism and incidence of in-stent restenosis in patients on clopidogrel: a matched case-control study. Drug Metab Pers Ther 37(2):155–161

Paudyal V, Fialova D, Henman MC, Hazen A, Okuyan B, Lutters M, Cadogan C, Alves da Costa F, Galfrascoli E, Pudritz YM, Rydant S, Acosta-Gomez J (2021) Pharmacists' involvement in COVID-19 vaccination across Europe: a situational analysis of current practice and policy. Int J Clin Pharm 43:1139–1148

Pedersen CA, Schneider PH, Ganio MC, Scheckelhoff DJ (2019) ASHP national survey of pharmacy practice in hospital settings: monitoring and patient education-2018. Am J Health Syst Pharm 76:1038–1058

Pedersen CA, Schneider PH, Ganio MC, Scheckelhoff DJ (2020) ASHP national survey of pharmacy practice in hospital settings: prescribing and transcribing-2019. Am J Health Syst Pharm 77:1026–1050

Pedersen CA, Schneider PH, Ganio MC, Scheckelhoff DJ (2021) ASHP national survey of pharmacy practice in hospital settings: dispensing and administration-2020. Am J Health Syst Pharm 78:1074–1093

Pham JT, Azzopardi LM, Lau AH, Jarrett JB (2019) Student perspectives on a collaborative international doctorate of pharmacy program. Pharmacy 7:85

Rajiah K, Sivarasa S, Maharajan MK (2021) Impact of pharmacists' interventions and patients' decision on health outcomes in terms of medication adherence and quality use of medicines among patients attending community pharmacies: a systematic review. Int J Environ Res Public Health 18:4392

Sammut Bartolo N, Ignas L, Wirth F, Attard-Pizzuto M, Vella Szijj J, Camilleri L, Serracino-Inglott A, Azzopardi LM (2020) Public perception of generic medicines in Malta. JPHRS 11(3): 295–298

Scala D, Mucherino S, Wirth F, Valentina O, Polidori P, Faggiano ME, Iovine D, Saturnino P, Cattel F, Costantini A, Makoul G, Azzopardi LM, Menditto E (2022) Developing and piloting a Communication Assessment Tool assessing patient perspectives on communication with pharmacists (CAT-Pharm). Int J Clin Pharm. https://doi.org/10.1007/s11096-022-01382-y

Schumock GT, Meek PD, Ploetz PA, Vermuelen MS (1996) Economic evaluations of clinical pharmacy services. Pharmacotherapy 16(6):1182–1208

Scott S, May H, Patel M, Wright DJ, Bhattacharya D (2021) A practitioner behaviour change intervention for deprescribing in the hospital setting. Age Ageing 50:581–586

Serracino-Inglott A (2021) How to think like Francke for a global vision in challenging times. Am J Health Syst Pharm 78:606–612

Seychell M, Hackbart B (2013) The EU health strategy- Investing in health. Public Health Rev 35:4

Siaw MYL, Toh JH, Lee JY (2018) Patients' perceptions of pharmacist-managed diabetes services in the ambulatory care and community settings within Singapore. Int J Clin Pharm 40:403–411

Slazak E, Cardinal C, Will S, Clark CM, Daly CJ, Jacobs DM (2020) Pharmacist-led transitions-of-care services in primary care settings: opportunities, experiences and challenges. J Am Pharm Assoc 60:443–449

Sternschein R, Hayes MM, Ramani S (2021) A model for teaching in learner-centred clinical settings. Med Teach 43:1450–1452

Strand MA, Bratberg J, Eukel K, Hardy M, Williams C (2020) Community pharmacists' contribution to disease management during the COVID-19 pandemic. Prev Chronic Dis 17:E69

Stranges PM, Jackevicius CA, Anderson SL, Bondi DS, Danelich I, Emmons RP, Englin EF, Hansen ML, Nys C, Phan H, Philbrick AM, Rager M, Schumacher C, Smithgall S (2020) Role of clinical pharmacists and pharmacy support personnel in transitions of care. J Am Coll Clin Pharm 3:532–545

Sule A, Horak P, Makridaki D, Kohl S (2021) Hospital pharmacy specialisation. Eur J Hosp Pharm. https://doi.org/10.1136/ejhpharm-2021-002975

Sutton RT, Pincock D, Baumgart DC, Sadowski DC, Fedorak RN, Kroeker KI (2020) An overview of clinical decision support systems: benefits, risks and strategies for success. NPJ Digit Med 17. https://doi.org/10.1038/s41746-020-0221-y

Thomson K, Hillier-Brown F, Walton N, Bilaj M, Bambra C, Todd A (2019) The effects of community pharmacy-delivered public health interventions on population health and health inequalities: a review of reviews. Prev Med 124:98–109

Tung EL, Thomas A, Eichner A, Shalit P (2018) Implementation of a community pharmacy-based pre-exposure prophylaxis service: a novel model for pre-exposure prophylaxis care. Sex Health 15:556–561

Ulrick BY, Meggs EV (2019) Towards a greater professional standing: evolution of pharmacy practice and education, 1920–2020. Pharmacy 7:98

Ungaro S, Wirth F, Azzopardi LM, Serracino-Inglott A (2015) Point-of-care testing for urine analysis and microalbuminuria for diabetic patient management. Point Care 14:71–72

Vella M, Grima M, Wirth F et al (2015) Consumer perception of community pharmacist extended professional services. JPHRS 6:91–96

Vella J, Attard Pizzuto M, Sammut Bartolo N, Wirth F, Grech L, Pham J, Mactal Haaf C, Lau A, Serracino-Inglott A, Azzopadi LM (2021) A three-year post-graduate Doctorate in Pharmacy course incorporating professional, experiential and research activities: a collaborative innovative approach. MedEdPublish 10:93

Villeneuve Y, Courtemanche F, Firoozi F, Gilbert S, Desbiens MP, Desjardins A, Dinh C, LeBlanc VC, Attia A (2021) Impact of pharmacist interventions during transition of care in older adults to reduce the use of healthcare services: a scoping review. Res Soc Adm Pharm 17:1361–1372

Weeda E, Gilbert RE, Kolo SJ, Haney JS, Hazard LT, Taber DJ, Axon RN (2021) Impact of pharmacist-driven transitions of care interventions on post-hospital outcomes among patients with coronary artery disease: a systematic review. J Pharm Pract. https://doi.org/10.1177/08971900211064155

Westein MPD, de Vries H, Floor A, Koster AS, Buurma H (2019) Development of a postgraduate community pharmacist specialization program using CanMEDS competencies and entrustable professional activities. Am J Pharm Educ 83:1354–1365

Wirth F, Tabone F, Azzopardi LM, Gauci M, Zarb-Adami M, Serracino-Inglott A (2011) Consumer perception of the community pharmacist and community pharmacy services in Malta. JPHRS 1:189–194

Yee GC, Haas CE (2014) Standards of practice for clinical pharmacists: the time has come. Pharmacotherapy 34(8):769–770

Yemeke TT, McMillan S, Marciniak MW, Ozawa S (2021) A systematic review of the role of pharmacists in vaccination services in low- and middle-income countries. Res Soc Adm Pharm 17:300–306

Yeoman G, Furlong P, Seres M, Binder H, Chung H, Garzya V, Jones RRM (2017) Defining patient centricity with patients for patients and caregivers: a collaborative endeavour. BMJ Innov 3:76–83

Yu YM, Kim S, Choi KY, Jeong KY, Lee E (2019) Impact of knowledge, attitude and preceptor behaviour in pharmacovigilance education. Basic Clin Pharmacol Toxicol 124:591–599

Part V
Practical Tips and Tricks

Chapter 17
A Successful Career in the Life Sciences Industry: How to Write Your Strongest Resumé and Ace that Interview

Sofie Paeps and Charlotte Peters

Abstract We all remember that white sheet of paper that must become the perfect resumé. It is a young graduate's nightmare, wondering what information could possibly be interesting, which experience to mention, when you only have had one or two student jobs.

Next to this, we definitely remember the first interview: the sweaty hands, the indecisiveness on what to wear and which smart questions to ask.

This chapter has been written by two recruitment professionals, who have spent a lifetime working in the life sciences industry, scouting for talent, interviewing hundreds of scientists and guiding and advising them in their careers.

HR One Group is a boutique recruitment agency, based in Belgium, but active in EMEA, the USA and Asia. We strongly believe that it is essential to advise candidates freely and ensure smooth recruitment processes. Well-prepped candidates are the key to successful hires. Companies benefit strongly from this preparation.

It is in HR One Group's DNA to bring out the best in people and to offer hands-on advice on what to expect when applying for a job.

With a passion for people, their personalities, skills and competences, we have gained great insight in the best practices for acing your interview and getting your aspired dream job.

This chapter offers practical guidelines and covers the most important aspects of a recruitment process, even though it will not provide answers to all situations.

A recruitment process remains a truly unique journey for each and everyone. Nevertheless, these guidelines can help you keep on track while reducing stress levels, anxiety or fear of failure. It will bring simple suggestions and answers to an array of questions that all candidates have.

· S. Paeps (✉) · C. Peters
HR One Group, Herent, Belgium
e-mail: sofie.paeps@hronegroup.com; charlotte.peters@hronegroup.com

© The Author(s), under exclusive license to Springer Nature Switzerland AG 2023
J. R. Thomas et al. (eds.), *Career Options in the Pharmaceutical and Biomedical Industry*, https://doi.org/10.1007/978-3-031-14911-5_17

We wish you all the best and remember this: be authentic, be yourself, and add a little touch of magic.

17.1   The Academic Paradox!

The world has never been a more exciting place to be a scientist. The career market is expanding and the war for talent has reached new heights. The life sciences industry is growing extensively and has been one of the biggest employers for talent in recent years.

For scientists, this means that the sky is the limit and career options are endless.

Nevertheless, this reality can be scary. Navigating the wide options in the life sciences industry, which expand over R&D, labs, biotech companies, big pharma, generics, medical devices, medical technology, diagnostics, hospitals and healthcare institutions, can be daunting for any job applicant.

For a scientist in training, academia will offer excellent scientific education, but there has never been a focus on the essence of job interviewing, resumé writing and finding the right career path. Scientists are expected to find out for themselves what they love and where their skills and competences would thrive best.

Whereas some companies attract the more introverted, self-driven, scientific experts, others are keen on getting in the more extraverted, team performing and versatile types.

This paradox is present across the entire scientific community, and in this chapter you will find hands-on advice on the following key aspects:

1. Understand who you are
2. Write that personal resumé
3. Ace that interview

17.2   Understand Who You Are

Your natural academic or laboratorial habitat might refrain you from understanding who you truly are, before starting a career in the life sciences industry. Thus, understanding how you interact with people and who you really are seems to be key to a successful career choice. It is essential to understand your natural ability to interact with people, your stress levels, your personality type, before applying for a job.

17.2.1 Ask Your Community: Who Am I?

The simple question—how do you see me?—is not as common as you might think. Who am I, to the eyes of my friends, family, peers or professors, is the most revealing question you could begin with. Do the test and ask your counterparts to be as frank as can be.

Ask your peers what they think of you. Be vulnerable.

What are your strengths and weaknesses? You might be the brightest scientist but an individual that has a hard time to interact with people. You prefer working on your own. You like odd hours; you might be a night owl or an early bird. You never had to wait on other assignments to continue your personal paper. You might be demanding for yourself and hard to interact with people, quite stubborn, open to help others, feeling the need to educate others, etc.

Understanding your true nature, your strengths and your flaws, your personal competences and personality traits are key in the first step to finding the job of a lifetime.

So, how to do this?

- Make a list of all your strengths/weaknesses.
- Make a list of all your personality traits:

  - Organized ↔ chaotic
  - Punctual ↔ deadline cruncher
  - Team player ↔ individual contributor
  - Concise ↔ loves to explain
  - Academic writer ↔ academic trainer
  - Gets energy from people ↔ gets energy from books
  - Loves to travel ↔ loves to stay at home
  - Likes individual contact ↔ loves to hang out with big groups of people
  - Loves to solve problems ↔ loves to analyse problems
  - Loves to prepare a presentation in the background ↔ loves to present before a large audience
  - Loves to meet new people ↔ loves to invest in long-term friendships
  - Stringent way of interacting with people ↔ easy to get along with

Link your personality traits to constructive adjectives:

Whatever personality you have, there is a key quality that will help you to sell yourself.

Your essential personality trait relates to an argument in favour of a job. Every personality trait you have relates to an argument in favour of your career:

1. You are demanding of yourself—a company could find this very attractive because it means you will go the extra mile
2. You like to work in team—you are a team player
3. Reading through academic, medical scientific texts—you are a strong medical writer/analysis

4. You like to explain complex matters in a simple way—educate on a scientific topic—you have the ability to train a team of non-scientists
5. You like detail and accuracy—you are accurate and detailed oriented
6. You can comply with tight deadlines—you are flexible and on time
7. You love sports—you are fit
8. ...

Remember all your personality traits. These are key for your resumé later on. You will find herewith a non-exhaustive list of adjectives describing personality traits that might be helpful when preparing your self-reflection:

Openness
Flexible
Trustworthy
Curious
Creative
Need for achievement and recognition
Accessible
Inspiring
Challenging
Charismatic
Dedicated
Disciplined
Eloquent
Empathetic
Energetic
Flexible
Focused
Helpful
Innovative
Intuitive
Decisive
Sociable

17.3 Write that Personal Resumé

Your resumé ideally covers a number of crucial aspects: your coordinates, professional experience, professional objective, education and extra competences.

When elaborating on your experience, make sure to keep some elements in mind:

– Make it chronologically—stating the last achievement first.
– Be concise—jot down the highlights and focus on achievements and concrete results.

- Write what matters for the job—make sure that the information you write in your resumé is relevant for the position you apply for.
- Think about the 'KISS' principle: keep it short and simple. Make it a one-pager or max. a two-pager. This will allow you really highlight the most important aspects of your experience.

17.3.1   How to Reach You

Make sure you put essential information on how to reach you on your resumé. Important elements are name, phone number, e-mail and address.

17.3.2   What Do You Want?

What job are you applying for or what position do you aim for? Make a clear statement on your resumé on who you are and what you would like to achieve.
    Some examples:

I am a scientist, with a passion for . . . .
Flexible, trustworthy, accurate, sociable and easy to get along with. . . .
Independent contributor and able to work with short deadlines, who loves to work behind the scenes on projects that need to be pushed forward.

17.3.3   Your Professional Experience

If you have professional experience, start with your latest position.
    Mention the name of the company, your position and the year/months:

For example, PharmLab—lab technician, 2021–2022

    If you have no experience, do mention your summer jobs, student job, lab experience, writing assignments and conference participation which show that you have engaged in a significant position:

For example, tour organizer—The city of London, summer 2020.

17.3.4 Your Education/Academic Background/Scholarships and Grants

Make sure to list your degrees and universities chronologically:
Last comes first!
Go back as far as your high school degree
Make sure to add scholarships and grants
International exchange programmes are interesting for the reader:
AFS (Ambulance Field Service) or EF (Education First)
Erasmus
FWO (Research Foundation—Flanders) scholarships and grants.
Do not hesitate to mention your achievements in this field.

17.3.5 Language/IT Competences

Keep declaring your language level short and clear:

– Mother tongue
– Excellent knowledge
– Good knowledge
– Basic knowledge

For IT competences:
Add lab- or job-related experience and knowledge.

17.3.6 Publications

You can add your publications on your resumé. If they are relevant for the position you apply for, state them on your resumé. If you have plenty of them, you can also choose to mention 'Publications on Request' or add them as an annex to your resumé.

17.4 Ace That Interview

In today's world, you most likely will have to go through a number of interviews in order to get a job. This is a crucial stage in the process to get to understand who your direct manager will be, your peers, your colleagues and other important stakeholders. Whether these interviews are online or face to face, there are similar important elements to think about.

17.4.1 Come Prepared to the Interview

It is crucial to come prepared to the interview: read the company's website. Read the job description thoroughly. Perform some research on the business the company is active in. Google or look up the person you will meet on LinkedIn. This will help you understand his/her background and experience. Prepare some interesting questions: what are the values of the company? What is your company known for among its employees? Why are employees happy to work at your company? Why did you ever make the move to the company? Print out your resumé and bring it along.

17.4.1.1 Appearance Is Key

Whether your interview takes place in the virtual or the real world, make sure to dress in a professional way. During an online interview, think about your background and look into the camera. If you have a second screen, make sure your head keeps turned to the screen with your camera in. In real life, look to the person in front of you. Give a firm handshake.

17.4.2 What Type of Questions to Expect and What Questions to Ask?

Tell me about your achievements.
What are you good at?
What do other people say about you?
What is a personality trait you would like to improve on?
If you could create your own job, what would definitely be in it?

Typical questions such as 'describe a project for which you were responsible' and 'what are your most common personality traits' are answered more easily when you did some thinking beforehand. It is important to keep some examples in mind.

Prepare a few smart questions yourself. Never go to an interview without questions.

It shows interest and dedication.

Some questions can be general in nature, others more specific.

Questions on company culture, people and the organization are good icebreakers:

- What is the company's DNA?
- What is the company's short- and long-term aspiration?
- What type of people thrive well in this organization?
- What are you looking for in a candidate?
- Which roles are available in the organization?

More specific questions related to the position:

- What's a typical day like in this position?
- On which elements will I be assessed after 3–6 months in the position?
- Which achievements will we celebrate after 1 year in the role?
- Which people are successful in this position and why?
   Be careful!
   Never ask questions about holidays and salary first. Make sure to embed them in the larger context:
   For example, you can ask what a typical remuneration level is for this position in general.

17.4.3   Follow Up on the Interview

Make yourself stand out in the crowd, by thanking your interview panel, for their time and effort. Do keep it short and simple.

Dear . . .,
Thanks very much for your time and effort during yesterday's interview. The position of medical science liaison in your company is very appealing to me, and I am looking forward to the next steps. Do not hesitate to contact me for any additional questions.
Kind regards,
. . .

If you have not heard back, call them in the next days.

17.5   Be Authentic

Dear scientist, we understand that your professional journey is about to embark. We wish you a long and happy career. Know that the path to that career will be covered with hardships, happiness, hurdles, hard work and hopefully fulfilling experiences.

In a world where a lot is written on how to be successful, please stay authentic. This is the best advice we can give you, authentic in your values, authentic in your choice for a position and authentic in your relationships with your colleagues. Be yourself always is the best you can be. Never compare yourself with others. Only compare yourself with your best self. Be the better version of yourself every day.

And last but not least, stay in touch. No better professional as a connected one. Talk to you soon.

Chapter 18
Skill Building for Career Advancement: Public Speaking and Networking

Hynda K. Kleinman

Abstract Public speaking and networking are important skills for obtaining a position in a pharmaceutical company and for career advancement. This chapter offers advice on how to overcome your fear of public speaking, present a dynamic and interesting talk, improve your oral and visual presentation, introduce yourself, and expand your network of colleagues. A considerable amount of time over years must be invested in this self-training and effort, but the benefits are huge and long-lasting throughout your entire career.

18.1 Introduction

This chapter will focus on improving your speaking and networking skills to increase your chances of getting and holding a position in a pharmaceutical company. As exemplified in the other chapters in this book, there are many different opportunities for various kinds of positions within the pharmaceutical industry that will build on the training that you already have. Many recent graduates feel that they do not have the experience for many pharma positions. However, your advanced training has given you basic skills for such a career in many different jobs in the pharmaceutical industry (Table 18.1). You have learned critical thinking and have acquired analytical skills in interpreting your data and that of others, including papers in the literature. Your oral and written communication has improved with the numerous presentations during your training. Various collaborations and your ability to work independently are highly valued by companies. Likewise, specific skills like statistical analyses, computer skills for presentations and searches, problem-solving skills, and ability to learn new techniques also strengthen your ability to succeed in various positions within pharma. This chapter will provide further advice on two important components of a pharma career, including public speaking/communication and networking. Excelling in communication skills and networking will not only help you get and retain the position you want but also

H. K. Kleinman (✉)
NIDCR, NIH, Bethesda, MD, USA

Table 18.1 Useful and important skills acquired during academic training that prepare you for all types of positions in pharma

Critical thinking
Analytical skills: Ability to understand complex papers and reports, data analysis, etc.
Oral and written communication skills
Work in a team or independently and with flexibility
Statistical analyses
Computer skills for presentations, searches, etc.
Problem solving
Initiating and successfully completing a long-term project (thesis)
Ability to learn new techniques, fields of science, etc.
Broad background prepares you for knowing and learning much in science outside of your training
Confidence that you can succeed and meet the challenges of working in pharma

further your advancement within the company. There is considerable useful and important information on the internet from journals, universities, professional societies, publishers, blogs, etc. about effective communication and networking that can help further expand what is presented in this chapter and improve skills. The readers are encouraged to consult these and many of the links embedded within the sites which have additional important and useful information. Some are listed at the end of this chapter.

18.2 Importance of Public Speaking

Improved communication skills will benefit you for your entire career and even in your personal life. Good public speakers can generate trust and empathy, excite and engage an audience, effectively share knowledge and ideas, and motivate a team. Public speaking is important for job interviews, presenting at conferences and seminars, mentoring, teaching, negotiations, etc. Audiences want to be stimulated, inspired, and glad that they came to your presentation. The good news is that these communication skills can be learned. The bad news is that most people have a fear of public speaking. This fear can be overcome with understanding the causes(s) of your fear, practice in public speaking, and following certain "rules" that will provide you with confidence in what you are saying (Table 18.2). Overcoming fear of speaking takes time, but being a good communicator is highly valued by pharma.

Table 18.2 Advice for overcoming your fear and for successful speaking and communication

A. Advice on what to do. Plan to
Know your subject thoroughly. Practice your talk multiple times out loud on your own and then in front of your friends
Know the size of the room and expected number of attendees. Know the level of training/ knowledge of your audience to focus the content
Use positive affirmations to build confidence (I know more about this subject than my audience)
Voice: Pay attention to the tone, volume, speed, and inflection of your voice. Vary the rate of speaking and the volume for emphasis—be enthusiastic!
Keep you posture in the "high-power" pose (stand up straight and tall). Use appropriate body language and natural gestures
Smile and look for people in the audience who smile back
Tell a humbling story about yourself or your science
Be empathetic and show you understand and share the feelings of others
Make eye contact with the audience
Use visuals as most people are visual learners
Walk away from the podium—do not stand behind it and walk the stage while facing the audience and speaking
B. Advice on what not to do. Do not
Talk too quickly, softly, only to the front row, or to the slide screen
Use a monotone or single speed of speech
Focus on a single topic
Use jargon
Use slides that have small lettering, thin lines, too much information or too little, poor contrasting colors, red for emphasis (10% of all men are red color blind and will only see gray); do not animate text
Speak with a frown or have a sad or angry face
Be impolite or lose patience with audience questions

18.3   Skills and Advice for Public Speaking and Communication

Overcoming Your Fear of Public Speaking Knowing why you fear public speaking (bad previous experience, low self-esteem, introverted personality, etc.) will help you to take corrective measures. There are many things you can do to overcome your fear of speaking and become more confident in your speaking skills (Scientifica 2021; Forsey 2021; Barnes 2010a; Fleming 2018) (Table 18.2):

1. Give yourself mental positive affirmations like "I know this subject better than anyone in the audience," "I am confident in what I will be saying," "I know this will be a good talk," etc. Athletes used positive affirmations (and visualizations) all the time both mentally and in public.
2. Be fully prepared. Practice your speech alone and then in front of friends. This relieves the stress level, eliminates problematic phrases and ideas, and can help

you anticipate the tough question. It also helps with some needed revisions and the pronunciation of difficult words.

3. Know the size of the room and expected number of attendees. Fear of the unknown can be problematic especially if you walk into a room and the size is not what you expect.

4. Get a good night's sleep. Sleep creates memories, maintains our immune system, regulates molecules that increase energy, relieves stress, etc. Do not use a computer or phone or exercise before going to sleep.

5. During your speech, have tall posture. Standing in the "high posture" pose reduces cortisol (the stress hormone), and increases testosterone (dominance hormone). Do not stand behind a podium but rather walk back and forth across the full length of the stage so you can engage the whole audience.

6. Pay attention to the tone, volume, inflection, and speed of your voice. First impressions are important, and you want your voice to be easy for the audience to hear, understand, and demonstrate your confidence in and command of the content. You also want to convey your enthusiasm/passion for what you are talking about (Larkin 2015). Be positive in your tone and content. No employer will want someone who mentions their failures and dislikes.

7. Look at your audience and try to find someone who is smiling or nodding in agreement and paying full attention. This positive reinforcement will help to eliminate your nervousness.

8. Tell a personal story, such as how you found your advisor or project. This will get a reaction and engage the audience.

9. Be empathetic and convey your personal feelings to the audience. Empathy is tied to brain mirror neurons, a special class of neurons that support observational learning. These neurons allow us to experience what others experience. For example, if you are talking about a disease or medical problem (cancer, heart disease, aging problems, etc.), you may want to convey that you understand the pain and suffering of the patient and family.

10. Make eye contact often with your audience. This will help you feel that they are one-on-one with what you are saying. Do not talk to the projected slides unless you are pointing out specific items. Look at faces in your entire audience, not just the front row.

11. Use clear, simple, and appealing visuals to support your talk (Barnes 2010b). Most people are visual learners, so the use of visuals will reinforce your message. Visuals help you with cues on what you want to say and can be used for smooth transitions between slides.

Preparing the Visual Presentation The content of your talk should be prepared based on the composition of the audience and focused on what they would be most likely to understand and be interested in (Barnes 2010b; Alexandrov and Hennerici 2012). A talk for a graduate school audience is very different from that for a pharma. For example, for a graduate school audience, you might want to present the rationale and simplify the techniques and focus on the findings, whereas for pharma you might want to show your broad technical skills and emphasize your collaborative approach

Table 18.3 Tips for preparing effective slides for a scientific presentation

Choose sharply contrasting colors for the background—choose text with a blue background and light or white text for dark small or large rooms and a white background with dark lettering for well-lighted small or large rooms or a Zoom
Do not put too much information on the slide—keep the slide simple and the content readable from the back of the room
Lettering should be large enough to read from the back of the room and should be an easily readable font like Ariel or Times
Limit transition slides and the number of animations or movies—do not animate the text
Use only high-quality images
Select slide titles carefully to reflect the conclusions of the slide content
Limit the complexity of the tables and charts so they can be read and understood from the back of the room

and flexibility. Modify your talk *every time* you give it to update the content and customize it for the audience. You may have two or three different basic talks on your computer that you can select from to modify to fit your audience.

The following are some important technical points that will greatly improve your presentation and the audience's response (Table 18.3). The color of your slide background and lettering are very important. Colors project moods and emotional feelings with white being related to purity, reverence, cleanliness, and simplicity, while blue is peaceful, tranquil, trusting, confident, and secure. Black projects as heavy, formal, and technical. The size of the room may dictate the slide background that you use, so know how large an audience will be present and the size of the room:

1. If you are presenting in a *dark* and *large* room, then a blue background with white or light text is best. However, if you plan to keep the lights on for your entire talk (highly advisable) in a large or small room, then a white background with dark text is best. Be sure that you use contrasting colors for the background and text as much as possible and not too many different colors. Use colors to emphasize important points. Do not use red for lettering or a red background as 10% of all men are red color blind and a red background causes eye strain.
2. Keep the slides simple with minimal text. Do not show too many different sets of data on the same slide.
3. Make sure the lettering for the labels is large and *readable from the back of the room*. The lines in a graph should be thick and labeled.
4. Limit transition slides and animations as too much animation dilutes the message. Especially do not animate the text. You can use summary slides as your transition slides.
5. Use high-quality graphics. Do not enlarge pictures to the point where the image has some blurring.
6. The title of each slide should convey the take-home message of the slide. For example, a slide showing data on the effect of a hormone on cortisol levels should *not* be "Effect of hormone X on cortisol levels" but rather should be "Hormone X increases cortisol levels."

7. Use appropriate and simple reader-friendly charts. For a pie chart, limit to 4–6 slices and for bar graphs limit to 4–8 bars. Tables do not work well for talks unless they are very simple. Limit the number of tables.
8. Font is important with Times and Ariel being recommended. Use the same font for the whole presentation. Use the same size font for all of the titles on the slides and as much as possible the same size (smaller than the title) font for the text.

Additional Unwritten Advice Effective speakers have some tricks they use to prepare and present their talks.

1. Dress as much like your audience as possible as it will help them "connect" with you. If you are speaking to students, be casually dressed. If you are talking to pharma executives, wear more formal but simple clothing.
2. Look up information about who will be in the audience and who invited you. Not only gear the level of your talk to the members of the audience or to the person who invited you, but also try to mention either them, their work, or accomplishments in your talk. This signals that you took the time to inform yourself about them and also "connects" you to them.
3. Bring business cards to hand out before and after your talk.
4. Smile a lot before, during, and after your talk. No one likes or will hire someone who is depressed, unhappy, and potentially angry.
5. Make sure that your every word, tone, gesture, posture, expression, and slide show concern, regard, and interest in the audience.
6. Be polite and respectful to your audience! For example, if someone asks a question about something you already presented clearly, thank them for the question and answer it. Do not say "as I explained in my slide...." This can embarrass them and likely your tone will not be empathetic.

Some Tips for Zoom/Webex/Internet Talks and Interviews With Covid-19 and travel costs, many organizations are using Internet platforms like Zoom and Webex for communication (Table 18.4). Much of what has been said above regarding slides, etc. is valid for such a presentation, but additionally there are some important points which should be taken into consideration (Diner 2021):

1. Be sure your computer is updated and charged, and you have strong Internet.
2. Chose a quiet room and turn off both your cell phone (best to put it in another room) and notifications on your computer. Notify your family of the meeting so there will be no interruptions and loud talking.
3. Be sure the background in the room is simple, preferably a white wall. Be sure the lighting is bright and not glaring off your glasses. Do not have a bright window behind you as your face will be in the shadow.
4. Wear a solid color shirt. Too many colors or patterns or jewelry can be distracting.
5. Join the meeting a few minutes early to be sure there are no connection problems.
6. Put your name in the box with your face on the screen if it is not showing.

Table 18.4 Tips for Zoom/Webex/Internet meetings, conversations, and interviews

Use a laptop or computer, not your phone
Be sure that your computer is updated and charged and has a good Internet connection
Choose a professional uncluttered background
Find a brightly lit and quiet room; tell your household about the meeting
Silence your phone and turn off notifications on your computer
Practice using this communication form
Join the meeting a few minutes early to be sure everything is working
Add your name to the box with your face
Use your mute button while others are speaking
Wear professional attire; solid color top is best
Use appropriate body language
Be prepared to introduce yourself
Look straight ahead into the camera while speaking as if you are face to face with someone; you may need to put books under your computer so you are facing forward not looking downward
If presenting, know how to share the presentation, keep the slides simple and readable, know how to enlarge them, and ask your audience if they can read your slides
Ask questions of the audience during your presentation to engage them—this also can be used to help to transition to the next part of your talk
If it is a job interview, have your list of questions ready and ask them

7. Use the mute button especially when others are speaking.
8. Be sure that your face is eye level with the camera. You may need to put some books under your computer to raise it. Many people are looking down at their computer in these types of meetings and not facing their audience when they speak. Everyone should be able to see your full face, especially when you are speaking. Eye contact is important for your effectiveness.
9. If you are giving a presentation, know how to share it quickly. Be sure to know how to enlarge the presentation on the screen so it is reader-friendly and check that everyone can read it.
10. While speaking look right into the camera (face to face). Ask the audience a few times if they have any questions to engage them.
11. Sit up straight and tall in an attentive pose.
12. Focus *only* on the meeting. Do not check your messages or look at anything besides the screen.

18.4 Importance of Networking

Networking is an invaluable skill that can advance your career and help you find a job, reagent or technique, new employee, etc. It is a skill that can be learned, and there are many ways to network both online and in public settings (Pain 2015; Joubert 2018; Gorian 2019) (Table 18.5). Networking requires both oral and written

Table 18.5 Networking strategies

Prepare business card, give them out freely, and collect the business cards of the people you meet (be sure to write on the back of the card when and where you received the card)
Update your curriculum vitae often and customize for the position
Join professional societies and volunteer to serve on committees
Be visible and meet people—go to meetings, seminars, posters, lunches with visitors, etc.
Go to the exhibitor shows at meetings and talk to the representatives in the booths
Invite scientists to speak at your institution
Present your findings at meetings, seminars, etc.
After a seminar given by another scientist, stand up tall, identify yourself, ask questions, and speak loudly and slowly
After attending a talk, go introduce yourself to the speaker and talk to them
Stay in contact with all your graduate student colleagues, advisors, mentors, professors, family, etc. thru email and social media
Join social media platforms like LinkedIn, ResearchGate, Twitter, Facebook (Meta), Instagram, etc.—allows you to find people and people to find you
Interview with school magazines and local newspapers

communication skills. It takes practice, initiative, and overcoming your fear of speaking and rejection. Most positions in companies or academia are not obtained by answering an advertisement but rather through someone you know. Employers do not want to waste time and resources with a well-qualified candidate who does not have good interpersonal relationships and interactions, does not listen to authority, shows arrogance, etc. Remember that the more people you network with and know you, the greater chance you will have of finding someone to write a good reference letter or refer you for an award or position. Do not be intimidated by those at a higher level. There are many tips provided below to help you network and to maintain your contacts for lifelong beneficial relationships as well as to expand your visibility.

Advice on Preparing for and Excelling at Networking Networking takes preparation and time and should be continued for your entire career. It is important to meet other scientists and be visible for your career:

1. First, make business cards and update you CV. The business cards should have your name, title, affiliation, and contact information all in simple lettering on a plain lightly colored or white card, no fancy script or pictures. The CV should have simple lettering and be as complete as possible. For a pharma job, you may want to list your skills (lab techniques, computer skills, languages, etc.) somewhere on the first page possibly right after your education and previous employment. For an academic position, you might want to emphasize your education, additional training, awards, mentoring, teaching, and publications. You should have different versions on your computer that is ready to share.
2. Join professional societies. Volunteer for committees.
3. Go to professional meetings. If you do not have the funds, ask the organizers for financial help. Many organizers have such funds available and/or can waive fees. Attend the talks and posters in your area of interest and also talks and

posters given by companies. Talk to the presenter with enthusiasm and give them your business card. If they give you a business card, write on the back the date and place you met them. Also visit the vendor booths and exchange cards. If appropriate, email these contacts and tell them how nice it was meeting them and/or do a follow-up on your conversation.

4. Go to seminars. Ask a question. Be sure to stand up tall, identify yourself, use your "power" body language, and speak loudly and slowly. Meet the presenter and exchange business cards. Give respectful praise and be polite.
5. Maintain an online presence so people can find you (and you can find them) thru social media: ResearchGate, LinkedIn, Facebook (Meta), Twitter, Instagram, etc.
6. Nominate yourself for awards or ask friends to nominate you. Awards on the CV/resume are usually important.
7. Be a "citizen" of your work environment by volunteering for special projects, panels, reviewing manuscripts, etc.
8. Solicit invitations to speak from your collaborators and friends. Also solicit and agree to do newspaper interviews.
9. Inform everyone about your accomplishments thru social media and email.
10. When you submit a manuscript for publication, always submit a photo for the cover. If your work is on the cover, frame it and hang it in your office for all to see.
11. Meet people in social and business situations and have your 1-min speech prepared.

The 1-min Speech or "Elevator Pitch" This introductory speech needs to be carefully prepared and rehearsed (Terry 2015; ALSO/Association for the Sciences of Limnology and Oceanography 2021). Practice it many times with different (imaginary) potential people you want to meet. The purpose is to allow you to introduce yourself and to answer the question "so what do you do?". Use this 1-min speech when you meet someone in the hallway at a conference or social event (or in the elevator) to explain who you are. It is a way to make yourself known and impress someone with your careful, clear, and short presentation. You can use the speech to add to your network; ask for a reagent, a job, and a cell line; ask an insightful question; introduce yourself to people you meet at conferences; etc. You want to be respectful of their time, polite, and use the skills above for public speaking such as eye contact, clear voice, smile, tall posture, appropriate body language, enthusiasm, etc. You can begin by politely asking if they have time to talk with you. For example, "Excuse me, I am a student here and would like to introduce myself to you. Do you have a minute to talk with me?" Then, begin your 1-min talk (Table 18.6):

1. Fully introduce yourself so they know your name, education level, current position, and if appropriate your present or former advisor.
2. Explain what you do and possibly what skills you have in terms of assays, bioinformatics, etc.
3. Next you want to explain what you are interested in terms of research area, learning new technologies or transitioning into another field or type of work,

Table 18.6 Guidance on the content of the 1-min talk

Who you are: Your name and position
Where you work and what you do
Why you are at the meeting or seminar: What you are interested in
Comment on their talk or work and/or if you want a position or reagent from them, tell them
Why they should care about meeting you
End by trying to "connect" with the person either thru mutual colleagues, interests, training, etc.
Look them in the eye, smile, and give them your business card

future jobs, etc. If relevant, also explain why you want to transition. For example, "I have worked in the basic science area and now want to apply my skills to translating lab work into therapeutics. Doing that is difficult in academia so I am interested in a job in pharma."

4. Explain why meeting them is important to you and to them. For example, "I have followed your work for a long time and it is finally nice to meet you in person. I will be looking for a job soon, do you expect to have an opening for someone like me? May I send you my CV?"

5. Share something you have or someone you know in common, like a colleague, growing up in the same part of the country, going to the same university, both using the same assay and working in the same research area, etc. For example, "My friend Mary was a post doc with you and always loved what she was doing in your lab. She will be happy to know that I finally met you."

6. Smile, look them in the eye, thank them for their time, and hand them a business card. Where appropriate, you may want to do a follow-up email.

18.5 Final Thoughts

This chapter is meant as an "outline" of the importance communication involving public speaking and networking for jobs in pharma (Fig. 18.1). There are additional in-depth resources for the topics of communication via speaking and networking online and available thru your professional societies, journals, and published literature. In addition, information on how to optimize your cover letter, prepare an abstract for a meeting, write a paper, get a grant, etc. are online for free and available at many university websites. Taking classes or training sessions in various aspects of pharma needs, such as intellectual property, quality control, clinical trial design, preclinical testing, regulatory requirements, etc., will add strength to your application for a position in pharma and possibly help you decide the type of position you would like in pharma. Take these courses and training when available at your university or at professional meetings. The following chapters in this book will also add information that will help you define the type of position you would like in pharma. Note that in big pharma, your position may be very focused in one area of

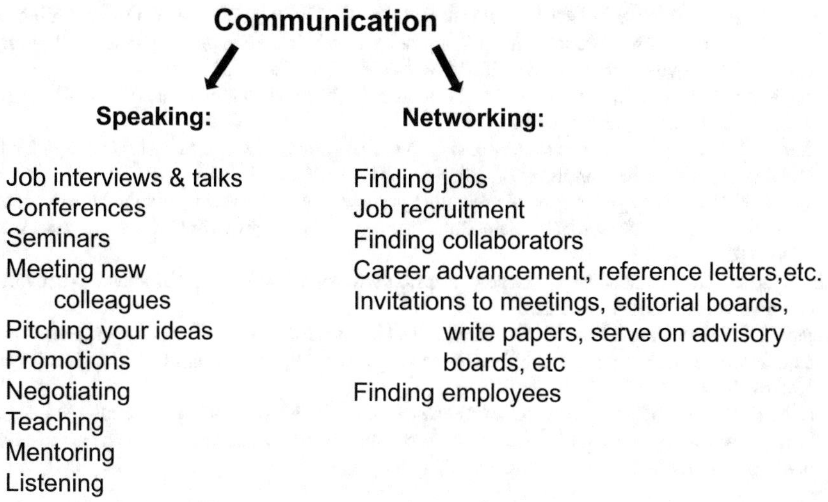

Communication

Speaking:

Job interviews & talks
Conferences
Seminars
Meeting new
    colleagues
Pitching your ideas
Promotions
Negotiating
Teaching
Mentoring
Listening

Networking:

Finding jobs
Job recruitment
Finding collaborators
Career advancement, reference letters,etc.
Invitations to meetings, editorial boards,
    write papers, serve on advisory
    boards, etc
Finding employees

Fig. 18.1 Career success is highly dependent on communication skills with public speaking and networking being key factors. Details of the benefits of effective public speaking and networking are shown

expertise, whereas in small companies, you may need to know several aspects, such as drug and clinical development.

Good communication through public speaking and extensive networking can be a solid foundation for a career in pharma. By carefully preparing yourself for communicating who you are, what you do, what you want, and what you can do, you will reduce your fears and gain confidence to meet the challenges of working in pharma. A strong and growing network of colleagues and professionals will greatly enhance your opportunities and career advancement.

References

Alexandrov AV, Hennerici AG (2012) How to prepare and deliver a scientific presentation https://www.karger.com/Article/Fulltext/346077. Accessed 20 Nov 2021

ALSO/Association for the Sciences of Limnology and Oceanography (2021) An introduction for all occasions: the elevator pitch. https://www.aslo.org/science-communication/elevator-pitch/. Accessed 1 Dec 2021

Barnes L (2010a) Public speaking for scientists 1: introduction. https://letterstonature.wordpress.com/2010/07/15/public-speaking-for-scientists-1-introduction/. Accessed 4 Dec 2021

Barnes L (2010b) Public speaking for scientists 7: powerpoint. https://letterstonature.wordpress.com/2010/09/19/public-speaking-for-scientists-7-powerpoint. Accessed 4 Dec 2021

Diner E (2021) 7 tips for giving the best virtual research presentation. http://www.slide-talk.com/7-tips-for-giving-the-best-virtual-research-presentation/. Accessed 1 Dec 2021

Fleming N (2018) (Hubspot) How to give a great scientific talk. Nat Events Guide 564:S84–S85. https://media.nature.com/original/magazine-assets/d41586-018-07780-5. Accessed 4 Dec 2021

Forsey C (2021) (Hubspot) Science-backed tips for mastering public speaking, according to 5 mental health professionals. https://blog.hubspot.com/marketing/science-public-speaking-tips#sm.000v7evuti52es011pw1w6plubwkw. Accessed 15 Nov 2021

Gorian R (2019) Networking for introverted scientists https://www.nature.com/articles/d41586-019-01296-2. Accessed 15 Nov 2021

Joubert S (2018) The importance of networking in science https://www.northeastern.edu/graduate/blog/biotechnology-networking-tips/. Accessed 20 Nov 2021

Larkin M (2015) How to give a dynamic scientific presentation. Elsevier. https://blog.hubspot.com/marketing/science-public-speaking-tips#sm.000v7evuti52es011pw1w6plubwkw.   Accessed 1 Dec 2021

Pain E (2015) How to network effectively. https://www.science.org/content/article/how-network-effectively. Accessed 20 Nov 2021

Scientifica (2021) 9 simple and effective public speaking tips for scientists. https://www.scientifica.uk.com/neurowire/9-simple-and-effective-public-speaking-tips-for-scientists#.   Accessed 15 Nov 2021

Terry M (2015) Scientists. Here's the best elevator pitch to sell yourself to a potential employer https://wwwbiospacecom/article/scientists-here-s-the-best-elevator-pitch-to-sell-yourself-to-a-potential-employer-/. Accessed 20 Nov 2021

Chapter 19
Training Opportunities for a Career in the Pharmaceutical and Biomedical Industry

Josse R. Thomas

Abstract This chapter aims to give young graduates and recent professionals a brief overview of the wide array of background educations and additional training opportunities that are available, and that can help to prepare yourself for a first job and a successful career in the pharmaceutical and biomedical industry.

The first part briefly summarises what academia has to offer as graduate programmes already more targeted towards the pharma and biomed industry, with the focus on life sciences, and as more advanced or more specific postgraduate education or training opportunities.

In the second part, training opportunities in the pharmaceutical and biomedical industry itself are reviewed, focusing on intern-, trainee-, mentor- and apprenticeship offers.

In the third part, other organisations are mentioned that offer training specifically targeted towards jobs in this sector, such as public-private partnership initiatives, professional organisations, regulatory authorities and specialised service providers.

The chapter ends with a selection of websites that can be useful to find your way in this wide variety of possibilities.

19.1 Introduction

The pharmaceutical (pharma), biotechnology (biotech) and medical technology (medtech) industries offer a wide variety of job and career opportunities for people with various professional backgrounds.

Undergraduate and graduate students have a broad array of possibilities to prepare themselves for a successful career in this sector. The wealth of opportunities is apparent from:

- The variety of preferred background qualifications, e.g. graduates in life sciences (such as pharmacy, medicine, biomedical sciences, biotechnology, etc.), basic

J. R. Thomas (✉)
PharmaCS, Merchtem, Belgium

sciences (biology, chemistry, physics), engineering (chemical engineering, bio-engineering, biomedical engineering), information technology, (big) data analysis, economics, law and others.

– The multitude of organisations that provide education and training, e.g. academia in the first place (universities, colleges and other higher education institutions), but also industry, health authorities, professional associations and service providers.

– The different ways of learning, e.g. traditional learning (on-campus/classroom courses, in person, all year round or during summer schools), distance or e-learning (online, webinars, video lectures, blackboard or Zoom sessions, massive open online courses or MOOCs, etc.) and hybrid or blended learning (a mixture or the best of both worlds).

– The number of possible outcomes, e.g. a degree (academic or professional), a diploma, a certificate or an accreditation.

As a result, students and young graduates are being overwhelmed by this multitude of possibilities. Therefore, the objective of this chapter is to provide a practical framework to help you to find your way in this jungle, not by being comprehensive (or even exhaustive) but simply by concentrating on the most wanted qualifications, and giving some examples that will hopefully facilitate your choice.

The focus will be on education and training opportunities for students and graduates in life sciences that might give them a better chance to start an interesting job or develop a successful career in the pharmaceutical or biomedical industry.

For more detailed information, the reader is referred to the list of Useful Websites at the end of this chapter.

19.2 Education and Training Offered by Academia

19.2.1 Targeted Graduate Master Programmes

Besides the more traditional graduate master programmes in life and health sciences offered by academia leading to the professional practice as pharmacist or physician, several universities currently also offer other first or initial master programmes more targeted towards biopharmaceutical and biomedical research and/or the corresponding industry.

One of the pioneers in this field was Leiden University in the Netherlands with its master programme in biopharmaceutical sciences (BPS), already offered since several decades when the Dutch government decided to limit the education of pharmacists to two universities, thus stimulating the other faculties of pharmacy to look for alternatives. The programme trains students mainly for a scientific career in drug research and development, and currently offers three sub-specialisations: biotherapeutics, drug discovery and safety, and systems biomedicine and pharmacology. The BPS training can also be combined with four other specialisations:

industrial pharmacy, business studies, science communication and science education. More information can be found on the corresponding website (see Useful Websites at the end of this chapter).

In Belgium, the Faculty of Pharmaceutical Sciences of KU Leuven pioneered several years ago with a Master in Drug Development, preparing graduates for a career in the biopharmaceutical industry. I personally had the privilege to contribute to the creation and roll-out of this master programme as visiting professor in clinical drug development at that time. In the first semester of the programme, students get acquainted with all the activities along the entire drug life cycle, i.e. discovery research, early and late development, and commercialisation. In parallel, they also get training on regulatory science/affairs and quality management all along the drug life cycle. Each one of the four parts of the cycle is treated in a 4-week module, with classic classrooms, workshops in teams and a flipped classroom at the end wherein real-world cases are to be studied, worked out and presented by teams of three students. The courses are provided by experts in their field, either faculty members or guest lecturers from industry or health authorities. From the second semester onwards, students have to choose between three sub-specialisations, i.e. drug discovery, drug development and drug commercialisation, with a number of the courses being taught in English. In the second master year, on top of a number of advanced courses, students have the opportunity to pass a 6-month traineeship in a biopharmaceutical company, and to prepare and present their master thesis. More information can be found on the corresponding website (see Useful Websites). Similar programmes are currently also offered by other Belgian universities, and several universities elsewhere.

In the Faculties of Medicine, a comparable evolution was seen towards offering a first master programme in biomedical sciences (BMS). This was mainly boosted by the growing insight that medicine is a lot more than an art or a practice, but that it is also driven by science. In addition, the Faculties of Medicine too had to deal with a limitation on the number of entry students, and were therefore also looking for alternatives. Nowadays, most universities offer a master programme in biomedical sciences, with a wide variety of sub-specialisations, e.g. wet-lab basic or translational research, clinical research, management, forensic research or science communication.

Similarly, other Faculties also offer graduate master programmes more specifically preparing students for a career in the pharma, biotech or medtech industry, e.g. Master in Biomedical Engineering or Master in Health Economics.

19.2.2 Postgraduate or Advanced Master Programmes

Most universities also offer different postgraduate programmes providing more advanced expertise and skills more specifically targeted towards a career in the pharmaceutical and biomedical industry. Some of these programmes lead to an advanced master, a specialty master, a master postmaster or simply an extra master.

Others lead to a PhD, while others rather provide a diploma or a certificate. In the plethora of offers, I will concentrate on a few much wanted extra qualifications or expertise in industry. Getting a PhD is left out of this overview, as most young graduates in life sciences are generally sufficiently well informed about the possibilities to obtain a doctoral degree.

Extensive information on worldwide education opportunities can be found on the website of the Norwegian Keystone Education Group, describing themselves as 'the leading online resource for people seeking the best education path for them' (see Useful Websites).

The majority of universities offer an advanced, specialty or specialised master programme in industrial pharmacy, originally more focused on drug production and drug quality (and leading to a certification as qualified person for batch release), but since several years also extended to other disciplines operating in the pharmaceutical industry (e.g. clinical research, quality management and regulatory affairs/science). In some cases the professional title thus obtained changed from industrial pharmacist to industry pharmacist.

Masters in Medicine (physicians or medical doctors) can choose to obtain a master or diploma in pharmaceutical medicine, offered by several universities. Some of these programmes are compliant with PharmaTrain standards, an EU-funded Innovative Medicines Initiative (IMI) with the aim to raise the standards in pharmaceutical medicine training, which is further discussed under Sect. 19.4.2. As an example, the PHARMED programme offered by the *Université Libre de Bruxelles* (ULB, Belgium), recognised by PharmaTrain as Centre of Excellence, is composed of seven modules: drug development (with the focus on the evolving healthcare environment), preclinical to first-in-human studies, clinical studies, data evaluation and biostatistics, registration and pharmacovigilance, health economics and biopharmaceutical market, and an elective module (either biologicals, ATMPs, medical devices or vaccines). A lot of these programmes are currently also open to other life sciences graduates, and are therefore sometimes also labelled as postgraduate in pharmaceutical (or medicines) development sciences.

Another interesting initiative is the Master's in Drug Innovation programme, offered by Utrecht University in the Netherlands, and covering the whole range of topics along the entire drug life cycle. This is an interdisciplinary programme 'open to graduates from a wide range of disciplines such as chemistry, biology, pharmaceutical sciences, biomedical sciences, medicine'. All needed information can be found on the corresponding website (see Useful Websites).

19.2.3 More Focused Training Opportunities

In addition to the initiatives already treated above that give students a more general idea of the many activities involved along the drug or product life cycle, other programmes focus on a specific activity or discipline involved in drug/product development and commercialisation. Some of these disciplines are highly in demand in the pharmaceutical and biomedical industry, and talented people with this extra expertise are for sure guaranteed an interesting job and a successful career, e.g. intellectual property and patent law, pharmacometrics (or systems biology/pharmacology, or modelling and simulation), clinical pharmacology, regulatory affairs/science, drug safety (toxicology, pharmacovigilance), quality management, health or pharmacoeconomics and marketing.

And again, also in this field, there is a plethora of specialised programmes, modules and courses available out there, leading to a degree, diploma, certificate or accreditation. It would take us too far to try to treat them all here, but I will pick one out, i.e. pharmacometrics (PMx), because this discipline is still relative young and booming; because specialists in this field integrate a rare combination of competences in life sciences, mathematics, data analysis and information technology; because experts with proficiency in pharmacometrics are highly wanted in industry; and because information on training opportunities seems to be less in the picture.

Pharmacometrics can be simply defined as the science of quantitative pharmacology. According to Nick Holford from the University of Auckland (New Zealand), one of the pioneers in this field, 'pharmacometrics involves the analysis and interpretation of data produced in preclinical studies and clinical trials'. Pharmacometrics uses models based on biology, physiology, pharmacology and epidemiology to quantify interactions between xenobiotics and human subjects or animals. Pharmacometrics and quantitative systems pharmacology (QSP) are two modelling and simulation (M&S) approaches that reach their full potential in model-informed (or model-based) drug development (MIDD or MBDD), a novel way to expedite drug development endorsed by drug regulatory authorities worldwide.

Probably the training with the best reputation in this field worldwide is the master's programme in pharmaceutical modelling offered by the Pharmacometrics Research Group (PRG) from Uppsala University in Sweden, still headed by Mats Karlsson the first worldwide professor of pharmacometrics since 2001. This group also organises yearly the Uppsala Pharmacometrics Summer School. Similar programmes worth mentioning are offered by the universities of Manchester (UK), Navarra (Pamplona, Spain), Leiden (the Netherlands, already referred to in Sect. 19.2.1), Auckland (New Zealand) and University at Buffalo (New York, USA). More information can be found on the respective websites (see Useful Websites).

19.2.4   Broader Additional Training Opportunities

Yet another and opposite possibility is to broaden your horizon further, and go for a second degree in a totally different but complementary discipline, e.g. engineering, information technology, marketing, management, business administration, law, health or pharmacoeconomics.

The broadest additional training, and probably the most widely offered and applied for, is the Master in Business Administration (MBA). Many renowned business schools offer this programme in order for graduates to get a better under-standing of the general running of a business, including study topics on entrepre-neurship, management, business strategy, business operations, marketing, finance and human resources. A lot of these schools offer post-experience or executive MBAs during weekends, allowing you to continue to work or study during the week. More detailed information can easily be found without further help.

In this context, it is also worth mentioning the recently co-developed postgrad-uate course by the Solvay Brussels School (the business school of the *Université Libre de Bruxelles*, Belgium) and a number of pharmaceutical industry partners, i.e. the Advanced Master in Biotech and Medtech Ventures, specifically preparing students to become an entrepreneur or a (senior) manager in start-up or young biotech and medtech companies. More information can be found on its website (see Useful Websites).

19.2.5 Inter-University and International Initiatives

Some universities team up to provide inter-university or international study programmes, also allowing student exchange partnerships, either within their own network of universities, e.g. UNICA, ULLA, Coimbra Group, The Guild, The edX Network, the International Association of Universities and many more, or within the EU in the context of Erasmus+ for instance. More details can be found on their respective websites (see Useful Websites).

19.3 Training Offered by the Pharmaceutical and Biomedical Industry

Many pharma, biotech and medtech companies offer various training opportunities for students, young graduates or staff members willing to progress. Most of these companies have an internal training department or academy.

As already mentioned, some master programmes foresee a short-term (up to 6 months) internship in industry as part of the course curriculum, so that students get some hands-on experience of the real-world functioning of a company or a department. In this case, the faculty usually partners with a number of companies to offer the students such a work placement. This type of partnership also provides for collaborative PhD studentships, where PhD students work (partly) in a pharmaceu-tical company under the mentorship of a company co-promoter.

Companies also offer intern-, trainee- and apprenticeships to graduates. Intern-ships are usually shorter-term placements allowing gaining already some work experience. The really short ones are known as sniffing internships. A somewhat longer rotational internship allows you to rotate between different functions within the same department or to rotate between different departments within the same company. Some internships are paid; others are not. Even if it is not paid, it will give you the opportunity to show your motivation to the employer. Traineeships usually last longer (6–12 months), are mostly paid (leading to quicker independence) and can more easily feed into a first full-time job, although this is not guaranteed. Apprenticeships are even longer-term assignments (1–3 years) and include a more structured training programme. They are always paid and can lead more straightforward to full employment.

Training departments of companies will also provide the so-called induction training for newcomers, introducing them to their new job within the organisation. In some instances, e.g. for sales representatives, this induction training can be very intensive, possibly culminating in a stressful examination at the end. In order to retain high potentials (HIPOs), companies will continue to invest in talented people, helping them to develop their competences and skills with a portfolio of specific internal training modules.

HIPOs might also get the opportunity to take a sabbatical, and attend a post-experience or executive MBA, or a middle- or advanced management programme in a renowned business school.

Finally, on-the-job training is also worth mentioning, as it is an invaluable method of getting fully acquainted with a new job under the supervision of an experienced manager or mentor who provides continuous guidance, advice and feedback to the mentee.

More detailed information can easily be found on the websites of many companies, often under the tab Careers. The Association of the British Pharmaceutical Industry (ABPI) gathers biennially information from its member companies on their links with academia, including training opportunities, and the results are available on its website (see Useful Websites).

19.4 Training Offered by Other Organisations

In this section, I will briefly overview other initiatives offered by a range of different training providers active in the pharmaceutical and biomedical sector, e.g. university spin-offs, public-private partnerships, regulatory authorities, professional organisations, non-profit organisations and private service providers. For each provider category, a few striking examples will be given. More information can be found on their websites listed in Useful Websites.

19.4.1 University Spin-Offs

Paul Janssen Future Lab is an initiative of Leiden University Medical Center (the Netherlands), operating as a non-profit organisation, and offering 'an international blended learning programme for tomorrow's leaders in biomedical science'. It currently offers four advanced modules: intellectual property, clinical development, clinical research regulation in the Netherlands, and market approval. A wide variety of teaching methods is used, requiring active participation and interaction, all focused on learning by doing.

The Drug Safety Research Unit (DSRU) is an independent registered charity associated with the University of Portsmouth (UK), principally concerned with pharmacovigilance. Its Education and Training department is a leading provider of training courses in pharmacovigilance, pharmacoepidemiology and related topics in Europe.

More information can be found on the respective websites listed in Useful websites.

19.4.2   Public-Private Partnerships (PPPs)

PharmaTrain is a PPP that started its activities in the European Union (EU) as an Innovative Medicines Initiative (IMI). It is currently a non-profit organisation under the umbrella of the PharmaTrain Federation. Its objective is 'implementing reliable standards for high-quality post-graduate education and training in Medicines Development'. It certifies a portfolio of training courses offered by different accredited training providers in Europe and beyond (mostly academic centres). The extensive list can be found on its website. The listed courses can either lead to a Diploma or a Master in Medicines Development, while some of them are part of a Continuing Professional Development (CPD) platform.

Eu2P is a similar IMI within the EU, announcing itself as 'the leading training programme in pharmacovigilance and pharmacoepidemiology in Europe'. It is a PPP of 24 academic, regulatory and industrial partners, and it offers short courses, certificate courses and master and PhD programmes.

Another IMI is LifeTrain with the motto 'driving lifelong learning for biomedical professionals', offering a framework for Continuing Professional Development (CPD) with information from four stakeholder groups, i.e. course providers, professional bodies, employers and individuals.

In the USA, TransCelerate is a similar PPP (academia, FDA, companies) who developed a set of minimum criteria to enable the mutual recognition of Good Clinical Practice (GCP) training offered by its different member pharmaceutical companies.

More information can be found on the respective websites (see Useful Websites).

19.4.3   Regulatory Authorities

Several regulatory agencies offer training opportunities aimed at university graduates, such as the EMA (traineeships for EU citizens, 10 months), the FDA (undergraduate, graduate and postgraduate training programmes, as well as visiting scientist programmes for foreigners), the Medicines and Healthcare products Regulatory Agency (MHRA, UK; apprenticeships) and the European Patent Office (EPO, trainee- and internships), to cite just a few examples. Ample information can be found on their respective websites (see Useful Websites).

19.4.4   Professional Organisations

Many professional societies active within the pharmaceutical and biomedical sector offer some type of education, training or certification, and even consider it as one of their key missions.

The Drug Information Association (DIA) is a global association of life science professionals that via DIA Learning Solutions offers a wide range of face-to-face, online or virtual training courses in 11 categories, from clinical development and operations, over project management and strategic planning, to value and access.

Numerous more focused professional societies propose an impressive catalogue of training opportunities, e.g. the Federation of European Toxicologists and European Societies of Toxicology (EUROTOX, also cited in Chap. 4), the Regulatory Affairs Professionals Society (RAPS, also cited in Chap. 11), the Organisation for Professionals in Regulatory Affairs (TOPRA), the Royal Pharmaceutical Society (RPS, also cited in Chap. 13), the Association of Clinical Research Professionals (ACRP), the Society of Clinical Research Associates (SOCRA), the International Society of Pharmacovigilance (ISoP), the International Society of Pharmacometrics (also ISoP) and the Dutch Society for Clinical Pharmacology and Biopharmacy (NVKFB). More information can be found on their respective websites (see Useful Websites).

A significant number of them allow successful participants to become certified or registered professionals in their field of interest. In many instances this certification/registration has to be renewed on a regular basis (often 5-yearly).

Most of these associations or societies also organise regularly congresses, conferences or workshops on hot topics that are worth participating in, as they allow a quick update on the state-of-the-art knowledge in a particular field, and are excellent venues for networking.

And again, between the many initiatives cited above, I will pick one out, i.e. the training and certification offered by the NVKFB in clinical pharmacology (CP), simply because it is the specialisation I personally opted for many years ago. The role of specialists in clinical pharmacology (and therapeutics, CPT) is to optimise drug therapy in humans, mainly by participating in the clinical development of new drugs and by promoting rational pharmacotherapy. Postgraduate training in CP was formerly mainly offered to physicians, later on also to pharmacists and more recently also to other graduates in life sciences. The NVKFB offers training opportunities and certification as clinical pharmacologist to internists, hospital pharmacists and 'others' (after candidate acceptance and a personalised programme). Certified clinical pharmacologists easily find their way into the pharmaceutical industry, especially in early clinical drug development, academic or commercial phase 1 centres (clinical pharmacology units, CPUs), or into clinical practice promoting rational prescribing of medicines.

The training programme focuses on foundational aspects (e.g. disease pathophysiology, pharmacology, clinical pharmacology, drug safety) with some clinical practice; on gaining specialised knowledge (esp. of clinical drug development, including clinical trial methodology, advanced data analysis and biostatistics, regulatory affairs and quality management); and on developing appropriate soft skills. Board certification can be obtained at best after 1-year full-time training, or after several years part-time. Afterwards, re-registration is mandatory every 5 years, with relatively tough requirements.

More detailed information can be found on the website of the NVKFB, and additional information and/or educational material can be found on the websites of the International Union of Basic and Clinical Pharmacology (IUPHAR)/Pharmacology Education Project/Clinical Pharmacology and the European Federation for Exploratory Medicines Development (EUFEMED).

EUFEMED recently developed a training course in human pharmacology, in close alignment with the PharmaTrain Diploma/Master programme in Pharmaceutical Medicine/Medicines Development Sciences, leading either to a certificate or a diploma.

See Useful Websites to access additional information from all the professional bodies referred to in this section.

19.4.5   Other Non-profit Organisations

Just to add two other organisations that offer excellent training in Good Clinical Practice (GCP), i.e. the European Forum for Good Clinical Practice (EFGCP), and the Global Health Training Centre (GHTC, offering GCP training as well as other courses).

See Useful Websites to access more detailed information.

19.4.6   Private Service Providers

Many private service providers operate in this field, but I will only cite two of them with PharmaTrain recognition, i.e. the European Centre for Clinical Research Training (ECCRT, Brussels, Belgium), offering a range of training courses in clinical research, either as classroom, e-learning, webinar or micro-learning sessions; and Learning by Simulation (LBS, Berlicum, the Netherlands), 'a unique condensed method of training to gain rapid understanding of what is needed in a complex process', offering three courses: drug discovery simulation, drug development simulation and biologicals development simulation.

See Useful Websites to access more detailed information.

19.5   Conclusion

As the pharmaceutical, biotechnology and medical technology industries offer a wealth of different job and career opportunities, it comes as no surprise that academia, the industry itself and other satellite organisations also offer a plethora of education and training opportunities preparing for this sector.

I hope that this overview, with the list of useful websites that follows, will help you to make an informed choice allowing you to successfully kick off your career in this attractive sector.

Acknowledgements   I want to thank Chris van Schravendijk, co-editor, for critically reading the manuscript, and for creating the Multi-URL QR codes allowing the readers of the Print Book to quickly access the Useful Websites. Also a special thanks to Erwin Dreesen, Assistant Professor in Pharmacometrics at the Faculty of Pharmaceutical Sciences at KU Leuven (Belgium) for helping me with information on training opportunities in pharmacometrics and systems pharmacology.

Useful Websites

This is a selection of useful websites where the reader can find more detailed information.

All accessed 31 March 2022.

Master in Biopharmaceutical Sciences, Utrecht University, the Netherlands
https://www.universiteitleiden.nl/en/education/study-programmes/master/bio-phar
   maceutical-sciences
Master in Drug Development, KU Leuven, Belgium
https://pharm.kuleuven.be/international/ffwenglish.html
Keystone Education Group
https://www.keystoneacademic.com/studyprograms?hsLang=en-us
PharmaTrain.
https://www.pharmatrain.eu/
PHARMED: Post-graduate Programme in Pharmaceutical Development Sciences, Université Libre de Bruxelles (ULB), Belgium
https://pharmed.helsci.be/
Drug Innovation, Utrecht University, the Netherlands
https://www.uu.nl/masters/en/drug-innovation
Master's Programme in Pharmaceutical Modelling, Uppsala University, Sweden.
https://www.uu.se/en/admissions/master/selma/program/?pKod=FPM2M
Systems Biomedicine and Pharmacology (MSc), Leiden University, the Netherlands.

https://www.universiteitleiden.nl/en/education/study-programmes/master/bio-phar
  maceutical-sciences/system-biomedicine-and-pharmacology
MSc Model-based Drug Development, University of Manchester, United Kingdom.
https://www.manchester.ac.uk/study/masters/courses/list/08749/msc-model-based-
  drug-development/all-content/
Summer Course on Quantitative Pharmacology, University of Navarra,
  Pamplona, Spain
https://www.unav.edu/web/pharmacometrics-and-systems-pharmacology/training
(Advanced) Pharmacometrics Courses, University of Auckland, New-Zealand.
http://holford.fmhs.auckland.ac.nz/teaching/
Pharmacometrics and Personalized Pharmacotherapy MS, University at Buffalo,
  New York, USA.
https://www.buffalo.edu/home/academics/degree_programs.host.html/content/
  authoritative/grad/programs/pharmacometrics-and-personalized-pharmacother
  apy-ms.detail.html
Advanced Master in Biotech and Medtech Ventures
https://exed.solvay.edu/en/11-program/1050-advanced-master-in-biotech-and-
  medtech-ventures
Network of Universities from the Capitals of Europe (UNICA), Student Webinars
https://www.unica-network.eu/event/unica-student-webinars-pharma-and-biotech-
  careers-in-europe/
European University Consortium for Pharmaceutical Sciences (ULLA, from the
  cities of its founding universities, i.e. Uppsala, London, Leiden, Amsterdam),
  Summer Schools.
https://ullapharmsci.org/events/summer-schools/
Erasmus+ programme
https://erasmus-plus.ec.europa.eu/
Association of the British Pharmaceutical Industry (ABPI)
Industry and academia links survey 2019
https://www.abpi.org.uk/facts-figures-and-industry-data/industry-and-academia-
  links-survey-2019/#
Paul Janssen Future Lab Leiden, an initiative of LUMC, the Netherlands.
https://www.pauljanssenfuturelab.eu/
Drug Safety Research Unit, associated with University of Portsmouth,
  Southampton, UK.
https://www.dsru.org/education-training/
The PharmaTrain Federation (formerly PharmaTrain)
https://www.pharmatrain.eu/
European Training Programme in Pharmacovigilance and Pharmacoepidemiology
  (Eu2P)
https://www.eu2p.org/
LifeTrain
https://www.lifetrain.eu/
TransCelerate BioPharma (GCP training and certification)
https://www.transcelerate-gcp-mutual-recognition.com/home

European Medicines Agency (EMA, EU)
https://careers.ema.europa.eu/content/Traineeship/?locale=en_GB
Food and Drug Administration (FDA, USA)
https://www.fda.gov/about-fda/jobs-and-training-fda/scientific-internships-fellow
   ships-trainees-and-non-us-citizens
Medicines and Healthcare products Regulatory Agency (MHRA, UK)
https://mhra.referrals.selectminds.com/
European Patent Office (EPO Headquarters, Germany)
https://jobs.epo.org/go/Internships/2867901/
DIA Learning Solutions (Drug Information Association)
https://www.diaglobal.org/en/learning-solutions
EUROTOX Education (Federation of European Toxicologists & European Societies
   of Toxicology)
https://www.eurotox.com/education/eurotox-faculty-programme/
Regulatory Affairs Professionals Society (RAPS)
https://www.raps.org/
The Organisation for Professionals in Regulatory Affairs (TOPRA)
https://www.topra.org/
Royal Pharmaceutical Society (RPS)
https://www.rpharms.com/
Association of Clinical Research Professionals (ACRP)
https://acrpnet.org/
Society of Clinical Research Associates (SOCRA)
https://www.socra.org/
International Society of Pharmacovigilance (ISoP)
https://isoponline.org/
International Society of Pharmacometrics (ISoP)
http://go-isop.org/
Dutch Society for Clinical Pharmacology & Biopharmacy (NVKFB)
https://nvkfb.nl/
International Union of Basic and Clinical Pharmacology (IUPHAR) Pharmacology
   Education Project (PEP) on Clinical Pharmacology
https://www.pharmacologyeducation.org/clinical-pharmacology
European Federation for Exploratory Medicines Development (EUFEMED)
https://www.eufemed.eu/training/
European Forum for Good Clinical Practice (EFGCP)
https://efgcp.eu/
Global Health Training Centre (GHTC)
https://globalhealthtrainingcentre.tghn.org/
European Centre for Clinical Research Training (ECCRT)
https://eccrt.com/
Learning By Simulation (LBS)
https://www.learningbysimulation.eu/

QR-Codes for the Above Collection of Useful Websites

Part I: From the start until Sect. 19.2.4:

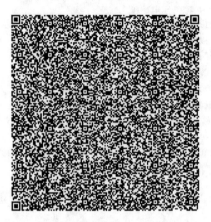

Part II: From Sect. 19.2.4 until Sect.19.4.3:

Part III: From Sect. 19.4.3 until Sect. 19.4.5:

Part IV: From Sect. 19.4.5 until the end:

Epilogue

The publication of this book has been a fascinating journey.

As Editorial Team we were fortunate to be able to collaborate with more than 30 enthusiastic authors, who—as insiders in the field—did not need much convincing to write a contribution.

They were all too well aware of the fact that recent graduates and young professionals still lack detailed information on the wealth of job and career opportunities that the pharmaceutical and biomedical industry has to offer. Despite the multitude of laudable initiatives deployed since several years by academia in collaboration with the industry to inform them better with brochures, lectures, online webinars, YouTube videos, industry days, job markets, career fairs, etc., there was the everlasting observation that something was still missing, i.e. bringing together the available information in one easily accessible source, a comprehensive book written by insiders.

This book exactly closes that gap, available as hardcover and e-book, both reasonably priced.

The 19 chapters are packed with concrete, specific, and practical information, complemented with insider advice, offering young graduates all that is needed to successfully kick-start their career in the pharma, biotech, or medtech industry. Even confirmed professionals in the field will find enough details and guidance allowing them to take their career to the next level, or to explore what other organizations in the broader biomedical sector have to offer.

Is it perfect? No. Unfortunately some of the contacted potential contributors had to decline, and three of the confirmed authors dropped out last minute. So there is room for improvement, either by publishing a supplement or future new editions. Anyway, we hope that the book in its present form will become a reference in its field.

And yes, the pharmaceutical industry is an attractive sector to work in or to work for.

© The Author(s), under exclusive license to Springer Nature Switzerland AG 2023   327
J. R. Thomas et al. (eds.), *Career Options in the Pharmaceutical and Biomedical
Industry*, https://doi.org/10.1007/978-3-031-14911-5

You will be part of the discovery, the development, the manufacturing, or the commercialization of life-saving innovative interventions, which is extremely motivating.

It is also a very dynamic industry, rapidly evolving, adopting new technologies early, where interdisciplinary teamwork is key, which are all contributing to professional and personal satisfaction.

However, there are a few things you should be aware of when you are enthusiastic, talented, and ambitious to build yourself a successful career in the pharma industry:

- First of all, a general one: it is a competitive world out there; pay attention to strike a good work–life balance. Everyone can be missed or replaced.
- Secondly, another general one: be aware of the Peter Principle, defined by *The Oxford English Dictionary* as 'the principle that members of a hierarchy are promoted until they reach the level at which they are no longer competent'. Very awkward.
- And finally, a more specific one for the pharma industry: avoid getting trapped in a golden cage. Although the industry pays well, it is not all about the money.

And with that, we hope you are ready for your first or next move.

We wish you all the best to become our next generation of inventors, developers, marketers, or entrepreneurs of innovative interventions to satisfy the unmet needs of future patients.

Josse R. Thomas, on behalf of the Editorial Team, 2 April 2022.

Printed in the United States
by Baker & Taylor Publisher Services